Charting a Course to Wellness

Treena and Graham Kerr

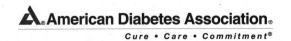
American Diabetes Association.
Cure • Care • Commitment®

Publisher, John Fedor; *Associate Director, Consumer Books,* Sherrye Landrum; *Editor,* Abe Ogden; *Associate Director, Book Production,* Peggy M. Rote; *Composition,* Circle Graphics; *Cover Design,* Koncept, Inc.; *Photographer,* Doug Evans; *Printer,* Port City Press, Inc.

Printed in the United States of America
1 3 5 7 9 10 8 6 4 2

Small Steps Press is an imprint of the American Diabetes Association.
Consult a health care professional before trying any of the suggestions in this publication. Small Steps Press and ADA assume no responsibility for any injury that may result from the suggestions or information in this publication.

☺ The paper in this publication meets the requirements of the ANSI Standard Z39.48-1992 (permanence of paper).

Small Steps Press titles may be purchased for business or promotional use or for special sales. To purchase this book in large quantities, or for custom editions of this book with your logo, contact Lee Romano Sequeira, Special Sales & Promotions, at the address below, or at Lees@smallsteps press.com or 703-299-2046.

Small Steps Press
1701 North Beauregard Street
Alexandria, Virginia 22311

Library of Congress Cataloging-in-Publication Data

Library of Congress Cataloging-in-Publication Data

Kerr, Graham
    Charting a course to wellness : creative ways of living with heart disease and diabetes / Treena and Graham Kerr.
        p. cm.
    Includes index.
    ISBN 1-58040-198-8 (pbk. : alk. paper)
    1. Diabetes—Popular works. 2. Coronary heart disease—Popular works. 3. Diabetes—Diet therapy—Popular works. 4. Coronary heart disease—diet therapy—Popular works. 5. Kerr, Treena, 1934—Health. I. Kerr, Treena, 1934- II. Title.

RC660.4.K47 2004
616.1'230654—dc22   2004045071

DEDICATION

When you love another person,
you do good to him,
and you do good to him
according to the best
that is in your nature. ❧

John at the Cross, 1421

Contents

Acknowledgments

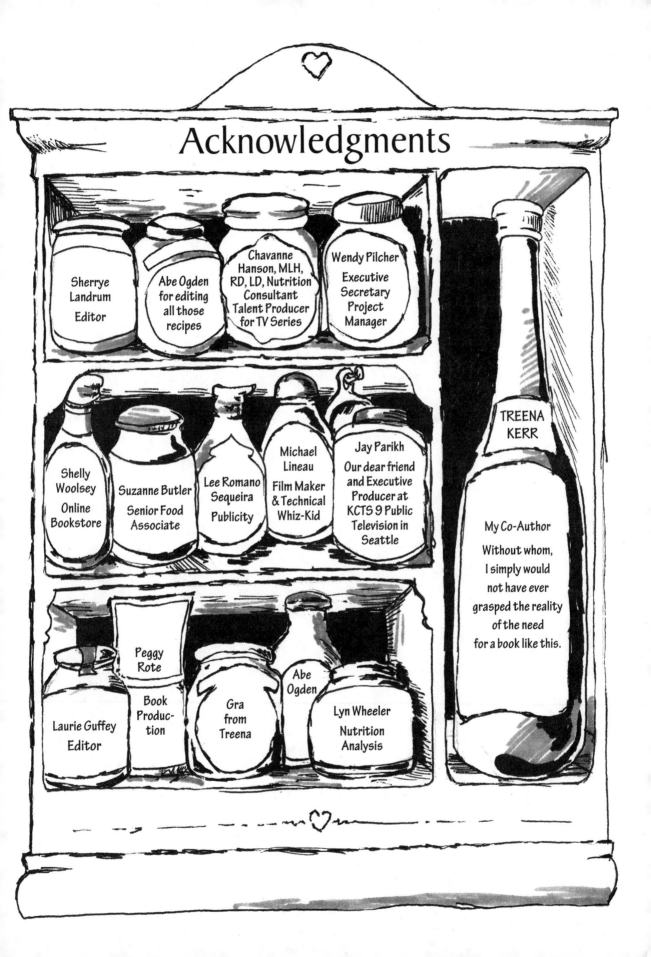

Sherrye Landrum
Editor

Abe Ogden for editing all those recipes

Chavanne Hanson, MLH, RD, LD, Nutrition Consultant Talent Producer for TV Series

Wendy Pilcher
Executive Secretary Project Manager

Shelly Woolsey
Online Bookstore

Suzanne Butler
Senior Food Associate

Lee Romano Sequeira
Publicity

Michael Lineau
Film Maker & Technical Whiz-Kid

Jay Parikh
Our dear friend and Executive Producer at KCTS 9 Public Television in Seattle

TREENA KERR

My Co-Author
Without whom, I simply would not have ever grasped the reality of the need for a book like this.

Laurie Guffey
Editor

Peggy Rote
Book Production

Gra from Treena

Abe Ogden

Lyn Wheeler
Nutrition Analysis

Introduction

When we got married, we had no idea where our life's journey would take us. It has been quite a trip with much of joy, some of tragedy, and enough dollops of surprising experiences to keep us engaged in living and wanting more. As we tell you our life story, we won't leave out any experiences because they were painful; we've learned much from these times. Actually, what we have learned from our lifetime (with food), acted out on many stages, is that you cannot change your lifestyle unless the changes fit you. With food, the changes that last are the ones that taste good to you. The changes you make have to fit you—your tastes, your likes, your style, your schedule, your needs.

Like every other family who is visited with a chronic disease—in our case, we got two, heart disease and diabetes—we went through a sequence of stages that are normal. We didn't know that. You may not know that. If we can help you get through the stages more quickly by sharing our story with you, we will be delighted.

If we can help you and your family to live longer, healthier, happier lives, then our lives are complete. We truly believe that we are here to help each other.

As Teilhard de Chardin once said, "We are not human beings on a spiritual journey; we are spiritual beings on a human journey." A large part of that human journey, perhaps the most frequently repeated part, is the daily food we eat and the effect on our health—both physical and emotional. The connection between food and health is real and powerful. We have more than 30 years of experience in this field that can help you be more powerful, too.

As proof of the power, here are the numbers that tell us how we are doing. Treena went from an A1C of 11.9 to a 6, which is normal. Her blood pressure went from high enough to cause a stroke and then a heart attack to normal. Her LDL cholesterol (the bad one) is 100 and total cholesterol is 184. Her weight is considered to be healthy because her other levels are all in the normal ranges. If you would like to turn up with numbers like these, the choices you make each day are important. Here's how we did it!

Why Tell You Our Story?

Because We Need Each Other's Love to Get Well

I've loved Treena since the summer of '45. It seems as though we've spent our whole lives together—and after 48 years of marriage, we have! I can remember very little about my life before knowing her and can imagine nothing better than sharing our remaining years.

Okay, so nothing is more certain than birth, death, and taxes, but what about the quality of life in-between—especially in our latter years? Did you know that more and more people are going to be living to the age of 100? If your mental image is of being creaky and old at 70—which we aren't by the way—then how will you spend those next 30 years?

Death has knocked on our door three times and gone away. These encounters were tough at the time; but they left us stronger and even more determined to get up every morning and to embrace and celebrate the gift of life and of love that we have been given to share.

We share a purpose these days, and we call it MYTC (more years to contribute). We truly desire to be "well enough" to look forward to whatever opportunities life may bring and also resilient enough to weather the storms, sadness, and the disappointments that will be part of the tapestry of our future lives.

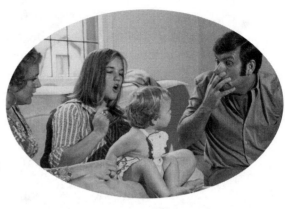

Treena, Tessa, Kareena, and Graham in Ottawa, Canada, during the filming of the *Galloping Gourmet*.

To be well for the "long haul" we've discovered one great truth. We need to have willing minds—one way or another. We must be willing to search for solutions to each new challenge. Willing to become partners in every sense of that word. Willing to allow each other into the deeper personal and private areas of our lives and to respect this as an invitation made daily and not an ongoing obligation. Willing to embrace lifestyle options as true choices and not rules and regulations. Most of all, willing to keep on searching for ways to extend our years together . . . without complications . . . even in the face of increasing age.

We have also found that our family isn't the outer limit of our concern. Of course they will always have priority and their well-being is what we call our cup measure of responsibility. One thing you may know about British people is that we like drinking tea out of a cup—with a saucer.

Our cup of family lifestyle experiences quite literally over-flows into the saucer to benefit our readers and viewers, both through these pages and all the other media in which we are privileged to serve.

Everybody nowadays seems to have a mission statement. Well, this is ours, and it really does involve you—deeply.

Our mission is: To serve creatively the people who are willing to make lifestyle choices that will last because those choices are enjoyable and rewarding.

We are now living in an era in which consumer lifestyle choices are making us sick—too much food of the wrong kind and not enough physical exercise for our remarkable bodies. The irony of this situation struck us full on years ago. How could our choices at our family dinner table help people in other places who do not have enough? Could we make choices that would benefit us and benefit those who needed help? For example, instead of a cookie for a snack, we switched to a frozen grape. They are both sweet, but the cookie can have 75 calories and the grape only 2. The grapes are a good deal less expensive to buy, and frozen ones take longer to eat. They are also a good source of nutrients that can't be found in a cookie. If we then saved the money we would have spent on cookies in a month, we could give it to others and receive a gift to our overall health, too—a double benefit!

You will read more about how we managed to go from indulgence to "outdulgence" and received the double benefit that can lead to deep and lasting friendships. Our prayer is that multiple wellsprings of truly creative change in all our lives will help to heal our damaged world. It begins with you and the two of us. So, with that vision in mind, let's get started!

CHAPTER ONE

Partners

It was the midmorning break. Most of my fellow students were out in the schoolyard on a crisp early summer day. I remained at the window, alone.

Michael Hall was a Rudolf Steiner Coeducational School, an extraordinary change for a product of the British Public School system of boys bred for battle at the end of World War II.

It was the summer of 1945 and peace was upon us, leaves were unfurling in the trees and pale sunlight cast vague shadows over the school grounds. A small crowd had gathered to watch a slim, dark-haired girl clicking a pair of castanets and stamping her feet in the gravel.

Until that moment girls were of no interest to me, only mildly irritating perhaps. But this girl was different. I snatched up my Box Brownie Camera, dashed out to push through the circle of students and asked, "Can I take your picture?"

"Of course." She struck a pose, arms held high, her eyes defiantly fixed on my camera.

I released the shutter—click.

How I wish I had that photograph to show you. It remains sharply etched forever in my mind, but I didn't have any film in the camera. But we did meet!

It was when I was midway through my eleventh year that I fell in love with Treena.

And here is how Treena remembers me.

YOUNG LOVE

A boy, a man to be, eventually.
I saw him once, eyes sort of green
With smile that captivated me
A girl, a woman yet to be.
All the girls thought him great,
But he loved me or so it seemed,
For he rescued me with crucial punch
At a beastly boy with an attitude,
Who tried my arm to break.
Thus my heart was fully won
moreover, has thus so remained.
furthermore, will until the end. ॐ

Treena's father was a portrait painter who moved often as new subjects called on his artistry, and before long Treena gave me the dreadful news of their departure to the Channel Islands, midway between Britain's South Coast and France. I was heartbroken . . . my first love was gone and so far away. I filled in an index card with dates and memories . . . a card marked #1 on the top right corner, and Treena was forever defined as "my type." Over the years I completed new cards and the numbers increased, but somehow, we stayed in touch as the years sped by.

At 19, Treena won the very first "Miss Jersey Battle of the Flowers" contest that included, as its prize, a film test at J. Arthur Rank Studios in London. *The Daily Mirror* newspaper covered the events, and I was amazed to see my first love as an emerging star. I read that she was now an actress well on her way to success. I wrote and she replied . . . and love was rekindled . . . briefly.

At 20 years of age, I was commissioned as a British Army officer and was stationed in Wales on the far west coast of England.

There I received a letter re-addressed multiple times and faithfully handed on by the British Post Office (bless them!). It was Treena. She had come back to live in England. Her parents had a place only 30-odd miles from my parents' hotel in Tenterden, Kent, in the southeast of England.

We agreed to meet. The intervening ten years had transformed a slim dark child into an extraordinarily beautiful woman. Within the hour I was hopelessly head-over-heels in love. My index cards now added up to #38 but she was still #1—*my type!*

One day later I proposed. Treena accepted. We were just 20—too young for both the British Army and my mother!

THE PROPOSAL

On a Sunday morn in November
Church bells rang, calling some to worship.
Two young people walked (oblivious to God)
Through fields of buttercups and celandines
Which appeared to give songs of praise
As they danced and swayed, unseen by the two.
They talked, laughed and joked, so unaware.
T'was England, so there were 'styles' to climb
From field to field; at one, the boy (guess who)
Carefully did lift the girl into his arms.
His feet sunk into fresh plowed earth
Made wet and muddy by night's rain.
"Now the question is" smiled the boy,
"Shall I drop you in this mud, or
shall I propose and by your saying yes
I will then carry you to dry land!
And we will wed next year . . . so . . . ?"
The girl was me, I laughed "Okay, Yes!"
Thus our lives were sealed . . . .
Among buttercups, celandines, and mud. ॐ

THE WEDDING SWING

And thus the day began, breakfast
My love and I together,
The ritual of not being seen
A superstition, not for us.
Afterwards we walked across the street
To play on high upon the swings.
We started feeling queasy—no more play!
So returned to the hustle-bustle of the day.
My darling's parents ran a thirteenth century Inn,
So all the friends and 'regulars' in the bars,
Joked and teased and bought us brandies,
Saying they would calm our wedding nerves.
We drank the brandies, stomachs calmed.
My mother waited up the ancient stairs
to help me dress (Bought by friends)
Mother told me I looked sweet, yet
Resentment, feelings of hostility transmitted
from my father's face and words.
As he walked me up the aisle
He whispered this encouragement to my ear
"I give this marriage six months at the most."
Graham, handsome in dress uniform, sword
Chattering in the scabbard at his side,
Gave me an all embracing smile of trust and love.
Daddy was wrong, We were a happy two
For we said "I do". . . 48 years ago.
On our 21st anniversary we made new vows
In the very church which we had vowed before.
We had come to Christ, you see, and felt it right
To marry once again in His Father's sight
Without the fuss and pain or strife
On that 22nd day of September 1955. ॐ

These were the days before written prenuptial agreements, but we had to have our own verbal understanding. I, frankly, didn't believe I had what it took to be the husband of a movie star! So, in the small back garden of our family hotel whilst stubbing away at the lawn in my awkwardness, I spoke out: "I need you to know that I don't think our marriage will last if you become a star. Would you give up that career to marry me?"

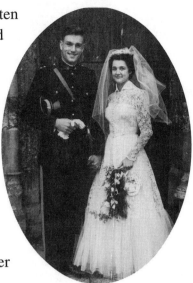

TREENA: I was so in love, without thought, I said, "Yes of course."

One by one obstacles were overcome, and on September 22, 1955, we were married.

Partners

This was the starting point of our formal partnership—one that would carry us through our Army days into the hotel business and parenthood. We moved from England to New Zealand and Australia. Treena's early theatrical experience was called on when the Royal New Zealand Air Force ordered me to go on television in 1960. There were only about 50 television sets in the city of Auckland. I'm probably the only person you'll ever know to have had a 100 rating (try and forget the 50 sets).

Treena made it crystal clear that a television appearance *demanded* more of me than a simple recipe. I was eager to please her and rehearsed a "funny" situation with my producer.

The dreaded night of the telecast—Wednesday at 8 p.m. between *Peyton Place* and *The Avengers* (location is everything)—my show came on, titled *Entertaining with Kerr*. This was a play on words . . . Kerr is pronounced "care."

The "funny" moment arrived, and Treena screamed!

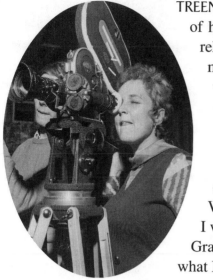

TREENA: Graham has been gifted with a natural sense of humor, and you just have to let him be, NOT rehearse him. He was SO awful, even the memory makes me shudder. He knew exactly what he was doing, as far as cooking and the recipes were concerned. I tried to tell the producer of these first shows to remember that he was not an actor but a communicator. As far as I was concerned, they would ruin him if they insisted on making him rehearse being spontaneous. When I saw Graham's wonderful humor ruined, I was rather forceful in my opinion, which made Graham yell in disappointment. Little did I know what I was letting myself in for.

GRAHAM: Okay, so I was now the world's most utterly boring man, quite a title for a 26 year old! I responded as only a wounded male can do: "Okay, if you are so clever, why don't you produce the show?"

So, when we went to make the *Galloping Gourmet* show in Canada, she did produce the show. Over the next few years, I was coached by Treena and warned not to look at a single episode.

TREENA: I cautioned him, in fact I "forbade" him to look at his shows. Why, you may ask? Because he would see things in himself he didn't like and things that he would think great (and thus remember) and gradually change himself into a phony Graham. To this very day, he probably has seen only about 10 programs out of nearly 2,000. What you saw in the past and what you see now is really who he is.

I also kept at him to "look up" into the camera and not look down. This is why he often cuts things up without looking, and this always gets a round of applause from the audiences. Ours was the first cooking show to have an audience and three cameras. I liked to keep Graham on his toes by surprising him—things were not where they were supposed to be or the phone rang in the middle of the show. It was my idea that he start the show by jumping over a chair while holding a full glass of wine. There was never a dull moment, ever!

Success, Stress, and the Accompanying Spiritual and Dietary Risk

If you aren't eaten alive by the speeding tiger of opportunity, you might just as well grab it by the tail. We were both mauled and what tattered remains we had left grasped and held on tight for what became a violent, unrepeatable ride.

For this story, it is enough to say that our sudden success at so young an age found me completely unprepared, and so I stumbled badly and fell against my beloved Treena. The collision was so painful that the open wounds, though tended daily, refused to heal. No matter how hard I tried, I failed to win her lasting forgiveness. We kissed and made up, but then my skeleton re-emerged from the closet, and once again our lives fell apart.

All of this was happening during the development and recording of the *Galloping Gourmet* series. The show was enormously successful and literally changed the way food was perceived by millions of people worldwide.

The *Galloping Gourmet* was based upon a slim volume written by Len Evans; at that time the wildly popular "cellar master" wine writer and myself. Qantas Airlines gave us a free round-the-world ticket if we would write a book about the experience. It was titled *The Galloping Gourmets* (plural) and an idea was born.

I was able to travel the world in search of the finest gourmet experiences; this time with Treena as the show's producer. We signed a contract for 650 shows to be made at the inconceivable rate of 195 shows each year. Up until that time the most that had been required of us was 39!

TREENA: As I remember it, we were in the American Club in Australia, and a friend of ours, a newspaper journalist named

Arnold (who was among quite a few to interview my darling) showed me the "fruit machines," which I had never seen before. He told me how they worked; so I put in 25 cents, and it went clink, clink, clink. I won. Winning $40 in quarters makes a wonderful, metallic waterfall sound, which accompanied Graham as he signed the big contract. He was mortified, but I was $40 richer!

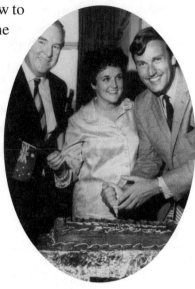

Professional Partners Go Galloping

TREENA: Of course, never having produced anything, knowing absolutely nothing about television, and being responsible for an international television show, I was faced with rather an awesome task, especially as there were very few female producers in the industry in 1968. I am so proud that I was one of the first.

How did I cope? Very simply . . . I acted my way through the whole thing and would give some piece of equipment a name that no one had ever heard of, including me. I simply pretended that was what we called it in Australia. I'm certain I didn't fool anyone . . . except myself.

Graham moved very fast, like an ice puck, and because of his agility, I insisted on an ice hockey crew, after all, we were working in Canada. I wanted a team spirit, a family feeling; so I demanded that we had the same crew on every show. This was not the way things were done. The studio changed crews everyday. But, not on our show, they wouldn't! Being pregnant and jumping up and down won the argument. In fact, we were blessed to have the same wonderful crew all through the *Galloping Gourmet* days.

I was told to cut the comedy—imagine—but I thought cooking programs were boring and frankly, took no notice of the advice. I had the best studio crew ever. When all is said and done, the crew can make or mar a program, and in spite of outside influences, we, the crew and I, with Graham of course, together made the

Galloping Gourmet what it was. Also I became an honorary member of NABET (North American Broadcasting, Electricians, and Technicians Union). This will always be a treasure in my heart.

Executive Producer Vern Ferber was wonderful and let me do my thing. I also had a great assistant producer, Muriel Green, director Marian Dunn, and technical producer Gerry Bouchard who, along with the crew, would push and encourage me to fight for what I felt was right. I used whatever I needed to win, swearing or shouting, and if that didn't work, I cried. Being pregnant was enormously helpful, too. I never remember losing a battle.

If Graham and I would argue, we did it through the system. I would shout at the TV monitor and Graham would respond through the studio camera. The studio director, Stevie Watts, would mediate in a diplomatic way. He was and is a true friend to us both.

How was I nominated twice for daytime producer of the year? I don't know! Did I enjoy producing? No! The responsibility was tough and not only did I nearly lose my femininity, but our baby—who is now married with two lovely daughters of her own.

My greatest joy was when the adviser who had told me to cut the comedy got to eat his words—even though he didn't know it. This happened on the day a *Galloping Gourmet* program was being shown for the first time at a sneak preview for the media from England, Canada, Australia, and America. When the program ended, there was silence . . . then as one, they rose and gave the show a standing ovation. (Unheard of, I hasten to add.) Well, my erstwhile adviser sidled up to me and whispered, "A nice compromise with the humor, Treena." I don't think he knows to this day that I never compromised at all.

Indulgence Daily

GRAHAM: It was sink or swim. We swam and swallowed a lot of water . . . and wine! Our risky diet was composed of dishes that would have audience appeal. These were both the famous and the infamous, but all had one virtue in common . . . they were designed to delight from the neck up. In short, they were sensual treats.

We dined multiple times a day at the world's finest restaurants. In one day in Paris, we ate in seven restaurants! We ate, slept, flew—ate, slept, flew, and then tested, rehearsed—tested, rehearsed—and wrote a companion cookbook. As I tested, Treena edited the film we'd shot on location and tried to find jokes for me to tell at the top of the show.

Now and again we saw our children. Our oldest, Tessa, was twelve; son Andy was eight; and Kareena was newly born between episode 65 and 66.

This was, of course, ridiculous, but it truly is the nature of the beast. I was consumed with the need to *do it right*. I insisted that we fly to a recipe's country of origin to ensure that I knew how it tasted at its cultural best and so, we spent our 34th through 36th year galloping and eating richly as we rode. Oh, . . . and trying hard to mend our emotional fences as our lives increasingly spun out of control.

Treena instituted a grading system for each program. I'll let her explain why.

TREENA: The grading system for each program was my way to keep the crew on their toes as well as Graham; they, too, wanted him to get A+. When I gave a lower grade, they all moaned at me. However, everything had to be the tops with jokes and humor during cooking. Sometimes when Graham was thrilled with the dish, I would give a C because it was a yawn. Grading certainly worked for all involved. Yes, even me.

GRAHAM: Of course I longed for an A+, especially when Friday came around, and we had the potential for a pleasant weekend together. If the week ended with a B, you could virtually kiss the break goodbye.

Sailing Away

Along with Treena's grades, I began my over-the-bed chart. We are told that Hollywood types install mirrors above their beds, but

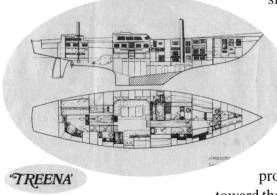

"TREENA"

since we were in Ottawa and didn't much like the idea anyway, I tacked up the plan layout of a 71-foot ocean cruising ketch that was being built in Southern Ocean Shipyards in Poole, Dorset in southern England.

For me it was a 71-foot carrot dangled in front of my nose . . . prompting me from episode to episode toward the finishing line of Episode #650. I colored in each section as we earned enough to pay for it.

TREENA: For me it was pressure and a nightmare. Just imagine having 650 little squares over your head every night, in the shape of a sailing boat, each one to be filled in with black pencil after taping that night's 2 or 3 shows. Then counting how many white squares we had still to fill. It looked impossible, and it was taking so long. Also, I hated sailing. No it wasn't funny!

GRAHAM: With 195 shows to go, we set off on our most ambitious plan ever. We would circumnavigate the U.S. in an RV filming on location from city to city the great dishes of the world that had been brought here by immigrants and changed by our culture's environmental pressures. We were to act out various scenarios in each location.

On day two, our professionally driven Winnebago was rear-ended by a vegetable truck. Yes, really . . . a large vegetable truck that didn't see us in a light fog. It hit us hard and although we tried to patch episodes together with guest stars like Liberace, Stiller and Meara, Gail Greene (food critic), Maitre Chef des Cuisines Silvano Trompetto (Savoy Hotel London), it just didn't work.

I was partially paralyzed, and Treena was badly hurt and traumatized emotionally by the accident. We called it a day, with about 500 episodes in the can.

Taking Stock of the Situation

We were not doing well. My cholesterol at that time was 265. I had gout and kidney stones. Treena developed what appeared to be lung cancer, but when her lung was partially removed; it turned out to be a tuberculosis focus. To find this out, she had to endure a major operation called a thorondoctomy, which needed 82 stitches and left an enormous scar. During her recovery she discovered a painkiller called Darvon, and her medically prescribed addictions began.

We built our dreamboat, the one I'd hung above our bed in Ottawa and marked off half inch "slices" representing the episodes we needed to record in order to afford it. Eventually the insurance settlement from the truck crash helped us with the final costs, and we were ready to set off to circumnavigate the world as a family.

All was not well. The yacht was splendid, but we were still scrambled in our relationships. I was amazed that our long-struggled-for dream didn't immediately solve the early mistakes I'd made.

May 18, 1972, was Treena's birthday, and we had reached Antibes in the south of France. We'd been here before on one of our production trips and had had a wonderful meal at the Bon Auberge. We went back to celebrate, and oh, how we celebrated!

TREENA: It was my 38th birthday—never to be forgotten. Lobster Bisque with double cream in a fried bread croute. A huge steak with red wine sauce and beef marrow and a large chocolate birthday cake, filled with chocolate cream and raspberry sauce. We drank champagne all night. We had a loud and joy-filled time with our friends the crew. Until . . . .

GRAHAM: On our return to the boat there was a major storm in progress and all 66 tons of our floating home was heaving up and down at least a foot and a half at our mooring space. That night indulgence encountered nature, and we were all seasick.

That's how I know exactly when we started to change our gourmet lifestyle to one that I call reasonable and moderate.

We sat around in the more stable main cabin on May 19 and agreed that the extremely rich, high-fat . . . well, high-in-everything dinner had greatly increased our reaction to the storm. We made it our goal over the next 22,000 miles to reduce excessive amounts of fats and refined starches in our meals. In their place, we ate fresh fish, poultry, and as much fresh fruit and vegetables and whole grains as we could find. It was a major change in our diet, and the results on our physical health were truly remarkable.

But we still suffered emotionally, and Treena's prescribed medications had become a fragile safety net.

Ports and oceans passed by as we aimed for the sunny seasons. Eventually, we arrived in the Chesapeake Bay in the fall of 1973, where we ran hard aground at the junction of Peachblossom Creek and the Tred Avon River—a few miles from Oxford, Maryland.

After two years on the move covering an average of one thousand miles a month, Treena was beginning to yearn for a stable dwelling place.

"Darling, look at that lovely house," she pointed across the river to a three-story white colonial mansion with a row of pillars, gabled roof, rolling lawns, a long new dock, and at least 600 feet of water frontage.

"Sure, yes, it's lovely," I replied, thinking that it looked like a small Tara from *Gone with the Wind*.

Much later, with Treena still admiring the house and the boat being still hard aground, I proposed, just for the fun of it, to row ashore and make the owner an offer.

"Don't be surprised if I get chased across the lawn with a gun," I joked as I paddled off to the long dock.

Of course I wanted to complete our circumnavigation, and it was only a joke!

"Do you have a shotgun?" I asked the somewhat surprised homeowner.

"Yes, a duck gun," he explained.

"Could you chase me down the dock with it?" I asked.

"Why should I do that?"

"Well, I'm going to make you a ridiculous offer for your lovely home, and it would be fun for my wife to see your reaction," I explained.

"Okay, but first let's have the offer." He seemed serious.

"Oh, do we have to do that? I really can't offer what it's worth . . . it's really just . . . fun," I added awkwardly.

"Price first . . . fun later," he replied firmly.

I named my price.

"You're right . . . it is a ridiculous offer," he paused, "but you happen to have come on an extraordinary day. How soon can you get me cash?"

After calling our accounting firm in New York, I said quietly, "Tuesday next."

He reached over his desk and shook my hand.

When I got back aboard Treena said, "Well, I didn't see anyone chase you off with a gun, wasn't the owner in?"

"No," I replied, "not anymore . . . it's yours."

TREENA: "It's mine? You mean it really is ours? You've bought it! He accepted? Can you believe that?" I turned to the guys and saw sad faces, and then realized my new beginning was their farewell. But you know, all I really cared about was getting to take a real shower for as long as I liked. To have clothes that weren't damp, having a home that didn't move or heave or tip from side to side. My feet were finally on terra firma again.

To show my pleasure I made all the curtains for the 8-foot windows to let the house know that it was cared for. Seventy-four curtains I made and lined by myself. I tell you the air was very blue during this period. Took me six weeks from six in the morning to five thirty at night! The man from whom I brought the curtain materials said I would never do it as well as his professional staff could do. I showed him, and he was more than a little surprised and very complimentary. I was challenged, so what was I to do? I did it!

From Ship to Shore

And so, in the fall of 1973, in our 39th year, we began the lengthy process of becoming American citizens.

I never found out what prompted that sudden sale, but very soon we discovered a major drawback to the house . . . it cost over $10,000 a year simply to heat and cool the place! Quite apart from the cost of a coat of paint, curtains for the 74 windows, and the nine acres of grass that hung heavily on our son Andy's head—it was growing much faster than he was.

The change from ship to shore didn't stop our downward drift to the emotional bottom. Treena's medications were steadily increased, as was the concern of our physician who thought the time was coming for her to be hospitalized for "an indeterminate period of time for her own safety and your family's."

We had tried all kinds of remedies, both emotional and spiritual, and for brief periods these held promise . . . only to be abruptly shattered by another uncontrolled outburst.

I had thought long and hard about the reason for her collapse . . . and it seemed unavoidably clear . . . it was me. I had asked her to give up her talented future . . . for me. I had asked her to produce both children and hundreds of television shows. I had failed her as her husband . . . it was me she couldn't forgive.

And so, with the late fall leaves swirling around us, I took the deepest breath of my life and proposed the unthinkable.

"I believe that I am the source of your deepest troubles and that the solution is for you to be free of me . . . to have every help in regaining your lost career . . . . I'll help all I can . . . but, well . . . you really don't need me anymore." I'd run out of breath, I'd heard my own words, and my heart was unbearably heavy.

"I'll go upstairs and think about what you've said," she touched my arm lightly and slowly went up to our bedroom.

I sat by the study windows watching storm clouds gathering over the bay beyond the river. The wind began to tease the water and stir the fallen leaves.

I felt her hand on my shoulder; it rested there for a moment as she handed me a sheet of paper. She'd written a poem and given it a clear title, *To love as one*.

TO LOVE AS ONE

To be aware
and love in faith
is all one should desire
to try,
and learn,
and rectify,

some seeming wrong,

this should be done.

yet, do not be alone,

for when two love

one is half

if left,

or leaves,

the arms of one

whose life is stressed.

i prefer to be complete

and walk with you,

along the street

toward the other half of self.

to learn with you

to help,

to understand,

the way we lost ourselves.

we have the right,

to right the wrongs

to each we've made.

no one, alone is wrong,

no one, alone is right;

in marriage, we are one,

and love is ours—not flight! ❧

I stood and took her in my arms . . . . I knew it was settled once and for all. Somehow we'd make it. But the way we'd succeed was so utterly and completely unexpected. It came as a simple knock on our front door.

God Works in Mysterious Ways

Ruthie Turner was a member of a small inner-city church in Wilmington, Delaware. Her pastor had told her that the church wasn't large enough to send her to Haiti where she wanted to serve as a missionary. He told her to find some rich folks who lived on the waterfront and to offer herself as a maid and put her wages in a savings account until she had enough for the trip.

She arrived at our door and knocked. Ruthie became a part of our lives in our darkest hours . . . she'd arrived in an unplanned mission field. At weekends she would return to Wilmington about 100 miles to the north, and there she asked for prayers . . . for herself and for Treena.

As the pressure mounted and the days darkened into winter, Treena's need grew more and more profound. Her physician warned that we were almost out of time . . . a decision had to be made . . . soon.

Unbeknownst to us, Ruthie had recruited her church as a prayer team who committed to pray for her 24/7 so that she was never left unattended, as one after another church member fulfilled their one-hour time slots.

After several weeks they decided to increase their commitment to include fasting. The extraordinary nature of their commitment was that they had never seen Treena and knew nothing of how I'd earned my living . . . they simply felt called to pray for a white lady living in a big white house who was having a real bad time.

GRAHAM: I knew nothing of all this, having been back in Ottawa recording a new series of television shows called *Take Kerr* (another play on the word "care"), which eventually wound up with CNN in its early days of 1974-1975.

It was here that I first experimented with healthier cooking in what I called "mini-max" recipes. This stood for minimum risk-maximum flavor. I began to break foods down into aromas, colors, and textures.

When I came home, it was almost Christmas, and the house was wonderfully quiet. Treena was more at peace than she'd been for months. I put it down to the season and was grateful for the respite.

After the best Christmas I had ever had, son Andy and I were in Safeway buying ham for the New Year's Eve when a lady behind me said she'd been baptized "in the same way as Treena."

DECEMBER 17TH 1974

i went to Bethlehem to find

a solace for my tortured mind.

with trepidation known to child,

i lingered, nervous, somewhat tired.

a pastor tall and black did walk

to greet me with a loving smile –

"my name is Pastor Friend," he said

and prayed for my unwary soul,

he said "the angels will rejoice

with Christ and me this very night."

as the congregation prayed

i fell surprised upon my knees –

then, wrenched from deep within my shame

a cry of hope was born throughout my frame;

"forgive me Jesus," cried my heart,

repentant tears of sorrow, filled my eyes,

burning tears began to fall,

then turned into a water-fall.

friends, Ruthie and Michelle,

and daughter Tessa too –

watched and waited silently.

i stepped—dressed in Ruthie's gown of white –

into the concrete bath of blue –

filled with ice cold water too!

thus, i was baptized, cleansed from sins.

although i didn't realize how or why

a course was set to now live by.

the pastor, Chester Friend, did ask,

"how would you like to tarry now

and wait upon the Comforter."

"I might as well as I am here"

"what do i have to do?" i asked,

"just kneel and thank our Jesus Christ

for the gift, He wants to give."

so there i knelt with eyes shut tight

saying "thank you" to the name

i cursed and swore just hours before.

suddenly upon closed eyes

a strong light shone, a blinding light.

i opened eyes to see

a man of brilliance standing there,

with joyous smile upon His face.

there upon my heart, i saw Him place

His gentle Hand; instantly, i was filled

with knowledge from within. i had His

Joy, His Peace and Holy Grace.

and from "my living hell," Hope took its place. ❧

I thought this hugely amusing until I gathered a household of family and builders to share the joke.

Treena looked up at me with those incredible shining eyes and quietly said, "I was."

My immediate impression, other than embarrassment, was to wonder if this would wreck Sundays and whether there was enough room in our 10,800 square feet for someone with as big a reputation as Jesus Christ!

Over the next week or so, I settled in to watch this latest attempt to repair the years of damage. I wondered how long this spiritual foray would last.

TREENA: My life HAD changed. I had changed; all because Ruthie and her church had prayed and fasted for me. I had a vision of Jesus, and He touched my heart with His hand. How could I not be changed? I threw all my medical drugs, uppers and downers, straight into the "loo." It was a rainbow of promise. My heart was light; my soul full of an amazing joy. I felt the Lord tell me to put a golden zipper over my lips, to be a witness without saying a word to Graham. This is how He said it to me, through my shiny new Bible. "Set a guard over my mouth O Lord, keep a watch over the door of my lips." Psalm 141:3

I had also read that we were to pray in the closet to the Father. Thus Ruthie, Kareena (aged 6), and I would pray among the brooms for Graham's salvation. If we happened to be talking about it when he came into a room, we would discuss the weather very "earnestly."

GRAHAM: Our physician paid a house call and sat on my couch in the den.

"Graham, I'm a Roman Catholic and that means I believe in miracles, but I've never seen one that I could not somehow explain medically," and then he paused, looking me straight in the eye while his filled with tears, "until now. You see . . . Treena is a miracle . . . she's completely well, literally overnight . . . to suddenly drop all medication . . . especially Valium, should mean a possible coma . . . but she's saner than I am . . . not that that means much," he ended with a nervous laugh.

"I truly believe that God has chosen to break into your lives, and you need to know it." I thanked him and went out in the garden to try to deal with the huge implications of this diagnosis. I wound up having a brief discussion with a large tree—it didn't talk back. I wanted to share in the miracle; if anything I felt left out and so I asked for one—just for me. I have come to believe that, regardless of whatever personal or selfish motive may be behind our deeply felt cry for help, God does in fact hear and actually acts then . . . it's just that we may discern nothing until much later.

That's what happened to me. I remember turning to the house, it needed painting . . . the cars, wrong colors . . . the boat, not being used . . . my career, without real reward. Suddenly everything that drove me, every possession that rewarded me—the James Bond Omega watch I wore . . . all these "things" suddenly lost their appeal. The manufactured lights had gone out. The only light that attracted my undivided attention was in Treena's eyes. All the rest gradually took on the look of highly paid slavery.

That was the starting point of my very own miracle. The fact was that it didn't feel good at all. Truthfully, I was miserable. For years I had worked really hard, but there were reasons and rewards . . . remember the 71-foot carrot hanging over our bed?! But now there was nothing . . . a lot of work and so little purpose.

On March 15, 1975, one month after my cry for a miracle, I too found my own place in the scheme of things. After a long, hard day in the studio, I got back to what is now the Four Seasons Hotel in Ottawa and, unable to sleep, found myself on my knees shouting at the ceiling.

"I want a personal relationship with you like Treena has, and I want it now!"

I'm here to tell you that God doesn't operate room service. Truly frustrated, dead tired, and I guess, angry, I lowered my voice and asked of the ceiling, "What do I have to say to you to get to know you like Treena does?"

The answer spilled out of my mouth without the slightest thought. I heard myself say, "Jesus . . . I love you."

I sat back on my heels and almost laughed out loud as wave upon wave of goose bumps flowed down my body. In moments I'd gone from flat-out exhausted to overflowing joy . . . an amazing experience that I've never been able to adequately describe.

Treena and I have taken this space to add our spiritual story because, had we left it out, we would have been lying by exclusion. What you do with it is your business. What we do with it is really part and parcel of the rest of our lives, but it doesn't need to dominate the rest of this book.

As Treena had prophetically written in her poem, we were off walking together down the street toward the other half of self, and in doing so we came to understand the way we lost ourselves and how to right the wrongs we'd made.

Unforgiving left—forgiveness arrived, and we were free to get on with our lives. We had turned 40, and the crisis we had endured for eight years was over.

A New Direction, or Several

Startling changes took place almost immediately. Our spiritual story received a huge amount of attention as we returned three times to try to explain ourselves on *Donahue* and other talk shows.

We were asked to compromise our faith . . . but that's another story for another time. In the end, we did not do so, but the back and forth took over a year, and finally we resigned from television and gave away all our rights and residuals, including the title *Galloping Gourmet*, which is why I refer to myself as the "former" Galloping Gourmet.

We sold our home (eventually) for the same price we gave for it. We auctioned off all our trinkets and rewards and left for the Colorado mountains to start a retreat for married couples facing divorce. A "place apart" in log cabins with sunken bathtubs and double beds . . . where they could give God one last chance at restoration . . . as He had done with us.

We built it but couldn't complete it. We ran out of money and were unable to raise a penny, even from the millions of people who had listened to our story. We took this to be another miracle and when prayerfully asking "Why?" were more than a little chagrined by what we felt to be the reply, "You never asked me."

This was how we came to live, in 1977, in Palm Springs at the home of a couple who understood.

FORGIVENESS

Forgiveness is no more a choice in this age of famine,
Bloody wars, divorce, denial and racial bigotry.
If you can win the wrestle, the hard wrestle to forgive,
Peace will tenure in its place, swallowing the negative!

We must forgive the misery—the memory of abuse,
The trauma suffered as a child—the hurts we hold so close.
Forgive injustice and the pain of being second-best,
The wounding of that hurtful word a parent said in jest.

"Forgive? You know not what you say! Forgive? It's not deserved.
Forgive! No way! More like their head upon a platter served."
No one can know the pain or the injustice done, it's true.
But to be free you must forgive, so Christ can you renew.

Stored sin becomes as cancer, inflaming sores that seep,
Self-pity steeped in matted sins that fester as you sleep.
Sins of bitterness encrust one's inner soul with weeping.
Self-pity loves itself so much it cannot be forgiving!

One's collected sins accept, though another was the cause.
The Forgiver will forgive if you repent and love His laws.
Look closely in a mirror. View your reflected self.
Look face-to-face and eye-to-eye. Now . . . forgive yourself.

Once done you'll find it easier other persons to absolve,
Those who abused, defiled, tormented body, mind and soul.
When the wrestle you have won, you'll feel clean and purified,
Because, dear friend, by "the forgiving" you'll be sanctified.

With peace of mind, new joy of life, depression soon will wane.
You'll not forget the past but will annihilate the pain.
From your deep-seated un-forgiveness, He's forgiven you
And freedom is His Gift, when you forgive as He has you. ✲

I began reading in depth about both good nutrition and hunger and found the statistics deeply troubling. According to UNICEF, there were 18 million children under the age of five who died because they did not get enough food or the right kinds of food.

At the same time, the Center for Disease Control released the information that as many as 600,000 North Americans were dying from eating too much food, and too much of the wrong kinds of food. This obvious injustice fundamentally changed my life and continues to this day to motivate me. Twenty-five years later the numbers are more accurate and the injustice remains just the same.

The sudden view of the pain caused by thoughtless lifestyle choices was difficult for me to handle, and we moved into an uncomfortable period of self-righteousness during which I tried to lay down the law in my home. (Some of you will recognize this as the Food Police stage.)

One day in 1978, I had been reading about the nitrite and saturated fat content in bologna sausage and went straight from this alarming (and well overstated) report to see my beloved Treena putting . . . yes . . . bologna into our son Andy's sandwich.

"You're not putting that in our son's sandwich," said I, pointing my finger at the sausage as it hung limply in her hand.

Suddenly, Treena snapped. She is, after all, a direct descendant from the Queen of the Romanian Gypsies. She flung the bologna in my direction. It makes quite a good frisbee. It fell at my feet. She then did something quite hard to replicate. She dealt the rest of the sticky pack like a Vegas card dealer . . . all over the floor.

She turned to the pantry cupboard, picking up random packets and jars and throwing them into the trashcan while shouting, "There's nothing in the world left to eat with you!"

We lived between Liberace and Kirk Douglas, and Treena has great voice projection. This obviously concerned me greatly since I still felt that I had a reputation as a gourmet that was in immediate danger.

Now I believe that men are really quite sensitive and have considerable discernment at times like this, and I definitely had the feeling that something was wrong.

"Tell you what," I cried out above all the din.

"What," Treena blazed back.

"I'll cook what you like to eat, and I'll eat what I like. We'll have two styles," I placated.

"Fine, fine, fine," she replied.

You always know when you've got a deal with Treena.

BOLOGNA

Bologna flew, flew, flew
Fury made this rare debut
"Can't eat this. Can't eat that"
Another piece graced this act.
As anger grew, more slices flew,
landing at Graham's feet, on cue.
Soon they were done, so cupboards next
Were emptied in the garbage bin.
I punctuated each item flung with "FINE!"
First one, then two, then three with
"There . . . is . . . nothing . . . left to eat . . . with you"
"Okay, okay, you have your way, I'll eat mine"
I had won, or so I thought, it wasn't true.
It was fine, fine, fine . . . until! ॐ

Adding Feathers One by One to the Scale

And so came our season of culinary compromise, one in which featherweight decisions were repeatedly slipped into our respective scales of justice. In and of themselves, they made very little difference, but when repeated day after day for eight years, they added up.

Tacoma, Washington, 1987: After nine years of trying to understand how to right the scales of injustice for the poor children, which included long-range development training in low input sustainable agriculture (LISA), I was suddenly called to account for our own scales that finally responded to our eight-year plan to have two cuisines.

"Graham, get down to St. Joe's Hospital. Treena's had a stroke."

I thumped the steering wheel in my car again and again as I drove through rain-streaked streets. "Why, why, why?" I demanded, as if I didn't know.

In a day or two she was released. Every test confirmed the stroke—but did nothing for Treena's unwillingness to accept the diagnosis. Her response swung between "They are all wrong" to "I've been healed." De-ni-al is not just a river in Egypt!

During the tests, we discovered that Treena was "borderline diabetic." Her fasting glucose was 140 mg/dl, which we now know is the diagnosis for type 2 diabetes, and it absolutely needs careful treatment.

We received no treatment or advice. That was the reality in 1987, and it still happens today to roughly 8 million people wandering around the U.S. with their type 2 diabetes undiagnosed or untreated. We had to wait until 1994 before her diabetes was finally recognized and treated—and that's when we learned that diabetes puts you at increased risk of having a stroke or heart attack.

Life returned more or less to normal until November 1987 when, during a leadership-training course at the University of the Nations in Hawaii, Treena had a heart attack.

Once again she didn't believe it. "It's indigestion" was her understanding of the pain.

The doctors in the ER didn't agree. We found ourselves in an air ambulance en route to Honolulu.

This event was our mutual epiphany, and is the reason we began to explore the creative lifestyle we'll share with you in Part II. It's taken us 17 years *so far*, so please be patient!

CHAPTER TWO

Search for
the Solution

It was my very first time in an air ambulance—everything was so matter of fact in spite of the drama. Treena lay quietly beside a battery of portable instruments wired to her heart. A machine beeped rhythmically, and green peaks raced over a small screen. We had a male nurse with us who monitored her blood pressure and made sure I was strapped in. We didn't talk, it was noisy and the short flight from Kailua on the Big Island to Honolulu was quite bumpy.

"Make your peace with her . . . she might not make it," the island doctor had said. I watched, my eyes going back and forth from her face to the little green line of peaks and valleys. We'd known each other for nearly 43 years; we'd been married for 32, and in spite of our own peaks and valleys, we were so happy together—would I lose her now?

The machine beeped. The green line continued to leap and fall. Why had I made it so difficult for her? So many rules: Don't eat this, don't eat that—no wonder she rebelled! At least I could have taken the best of what I knew about cooking and about healthy food and made it taste better for her, something she would love to eat! Thoughts and regrets raced through my mind as the machine continued to beep.

Treena was swiftly transferred to the critical care unit at Honolulu General Hospital. Again it was all so . . . normal . . . so organized . . . so . . . in charge. I waited with other family members to know if she would live or die. My mind continued to race over memories and a growing list of options. If she did make it . . . what would we do this time with our lifestyle?

I now had 16 years of experience and knowledge bolstered by searching through the science of lifestyle choice. I'd read conservative western medicine and fringe-eastern alternatives. It was a jumble until the 1978 U.S. Government White Paper on "Seven Goals." I'd worked on those goals for a whole year when I recorded *The Double Benefit* video series with Global Net News . . . so really I knew what to do, but Treena hadn't been *willing*. Her DOW (degree of willingness) was still resisting my earlier intrusion into her private space.

Would this heart attack change things?

TREENA: Yes this heart attack was to change a lot of things, in both our lives. While in the plane, I looked at my Gra (my special name for Graham) and he WAS grey! I knew that God wasn't ready for me; He had too much work to do in me yet. "Gra looks so awful" I was thinking. "WHY didn't I do as he said, he knew, HE ALWAYS KNOWS EVERYTHING. Because of my "don't want to know" attitude, we were going to count the cost, literally!

We had no insurance and certainly not enough for all the medical bills. "I'm sorry Lord, I will obey and do what Gra says to do in the future." Why was I so rebellious? Maybe it was because I didn't like being "sick"—that can still make me angry. One of those things the Lord had to work on. Then we landed and off we went in another ambulance to the wonderful people who would care for me.

Lifestyle Change?

I met Dr. "Got-Your-Car-Keys," our Japanese-American cardiologist, who explained that it was the best way to remember his name. He showed the two of us (I'd been joined by our son, Andy) an x-ray film of the angiogram of Treena's heart. He pointed out the narrowed artery and told us of the need for a bypass "within the next 10 years." He then turned from the screen and gave me that level stare that physicians must be taught to use when delivering really important messages.

"Of course . . . you could also try lifestyle," he suggested.

I listened, but what I saw was Treena in full spate, dealing bologna over the kitchen floor!

"I'm going to give you some books and ask you to try some of the ideas for three months and then we'll see what to do next." He was serene and in charge, and in some special way, he ignited a desire within me that flared high that day and has never diminished.

I would search for a solution. I hadn't lost her . . . we had more years to live together. They would be good years . . . we'd deal with this challenge and we'd overcome it . . . together.

⚬

Be Willing and ACT

Treena left the hospital two days later. Her total cholesterol was 365. We were still in the middle of our leadership training school at the University of the Nations, so Treena rested for two weeks and listened to the tapes. Notwithstanding all the upset, she still graduated with a B+!

In the early mornings we set out together on a gentle walk while the temperatures were still moderate. We had our own condominium unit, so I was able to cook all her meals. I read the books. I knew exactly what to do . . . it was all the tried and tested advice I had read and re-read. Nothing was different! Eat a low-fat diet, especially low in saturated animal fats, restrict salt, trim calories to about 1,400 per day, walk, stretch, and lose weight. It was so normal . . . so logical, and yet something was missing. How could I motivate her and get her DOW going?

It turned out that she had also been thinking creatively in the air ambulance and had decided to "do what he says." She chose to be willing . . . and there's no doubt in my mind that this won 50% of the battle.

The other half was won by what I now call a revolutionary idea—like the paper clip. Look at the twisted wire paper clip—it's so obvious and so simple, and yet it took 100 years to develop and perfect. Was this the case with ACT? ACT stands for Aroma, Color, and Taste—and it's where I started my search for a solution for Treena's special needs.

We both knew what needed to be done. We had been given the opportunity of three months to "try lifestyle." Now all we needed was to know how to put good science into practice!

It began with a large sheet of plain paper and the initials ACT. I asked her to tell me what she most loved about food under each of the headings.

It started slowly and not very helpfully.

"Under A, aroma . . . let's see," she paused . . . "I like bacon, a good Vindaloo curry . . . Bresse Bleu (that's a creamy blue veined full-fat cheese), roast lamb. . . . " The list went on and on as she reeled off the foods that had contributed to her health problems. I sighed. We kept at it and slowly but wonderfully the list grew as we added a much larger number of vegetables—peas, lentils, beans—all manner of fruit and herbs, spices, and, of course, the hot sauces. We wound up with more than 400 foods. These were not recipes. They were individual ingredients.

An unexpected fringe benefit began to surface—her list of most disliked foods. I had no idea that she loathed broiled sweet bell peppers (they are my favorite food!), eggplant, and okra. I had put peppers in many dishes I'd made for her in the past, and she'd never complained.

The T stood for taste and should have been obvious from the start! If we like how a food tastes, then we are more likely to eat it, right?

The method took place slowly over several years in which I cooked for Treena and then let our experience spill over onto television.

TREENA: I loved the dishes Gra was now creating for me; the vegetable sauces, brown rice, even green veggies tasted great with a little cayenne pepper or ground white pepper. (I love HOT stuff.) No more eating things I really didn't like. Moreover, not only that, Gra ate everything I was supposed to eat, too, and exercised as I was doing. Here I started to get an inkling of how to be obedient. However, I still had to learn the full truth the hard way!

The ACT list began a method that has evolved and continues to evolve to this day, as more and more people use it to pin down the foods they like to eat. We've added another T for texture,

which makes it TACT. We now c
Sheets and we've included it in th
available to download at www.g

What, Television Again?

Little did I know it, but the nex
the horizon roughly east-southeas ͑ ͑.

Bruce Reynolds had inherited Reynolds Film ͑
his father. Reynolds was a small but highly respected film com
pany based in Auckland in the North Island of New Zealand.
Bruce had an idea. He would connect with the *Galloping Gourmet*,
where I had begun my career in New Zealand, to see if I would
make a series of video programs for Japan about New Zealand and
its wonderful foods.

We began to talk. I really liked Bruce and in spite of Treena's
and my reluctance to ever be on television again . . . we agreed to
think about it. In our thinking, we contacted our old buddies in
New York who insisted that it be shot in Beta-Cam format so that
it might also be used on television in the U.S. and elsewhere.

What had begun as a simple but good idea with a small budget
. . . began to mushroom. Along with the idea for the show came
the *mission* to share what Treena and I were learning. Her cholesterol had dropped more than 100 points in the three months given
us by our cardiologist. He and we were delighted and eager to
share our early success.

The lifestyle mission began to mesh with our spiritual lives and
the program morphed into a full-blown production called *Simply
Marvelous* funded by a New Zealand foundation with global
expectations.

Early in 1988, with Treena in the midst of a blooming recovery and our prayerful release from our obligations to Youth With
A Mission, we recorded an initial 13 episodes in New Zealand, followed by 26 episodes in the British Isles in 1989.

The idea was intriguing. We would take well-known, well-
loved dishes of a region and tweak them so that the risks fell away
and were replaced by foods that added aroma, color, and texture to
the dish. In other words, we were doing a cultural, regional upgrade.

Treena did research and gathered information on camera, helped to interview the different people. We wanted her to be in front this time and not behind the camera. She did not produce the show, the only time in my career that she hasn't.

We had a wonderful time cooking for real people in their own homes—both for family and friends. I look back on it with great fondness—such neat people and a great crew and the food truly was excellent. But it didn't sell (it played eventually on the Food Network) because 39 wasn't enough episodes (remember the 195 required each year?) And, at that time (1988), the critical mass of information about food and health had not yet been reached . . . we were way ahead of our time!

The Low-Fat Era

As it happened we were running alongside a number of others who had seen the commercial opportunity of making "no-fat" foods, but they had stripped food of its essential balance and somehow rendered the packaging more tasteful than their products. Inevitably there was a predictable backlash and some widely respected, very popular food experts cried "foul" and declared (rightly) that "no fat meant no flavor" and that "you could eat anything if you ate it in moderation."

All of this is true . . . but then, like every oversimplified statement, it eventually runs off the rails of reason. How do you measure what is moderate? How for yourself as an individual with a specific need? Dietitians and medical researchers relied on science to provide the guidance. Gourmets and celebrity chefs and authors relied on their senses. The "war of the diets" had begun, and the lines were drawn.

❧

In 1993 I attended a meeting of the International Association of Culinary Professionals (IACP) in San Francisco. I had recently joined as a member and had won the Julia Child Cookbook Award for my Mini-Max Cookbook (Doubleday, 1989). Julia was speaking at a large luncheon for several hundred fellow-foodies and was firing some pretty heavy stuff at another San Francisco resident, Dr. Dean Ornish, M.D., the famed lifestyle researcher and author.

"I don't believe that anyone can eat a diet with only 10% of calories from fat" she thumped the lectern with considerable vigor. "In fact," she cried out, extemporaneously, "If anyone here is doing that I'd like to see him STAND UP!" she challenged.

I stood . . . apparently alone amongst hundreds who seemed to wheel around in their seats in shock. Julia was looking down at her notes. I remained on my feet . . . feeling acutely uneasy . . . "Where is this going?" I thought. After what seemed like an age, I sat down and Julia looked back up and continued, unaware of my "demonstration." She didn't know that I had stood, but the press did—and they smelled blood!

"Are you leading a rebellion against Julia?" one breathless media type asked urgently in a crowd of others eager to get the story.

"Not a bit of it," I replied. "Julia asked to see anyone who did . . . well, I do . . . for my wife Treena . . . so I stood . . . nothing more or less than being obedient to someone I love and respect."

And that was the end of it . . . well almost.

Julia and I met that night and over her Scotch, hamburger, and fries (she didn't like the Californian Fusion Cuisine served at dinner) and my de-alcoholized beer . . . we discussed our differences.

Julia, during the ensuing years, has come to accept what I do for Treena. She does not go beyond her definition of moderation couched as it is in French culinary method, and I have come to accept her position out of respect for her consistency and ability, and frankly, out of a desire for synergism. It was because of this averted conflict that I learned an important lesson about opposite opinions.

In the past I'd been embroiled in controversy over diet and cuisine, and each side went knuckle-to-knuckle with the consumer's head in the middle. The result was both newsworthy (for 15 minutes or so), painful, and ultimately, for the reader, confusing.

I'd tried another tack . . . that I now call a politically correct compromise . . . where I worked with people who took the opposite of my new direction. I found this also confused folks . . . who would say "Why is he doing that with them?"

It wasn't until Julia that I learned that you could fully respect the position of others without relinquishing your own place. I shall always be deeply indebted to her for her "inclusiveness."

I now focus my energies on trying to understand how best to serve people who want to make changes, and I don't waste my energy being critical of others. If I can make a solid contribution such as eating more vegetables, food safety, or smaller portion sizes, then I'll do it with all my heart . . . and if I can't make a contribution, I'll SHUT UP. We have too many opinionated pundits that do little but stir up controversy. There is no need to swell their ranks—especially in these troubled times.

It has been obvious that our direction had changed, and it was perfectly clear that I had chosen a path less traveled . . . it was certainly less popular and profitable. Unfortunately it offended some of those with whom I used to walk who felt my decision somehow implied a criticism of their continuing on in that other direction.

I am fully aware and unhappy about this misconception. I know of thousands of well-meaning food professionals who work sincerely and diligently to provide excellent dishes that go in exactly the opposite direction to mine. They have their careers and their families to support, and I embrace their right to pursue their own purpose in life. My wish is that everyone who cooks for others would creatively include recipes that "do no harm" (hopefully to anyone). As a result, you and I would have truly creative choices at every restaurant and in every family kitchen (please see Menu 2 at www.grahamkerr.com).

❧

Treena and I continued to search for heart health solutions. Our media efforts now included a show simply called *Graham Kerr* that lasted from 1990 through 1994. It was mostly seen on *Discovery*. We continued on public television until 1996 when we began our opus work . . . *The Gathering Place*, in which we spent more than five years researching, traveling, location filming (and eating), and eventually testing, rehearsing and recording.

Never before had we set out with such an ambitious idea . . . a global sampling of comfort foods from the U.S., Mexico, Caribbean, Pacific Islands, New Zealand, Australia, Japan, China, Malaysia, Seychelles, Sri Lanka, India, Jordan, Israel, Greece, Italy, England, Scotland, and Canada—more or less in that order. [You will find all these recipes in Part V of this book.]

We had "embedded" teams of local experts who graciously worked on multiple layers of research before we arrived. Our panel of experts included the field of cooking, agriculture, fishing, health, anthropology, and tourism. We were especially well served by members of the International Association of Registered Dietitians.

We wanted to see, make, and taste a dozen or so culturally popular dishes that used locally grown ingredients and, wherever possible, contributed to a healthy lifestyle (or could be modified to do so without doing damage to the taste, aroma, color, and texture).

We filmed, ate, talked, made friends, hugged, and moved on and on and on. Recipe files bulged as we went, but something else was happening as we searched, something we should have suspected, something that would kick open an entirely new door of lifestyle change!

CHAPTER THREE

The Daily Olympics of Life

Just before leaving on our worldwide adventure in 1994, we attended one of Dr. Dean Ornish's retreats in California. I was one of the speakers, and Treena went through the system on a special-fee basis. We listened carefully and were impressed with his extremely diligent research and positive results.

We decided to give his "vegan" vegetarian ideas a serious go. Basically Dr. Ornish suggested that Treena could eat pretty well as much as she liked providing that the total fat content was 10% or less and there was very little saturated fat—and that only from plants. What starches or carbohydrates she ate had to be whole grain.

While everyone's laboratory numbers (cholesterol, etc.) were reviewed before we began, I have the feeling that Treena's somehow slipped through the cracks—otherwise, I'm sure she would have received some additional advice. Treena's fasting blood glucose had always hovered around the 140 mg/dl level, which at that time was considered borderline type 2 diabetes.

I should add that at the date of this writing a fasting glucose of 110 mg/dl is a warning sign and is called pre-diabetes. At this level you can make some lifestyle adjustments and prevent or at least slow down the onset of diabetes. The same lifestyle changes could have been started at Treena's 140, but they weren't, so, by 1994, Treena had been living with untreated type 2 diabetes for 10 years!

With her blood glucose at 140, she should have been told about counting the amount of carbohydrate in each meal, but she wasn't. Interestingly, this would have had a great impact on the idea of fat percentage that had so upset Julia Child and was to be our next big hurdle.

If you want to lower your cholesterol, especially the "bad" LDL, you eat less fat, which is expressed as a percentage of your daily calories. For Treena, there was a subtle trap lying in wait. All it takes to get down to 10% fat is to add more carbohydrates to the day's menus. But if you increase calories from carbohydrates, it can spell trouble for blood glucose levels for people like Treena, and even more complicated in her case, it drove up her triglycerides, which in turn reduced her "good" HDL cholesterol.

Our door got kicked in. Treena's fasting glucose shot up to 286 mg/dl. Her AlC (a measurement that shows a three-month average of glucose stored in the red blood cells) was 11.9. Nearly 12% of her blood was glucose. And this disastrous turn of events happened while she was trying so hard to lower her cholesterol on a vegan vegetarian "eat as much as you want" diet. We were between a rock and a hard place (diabetes and heart disease) and had to see where we could go now in our search for what was, in fact, a brand new solution.

We discovered that a heart-healthy diet was not healthy for a person with diabetes. But we have also discovered that a diabetic diet is just about perfect for heart health, diabetes, and almost all other major diseases! A diabetic diet is good for everyone. Once more my enthusiasm flared. We could do this.

⋘

Education Really Helps

Our first steps took us to a diabetes educator who, bless her heart, seemed to be more impressed with my old *Galloping Gourmet* shows than Treena's blood glucose. We were hit with a barrage of books that were supposed to help us bring her "sugars" to a managed level. Unfortunately, the educator began where even angels fear to tread—with the negatives.

"If you don't manage your glucose levels, you could (she stressed *could*) go blind, suffer pain at nerve endings, face toe or foot amputation, or kidney failure. And then there's an increased risk of another heart attack and stroke!" She waited until after the word stroke to inhale.

One of our stellar guests on *The Gathering Place* was James Procaska, Ph.D, a famed psychologist who has written a remarkable book, *Changing for Good* (Avon Books, 1995), which explored the sequence of events that helped people with habits they needed to change. One of his absolutes was that if you begin the process with a negative, it is much less likely to have a positive outcome.

I've come to call this the Klingon factor after the alien space travelers in *Star Trek*. They are the warlike chaps (warts and all) who have a cloaking device that renders them invisible. So, the Klingon factor happens when a health care provider begins with a negative (or series of negatives in our case). Treena tried hard to listen . . . we both did . . . but frankly, all the well-intentioned advice simply evaporated. We just didn't get it.

Our food became "exchanges"—our carbs needed to be counted—her fingers needed to be pricked several times a day. We exchanged glances and looked upwards and rolled our eyes when the educator wasn't looking.

The moment we got home, I attacked the booklets we'd been given. We were 60 years old, reasonably intelligent, well versed in dietary change . . . but this was . . . awful! Once again, as with the heart attack booklets, we were getting excellent advice that just didn't fit us . . . especially the suggested menus. Does anybody eat like that!?

Our very good friend, Dr. James Castelli, the former director of the Framingham Research Project, loves to say that "a low-fat diet may not help you to live longer . . . it's just going to seem like it." Well, Dr. Castelli should have seen the meal plan proposed by our educator.

James Procaska suggests that you begin with positives that empower you (such an overused word) with the hope of a successful outcome through good management of blood sugars. We went off in search of someone else to help us. To have the door kicked open was one thing, but ours was hanging off its hinges.

❧

Help with a Shiny Helmet

Kitty Carmichael, RD, CDE, rides a motorcycle. When she does, she wears a practical shiny helmet. At work she changes into a long white coat. She's highly recommended; we are impressed. Perhaps now we'll get positive advice we can understand?

Treena shakes hands and launches into her feelings about diabetes. "After all," she explains, "number two must be less complicated than number one."

Kitty rose to her feet and thrust her face forward until her nose almost touched Treena's. They are almost the same height. "Treena," she said firmly. "I don't have diabetes . . . you do. I can't live it for you. You've got to do that. If you understand it's a chronic disease that isn't going to go away, then you're halfway there. The rest is to believe you can control its effects. You don't have to face serious complications."

"Ha ha, there it is," I thought, "she's gone positive." I had to admit she had me worried at her in-your-face response to Treena. Remember the bologna?

TREENA: I have to admit I was very upset when I found out I now had something else caused, in part, by trying to behave and follow the heart diet. Think of all that lovely smoked salmon I missed, the caviar which I like when I have a chance, all the luscious food I could have eaten and didn't, what a crock!

I have come to the conclusion that the reason I was so difficult over the years was my fear of people thinking I was making a fuss. I had always found it irritating when people made a fuss about nothing. I never believed there was anything wrong with me physically even if I was told there was. However, when beloved Kitty told me in her positive attitude that I DID have a chronic disease, I was surprised. "I do?"

"YES, YOU DO!"

Was I afraid? No not at all. I knew Gra and I could do this together. He didn't have it, but don't forget, he knows! Was it easy? You're joking!!! No, it was not, but I was soon to find the key to obedience.

GRAHAM: Well, Treena loved her. Kitty took one look at the glucose monitor (which shall be nameless) that we'd been given and dropped it into the trash. "Let's start over with this one." She opened the box, explained how it works, got a blood sample done in only five seconds, and we began a partnership in purpose with someone Treena calls her "little angel."

Treena kept her "scores" in the small logbook provided by the meter company, small enough for a purse, just big enough to avoid confusion—sometimes. Little logbooks didn't work for me. I'm in love with graphs. I enjoy watching progress over at least a full month, so I asked Treena if she'd mind if I kept a five-week graph of all her fasting levels.

Remember, this is her private space. It would mean logging what she ate, how much she weighed daily, and her blood pressure, pulse, and fasting glucose. If I wasn't careful, if I took it for granted, I could blow the whole deal and her DOW would drop back to near zero.

I've been careful not to push (most of the time) and in the process, we've named our graph *The Daily Olympics of Life* (DOOL). It's become a journal that makes a real difference. In a way, it's our accountability link, but more importantly, it's become a true partnership with me as the coach and Treena as the athlete who wants to do better.

The race we have to run isn't a one-time stretch for a record, it's a daily checking of a shared purpose . . . to have more years without complications, so we have more years to love and be loved. It's the gradual search for some featherweight idea that can nudge the graph line lower.

I've got enough DOOL graphs to lay side by side down our hallway at home. We walk alongside month after month, and although we are getting older, the numbers are getting better. We are not losing the battle. We've held our own, and now and again, we see the overall trend for the better.

Treena's last lab report shows a 5.3 AlC. (It had been 11.9.) An A1C of 5.3 is normal. During the past 17 years, she's lost 23 pounds, lowered her average blood pressure from 184/92 to 122/72. Her total cholesterol from 365 to 187 with an LDL of 109 and an HDL of 46.

If you are interested in using a journal like ours, we recommend the companion journal to this book called *My Personal Path to Wellness: A Journal for Living Creatively with Chronic Illness.*

(We changed the name in case some folks thought that a Daily Olympics was too difficult to even attempt.) See pages 490–491.

You can purchase this 4-month journal with health tips from 100 experts who appear with us on *The Gathering Place*. The journal is available at your local bookstore or by calling the ADA at 1-800-232-6733 or visiting the online bookstore at store.diabetes.org (no www is needed). It's 240 pages for $16.95.

Now I may be her coach on paper, but I'm her cook in the kitchen, and every day I cook for her a mighty featherweight (how's that for an oxymoron) provision. I'm making a contribution to her 150% lowered risk of another stroke or heart attack. When I really think about that and really appreciate her ongoing degree of willingness . . . I could run laps around the ceiling with pleasure.

Now just like Kitty said to Treena, may we please say to you: "We don't have your diabetes . . . you do. We can't live it for you. You've got to do that."

In Chapter IV, we'll list the featherweight choices we've made in our partnership in purpose. You will use some, discard others, and replace them with some of your own. Whatever you choose to do, remember: "it's a chronic disease that isn't going to go away. If you understand this, then you're halfway there. The rest is to believe you can control its effects. You don't have to face serious complications."

CHAPTER FOUR

Little Choices Add Up

I t's all about quality of life . . . and love. You shouldn't have to go through life alone, especially with a condition that needs consistent attention to manage it well. You need a partner . . . be it spouse, close family member, or friend. Your chances of successfully managing blood sugars and cholesterol and hypertension increase dramatically when you have a partner in purpose. So . . . before we get into what could happen day to day, a brief word to the partner.

Hi Partner!

It's always tough news to find out that someone close to you has a serious health problem that may not go away. And somewhat like the "owner" . . . you, too, will respond in different ways. It's easy to get angry—at least in the early stages. "Why does this have to happen to us?" In the midst of anger or upset, you may feel critical or occasionally impatient. None of these responses help, but they are human—and I've been through them all!

What did help was to discover for myself the meaning of the word care. My love for Treena was not in doubt, and to some degree, the anger, upset, criticism, and impatience grew out of love and feeling how unfair it was to have our love threatened or made . . . imperfect. So, let's sideline love for just a moment, and bring the word care to center stage, I'll try to explain. Just say these sentences and examine your feelings. Do they differ?

"I love you."

"I care about you."

In my case, the word love usually (hopefully) invites a response, "I love you, too" and that feels good. Again, in my experience, the word care is an expression of a feeling that doesn't need a response and, in fact, may have no expectation of getting one. Because of my interest in the way these two words felt, I tried an acronym to help explain the emotional difference. I used *Webster's Dictionary* to find these meanings.

C   Stands for the word CONCERN.
"To have one's mind filled with."

A   Stands for the word ALTRUISM.
"A selfless devotion to the well-being of another."

R   Stands for the word RESTORATION.
"To return (something) to its original design intention."

E   Stands for the word ENTHUSIASM.
Greek (en theos) "in God."

If you combine these words and meanings, you get a definition of the word care: "To have one's mind filled with a selfless devotion for the well-being of other people so that they may be restored to their original design intention in God."

No matter what is the source of your personal faith, I cannot believe that any Creator's original design intention was for disease. We can accept the results of fair wear and tear through age or accident and our eventual death . . . but disease that shortens life expectancy seems not to be "designed." We need to do something about it.

As I thought this through, I was helped by scripture: "I came that you might have life and have it more abundantly." It seemed to me that the original design intention was abundant life and that condition comes through an interdependent relationship of body, soul, mind, and spirit . . . leaving nothing out. So, I understood that while I loved Treena . . . I also needed to care for her, and that in doing so, I would begin to discover the meaning of abundant life— for both of us.

That is now my challenge to you, as the partner in a truly remarkable journey of restoration, that both of you return to your original design intention . . . abundant life . . . and have more years without complication in which you can make a contribution to love and life and laughter. It is possible.

Understanding the Basics

As partners in purpose, we have found five building blocks that provide you a foundation, no matter which lifestyle options you choose.

1. It's Options and Choices Not Rules and Regulations

We have learned this in the School of Hard Knocks . . . anytime you create a rule or regulation, you invite a rebellion. Clustered about every rule are several creative choices that probably fit your lifestyle needs. Never accept a hard-to-live-with rule without seeking out your options and choices. Your objective is abundant life, not rigid restriction.

2. Have a Degree of Willingness (DOW)

I've covered this on page 32 but must repeat it. Both of you need to be willing—on a daily basis—to jump back into the same foxhole. And willingness is really sensitive to you asking permission to enter each other's space, not assuming it as a right. A partner must never insist on anything. By all means, keep it fresh by gathering new options and choices, but be careful not to let them harden into rules and regulations. The journey is one of discovery. "Having more years to contribute" is an extremely creative and rewarding goal.

3. Measure So You Know

Our very dear friend Julia Child has been often quoted as having said; "You can eat anything if you eat it in moderation." She is, of course, absolutely right. What is left, however, is to have a way of measuring what is moderate . . . for ourselves.

Without a means of measuring, it is remarkably easy for each of us to judge almost anything we desire as moderate! Appetite is not unlike the challenge facing a gambler or a manic shopper with credit card in hand. Eventually the numbers will add up and remind us of our folly. Today we have a wide variety of measurements we can do on a daily basis, such as the one-cup measure in the kitchen or the blood sugar check two hours after a meal, that greatly help us to understand what is moderate. The big issue is to measure often, especially during the learning curve of creative changes so you can see how effective those changes are.

4. Take Your Medications

Some well-intentioned lifestyle experts lay heavy emphasis upon becoming medication free. This is, of course, highly desirable, and we all like the idea of living independently of chemical support. The trouble is when freedom from medication becomes the gold medal of achievement and anything less is some kind of failure. Through no fault of your own, your pancreas may just wear out, and you will need diabetes pills or insulin to keep your blood sugar levels near normal. This is how you continue avoiding those complications.

It is especially troubling as we age, and some of our systems may begin to be less efficient. At these times, regardless of your very best efforts, it is time to add medications, but not time to feel you failed! Treena and I have gone through this one and have come to accept our carefully researched medications as a real partner in our search for abundant life and more years to contribute (MYTC). You only have to see Treena's DOOLs spike when she misses just one pill to know what benefits we get from taking the medication on time every time.

As a brief P.S. . . .we are all aware nowadays of threats to our security and the need to keep an ample supply of important medications in a cool, dry place, just in case that supply line is ruptured. Take twice as much as you may need when you travel, too, in your carry-on bag.

5. The Search Is Never-ending for Creative Change

Medications and surgery are wonderful interventions for which we are sincerely grateful; however, neither should be an alternative to creative lifestyle choices. For example, no amount of medication can replace your body's need to exercise or to eat fewer saturated fat foods and processed carbohydrates.

Nothing should ever let you feel that you should stop searching the web and other references for the latest creative ideas that might unlock yet another door to abundant life. Now, let's get on with the sequence of changes that Treena and I have experienced since 1987 when we began our true partnership in purpose.

Sequence Not System

Years ago, I awakened from a deep sleep with four words constantly repeating, "It's sequence not system." It was so insistent and so disconnected from my immediate circumstances that I wrote it in my journal and carried on with life's pressing challenges.

I never forgot that instruction, and gradually, it began to make more sense. Systems such as diets are fashionable and fickle . . . often driven by media exploitation rather than careful evaluation. Systems are also adopted by people who need to try something they can blame if it doesn't work. A sequence, on the other hand, is like water running downhill. Each drop finds its own path of least resistance and gradually deepens the channel if the intention (the flow) remains constant.

Treena and I had tried most all the systems and failed. When we began to understand sequence, we saw it as a journey of individual discoveries—not a packaged tour! We could select our own menu of options . . . a process that some now call tailoring . . . a series of choices that lead to a lifestyle that fits perfectly.

We now have the benefit of hindsight as we look back upstream at the sequence we gradually discovered. If we felt that we had it exactly right for everyone . . . then we would be suggesting that we have a system for you to try. That is not our intent. You have to find your own way. But, in laying out our sequence, we hope to encourage you to discover your own, and perhaps, pick and choose from our life experiences if they seem to fit with yours.

The Feather Factor

Imagine for a moment an old-fashioned scale, with two dishes suspended by chains from a crossbar. Place a feather in the right hand dish . . . we'll call that a wise choice. Now add one to the left dish . . . for an unwise choice. This is something we all do multiple times every single day of our lives. Do we add more feathers to the left (unwise) dish than to the right? If we do, the possibilities grow that we will experience disease. Make different choices, and we may prevent disease or even reverse its effect.

The important truth about the featherweight of a single choice is that, in itself, it doesn't weigh enough to have a measurable effect. It's only when we repeat a negative choice again and again (habit) that the scales tip toward disease . . . and it seems to take an enormous number of positive choices to balance the scale and edge toward wellness.

With this picture of the scales in mind, you may be able to see that your future is best served by small consistent daily choices. As a result, you will make slow, gradual progress. Unless there is an urgent (physician ordered and supervised) reason to do something, for example, to lose weight rapidly, then we always take the gradual approach of one feather at a time. As my father used to say, "softly, softly catchee monkey!" So, let's deal with featherweight choices in sequence.

THE NINE STAGES OF CHANGE

STAGE ONE
Aware Yet Disinterested

You'd have to live on another planet not to know something about heart disease, high blood pressure, diabetes, and the risks of being overweight. We listened with half an ear. Awareness of lifestyle-related disease isn't high on the agenda of the young or ambitious middle-agers. In our case, it was simply too far off to happen to us, and yet, the simple truth is that the earlier you start making wise choices . . . the more likely is your long and health-filled life.

STAGE TWO
Relative Impact

My father had a cerebral hemorrhage at 50, followed by diabetes and repeated thrombosis. He died at 74 when I was 44—nicely middle-aged. Treena's parents both died in their early to mid-60s from coronary heart disease. There were no records of cholesterol tests or checkups for us to review either before or after their deaths. We just didn't measure very well back then.

The death of a parent or grandparent sounds a definite wake-up call. If these health issues run in the family . . . would they be repeated in us?

I had my cholesterol checked when I was mid-gallop with the *Galloping Gourmet* series. It was 260 . . . and judged *at that time* to be within normal range, which *of course*, it was not. I had a high uric acid level . . . which meant kidney stones (I'd had one painful bout) and gout. The doctor's report simply said, "I suppose this is an occupational hazard" (meaning my apparent liberal on-screen consumption of wine!).

Treena sailed on unchecked . . . we slept through the wake-up call . . . in fact several wake-up calls as the dish on the left side of the scales sank lower.

─────── S T A G E T H R E E ───────
Concern Leads to Enquiry

My level of concern had spiked with the seasickness and remedy of lowering fat and eating more vegetables and fruit. I felt so much better that I wanted to know why. I was looking for a reason why I was well . . . not for any disease-risk factors. Treena's annual tests kept getting worse; her blood glucose easily passing what we now use as the diagnosis for type 2 diabetes (126 mg/dl), and her cholesterol was also off the healthy (present day) charts. But the trend upward failed to activate our physician's concern.

─────── S T A G E F O U R ───────
Denial

It was during this stage of personal awareness that Treena began to practice a series of outward denials that seem to be pretty typical . . . let's see if any of them fit your experience.

- "It won't happen to me. I'm not an 'average statistic.'
- "I'm too busy to worry about it . . . if the doctor isn't concerned neither am I . . . it's his problem not mine."

- "I'm feeling good, so why look under the hood?"
- "My care team will think I'm fussing unnecessarily."
- "Type 2 diabetes is a small thing compared to type 1 diabetes." (It certainly isn't, by the way!)
- "People will reject me . . . thinking I'm a sick person."
- "I can't afford the treatment/medications."
- "Anyway, I don't believe it. They are all wrong."

Said Daddy to me when I was small,
"Be the best, Treena, the best of all.
The best student, swimmer, or crew
Always be better than the best of the few.
At all times be top, never scrape through!"
Said mummy, when I was really hurting,
"Never bother or fuss about a pain,
"Strive to be better, and never complain,
More often than not it's imagination.
And hypochondria is an abomination,"
This is what I learned was success.
If I knew, I couldn't do better or best
I'd not even try to do any new things,
I would let others down with my failings
Because failure can simply cause shame.
And I'd be the only person to blame."

TREENA: Thus, I learned to never believe when I was sick, never complain or moan. This was also a reason why I feared to try new things, in case I would fail. Funny thing, diabetes has helped prove that I can do anything well, if I just am willing and try. Fear of failure is a tiny bit there, but I do try new things and realize I do not have to be the best, and THAT is success. Yes, through diabetes, I am learning many things. I know it is a strange thing to say, but it's true. Not the least is obedience to the one who loves me, both above and close beside me. Acceptance with willingness is the secret and only you can do it, no one can do it for you. NO ONE. It's over to you to listen and obey. Take it from one who knows!

So, we had begun to be concerned . . . but denial was a stumbling block to real progress. I made changes, but Treena opted to continue feeding feathers into the left dish on the scales.

—————— S T A G E   F I V E ——————
Acceptance

The air ambulance and Dr. Got-Your-Car-Keys (page 32) got our mutual attention about Treena's coronary heart disease, and Kitty Carmichael certainly got our attention with her in-your-face challenge to Treena's last-ditch denial (page 44). So now we had acceptance of a real need, and we had interested physicians and a care team to help us with the science-end of things. We also received our One Touch Ultra blood glucose monitor, which became, for both of us, an instrument as valuable as a GPS for a sailboat or a stopwatch for an athletic coach.

The moment we grasped its real value we began our DOOL (Daily Olympics of Life) charts in which we recorded her fasting glucose levels taken before eating every morning. Since we had the chart going, we also made use of an accurate pair of bathroom scales. Yes, her daily weight was recorded. We also added the results of a small but accurate blood pressure cuff. In this way, we began to truly partner in checking our progress.

Since I do 90% of the cooking at home, it works out well if Treena's weight or blood sugar or blood pressure rises. I review what we ate the day before and bingo, we've often got a clear cause and effect.

As we began to fine-tune the measurements, we learned about postprandial testing. This is a blood check exactly two hours after the first bite of a new dish. This helped us know if this food was, in fact, a wise choice for her to eat. It is generally agreed that if the number is higher than 150 mg/dl at the two-hour point, then you may need to check the carbohydrate content, portion size, and the amount of fiber in it. Fiber—which is in fruits, vegetables, whole grains, and beans—is not digested, so it is carbohydrate that doesn't count. It also slows down digestion, so blood sugar doesn't spike after a meal.

We have found that we can reduce the amount of carbohydrate from starchy foods (rice, pasta, potatoes, pastry, tortillas) by 50% just by cutting the serving size in half. Then we add a vegetable we really love that is either green leaf (Swiss chard, turnip greens, collards, spinach, kale, cabbage) or high in water content (tomatoes, mushrooms, summer squash) or high in fiber (beans, peas, lentils) or cruciferous (cabbage, cauliflower, broccoli, Brussels sprouts). This will usually do the trick and keep your sugar levels where they should be and will help with your weight and blood pressure, too, which is good for your heart.

All that remains then, is to exercise that heart with a daily walk and to practice some gentle measured breathing (more of this later, see page 68).

Armed with our written record of DOOLs, we were able to have extremely useful meetings with our physicians and began to be encouraged about the future.

———— STAGE SIX ————
Possibility of Success

Our record keeping, together with constant checking, began to pay off. All of us could see the progress we were making. Treena's total cholesterol dropped to 184 with an LDL of 88. The treatment included her taking a statin drug, which is common, so we cannot precisely say how much of the drop from 360 to 184 is due to lifestyle and how much to medication. Since we have not made "lifestyle only" a goal, that's just fine with us. But we will also never stop trying to keep our numbers in good control and adding new feathers of choice to the right hand (wellness) dish on the scales.

It was during this stage that the idea of MYTC emerged—more years to contribute. This became our concrete goal. Notice that we didn't say we were going for "old age in good health." That was too ill-defined. What we know about type 2 diabetes is that, as a result of the effect of high blood sugar on blood vessels and nerves, a person develops poor circulation and nerve damage. This damage puts a person at risk of amputation of toes or foot or leg if a sore develops on the foot, of blindness, or of kidney failure. The damage caused by high blood sugar is made worse by weight gain and high blood pressure, and leads directly to coronary heart disease and stroke. All these are considered complications of diabetes. We also saw them as limits to our quality of life—to be avoided if at all possible by our daily attention to the choices we make.

Our definition of success is, therefore, to increase our availability for life by diminishing our risk. We have been told that the A1C measurement every three months, which records the concentration of glucose in the blood, is a good marker of progress (or otherwise). If it drops by just one percentage point, it can mean a 30% reduction in the risk of another stroke or heart attack. Treena's A1C has dropped from 11.9% to 5.3%, which is a 6-point drop. Multiplied by 30% for each one-point drop, we have 180% less risk of those complications. We know this can't go on forever, but frankly we are fascinated to see continual progress as we cross over the 70 years of age mark. (Is this middle age? Can I have another crisis? Is it finally time for a sports car?)

Of course a goal is all well and good . . . but every goal needs a motive, a reason to pursue it. Is it just to avoid pain and the inconvenience of disability? Is this enough to keep the constant connection going day after day?

We think not! In our case we'd see this as exceptionally self-focused, and we've been trying to avoid that trap for many years now. We took real time . . . a lot of it, to examine why we wanted to be alive and in good health. So, while this is extremely personal, we'll share our three basic reasons, knowing full well that yours will be different.

Motive 1: More Years for What?

This reason has become our grand scheme . . . the big picture . . . and has to do with purpose and passion. We went looking for the sort of reason that gets you out of bed wanting a day that leaves you feeling fulfilled.

TREENA: I'm a poet. I also love people, and enjoy being an "encourager" and seeing others grow and succeed. Gra and I have much to share with others that may help them live more abundantly.

To find fulfillment, touch the life of another!
And each new morn, pray for God's way
To bring new miracles to you each day.
Sometimes they are great and sometimes small.
Such as waking to the chirp of a birdcall,
And the scent of dew-drenched lawns,
With mingling perfumes that rise with the dawn
From fragrant wild flowers and roses in bowers
Nature's winds may blow or the sun may shine
Whatever the day, it will bring us a sign
If we're only willing to act and obey
That which is put before us today.
We should answer rings from the telephone
With the right attitude and gentle tone.
Because they don't know you have a deadline,
They're the fifteenth call you've had at that time.
We need to respond with a ready smile
To neighbors who need to talk for a while.
We can pray silent prayers, for those down on their luck
As we put an offering into their cup.
Ask the name of that person and from whence they came
Spend more than small change, that's the usual game.
Then maybe they'll feel like a person again.
There're so many openings which can make some heart sing
Which will bring us fulfillment and pleasure to Him. ॐ

GRAHAM: I've done so many different things in my life span that I'm tempted to continue to spread myself thin. Over recent months, however, I've tried to focus my energies into clearly defined projects that I see as my passions. The odd thing is that they are big enough that I don't expect them to be completed in my lifetime. I see myself more as a relay runner in a race that will be won by others down the line. My privilege is to be part of a team that, in many cases, has already run. All this to say that I'm a part owner, so I do the best I can while the task is in my hands. My task is to teach you the four ways to succeed at making significant lifestyle change:

1. Indiv-ity. To use individual creativity in the selection of lifestyle choices, especially by using the Food Preference Sheet (pages 81–95).
2. Fruit and Vegetables. To move from eating 3 servings to 9 servings per day . . . a 300% increase! There is detailed help and recipes in this book (page 75). Use the vegetable list on the back flap of this book to choose new ones!
3. Portion Sizes. To make individuals and restaurant owners aware so serving sizes are reduced from excessive to reasonable/moderate (RM). I offer Menu 2 as a method, which is a second menu, identical to the first, except that the nutrient analysis of each food is listed, too. Diners can make healthier choices with this information. Field testing of Menu 2 shows that most people do select healthier items.
4. Double Benefits. To help people "convert habits that harm into resources that heal" using the above three ideas and the worldwide web, for example, www.outdulgence.com.

Motive 2. More Years to Give and Receive Love

A brief review of my life in the early part of this book will confirm the fact that I've been far too busy for my own good. Too busy, I regret to say, to love unselfishly. (I'm trying hard to restore those "locust" years.)

I've been blessed to have been healthy, and so, I've been the one who has loved and cared for Treena during her periods of restoration. She has loved me through all my selfishness and immaturity. This "give and receive" has meant a great deal to us both, but it's really Treena who has always led by her example of giving. And yet, strangely it has been harder for her to receive. She'd best explain this for herself.

TREENA: Do you find it easy to accept another's help or their gift of time to you? I don't. I feel uncomfortable, a problem and trial, even with Gra. It is worse with family or friends. I realize it is easier to give than to receive, and that is the rub, as Shakespeare would say. Why should I deprive another of the pleasure I get when I give the gift of myself? Pride is the reason.

Have you ever washed another person's feet? That part is easy, it is having my own feet washed that I find difficult! I am trying to accept those helps or gifts with graciousness. Yes, I am slowly learning, very slowly. I recently broke my wrist in two places. I had to ask for help (yuk), accept, and be patient! Three big lessons from one broken wrist. Acceptance and grace go together and are a joy to behold in a person. Maybe it can be beheld in you . . . and me?

Motive 3. What We Are Looking Forward to . . .

After the other "outgoing" motives, this one is going to seem almost self-indulgent, and really, I suppose it is. We have some short-term and mid-term plans that we'd like to see happen and to enjoy them, we need to be well.

When our daughters and our son married, when our granddaughter married, when our other grandchildren and our daughter graduated—these were milestones in their lives but very significant and rewarding events for us, too. To be well means to be able to fully embrace each of these moments.

Beyond these high points, we have our annual vacation. For the last ten years, we have had several weeks aboard our 36-foot Nonsuch sailboat named *Dovetail*. Since we are the only ones aboard, we have to be well enough to manage it. After a couple of years gunkholing in Puget Sound's protected waters, we went through Treena's annual physical with her cardiologist. I asked him, "Do you think that Treena is up to a 2,400-mile round trip to Glacier Bay in Alaska?"

The cardiologist reviewed his own notes on the treadmill test, the lipids report, and our own DOOL charts and gave me that steady look . . . then he smiled broadly. "I can see no reason why not . . . you two have earned the right to do it . . . you've won your lives back."

The pure satisfaction of receiving his unconditional support was a wonderful moment . . . and now, even though our travels have changed again (we'll be driving on our next trips), we still look forward to our weeks on the road. We take each year one at a time. We assume nothing, but we plan in a positive way, and when we reach the due date, we relish every moment, and we are so grateful.

I want to retain my balance and strength, and because of this, I do daily exercise of stretching and push-ups with free weights. I don't need this kind of strength to write and be a public speaker, but without it . . . I really couldn't sail and drive and do the grunt work. So our type of vacation has become a daily motive that is really quite compelling.

———— S T A G E S E V E N ————
Engagement

Passion, purpose, goals, and motives are all well and good. They really are an essential part of any individual sequence. But we found that to engage in the process of making day-by-day change, we needed more understanding of what was actually happening to us. Specifically, we had to learn how to avoid setting unrealistic goals in frankly silly time spans, such as "I will lose 30 pounds in two weeks!" We needed to use common sense.

Our First Level Was Lifestyle Only

Dr. "Got-Your-Car-Keys" was the one who initiated us to the normal medical protocol in which the newly diagnosed patient is asked to try lifestyle change only. What is going on here is to see if you can make progress from your old unaware lifestyle to your new managed lifestyle without needing medication or surgery.

Except for emergency situations, this period is usually three months. We began our three months directly after Treena's heart attack in Honolulu when her cholesterol was 365. After three months it was down to 250, a dramatic recovery of over 100 points but not enough to avoid medication. We were, nonetheless, delighted in our success, and it gave us needed encouragement to keep searching for new lifestyle choices.

I have been told that, in some cases, it's better to start with a statin drug immediately and then—when the usually senior executive-driven-alpha-male—patient sees the satisfying 30-40% drop, he is encouraged enough to add the lifestyle choices.

Whichever option is taken, you'll notice that the intervention is based on numbers that preceded the change. Your starting cholesterol level is your baseline, and we believe you need to remember where your journey began, and that you keep a log of your progress, otherwise you will attempt real change without any way to measure it or see your reward . . . *not* a good idea!

Our Second Level Was Added Medication

Fortunately, our health care team knew their business and they explained that Treena needed to have an LDL cholesterol (that's the "bad" cholesterol that sticks to artery walls) of 100 or less and to do this we may well need a statin drug, which, at that time, was reasonably new but proving to be most effective.

Our physicians, then and now, felt that a new medication should be allowed to "prove itself safe" even beyond the exhaustive trials mandated by the FDA. They believed that one year on the mass market should be enough. We obviously agreed and carefully took on those new drugs in an orderly way, making detailed notes of both "feelings" as well as lab reports.

The other thing we did is called "compliance." Treena, with very few exceptions over the past 17 years, has taken her medications exactly on time. It amazes me that very effective medications are robbed of their ability to help or to heal because the patient simply forgets to take them. Of course one of our great assets is the daily journal. If she misses a pill, the results on her blood sugar and blood pressure are immediate and obvious, so in and of itself, the daily journal is a great accountability link.

Our Third Level Was Step and Check

Trying to do your best to make quite substantial lifestyle changes isn't easy, and I hope we are not giving you the impression that it is . . . any change can be upsetting! But, what makes it much more difficult is to attempt vast changes almost overnight and to discover that either it simply doesn't work for you, or that you can't stand it for one more day!

Better by far, we found, was to convert the BIG CHANGE into a series of small steps and then to check each step as valid. Here again we were able to make that check with the daily journal, see pages 490–491 sample journal pages.

After several years of experimenting, we literally stumbled over a new way of planning these steps, and to describe this, I need another brief metaphor.

Fording the River One Step Ahead

Please imagine, for a moment, a swiftly flowing river. You walk down the bank looking for a shallow spot where you can cross over . . . it's called a "ford." You find one, the water rushes past multiple stones . . . all look as though they may be stable enough to support your weight. The question is which ones do you choose?

The answer is to keep one foot on the shore and test the nearest stone with the other foot. Then, before putting your whole weight upon it, you look for the next stepping stone, and then make the transfer. And so you go, test, look ahead to the next stone, transfer weight, test, and so it goes until you are over.

You always look one step ahead . . . that's the way we've finally decided to work. Each small step is complete when we include the next one to try. We never move without two baby steps planned out in each of our lifestyle options. Which neatly brings us to the options themselves, and stage eight.

------- STAGE EIGHT -------
All Things Can Work Together for Good

Remarkable as it must seem . . . diets, on their own, really don't work. I say remarkable because that seems to run counter to the messages on every magazine rack you've ever scanned.

What has worked in our case, and I don't doubt in millions of other cases, is the synergism of several lifestyle options working together. I've listed those that we have included in our voyage so far. In Stage Nine, I'll go into each one with a little more detail, so you can see how we use the stepping stone idea of always one ahead.

Our Lifestyle Options

Option 1. Diet
Option 2. Exercise
Option 3. Sleep
Option 4. Stress management
Option 5. Faith
Option 6. Compassion
Option 7. Attitude

There is no special order of importance here, this is just how each option led the two of us to another over a period of ten years. As always, this kind of life change is best made by personal choice and not at the suggestion of another. We know that it's pretty normal for us mortals to want to do as much as we can as soon as possible and then live happily ever after . . . but that really is a fairytale. If you try too hard, it will more than likely result in burnout with negative consequences for your health.

—— STAGE NINE ——
Taking Action

Option 1: Diet

STEP 1: We completed the Food Preference Sheet on pages 81–95.

STEP 2: We estimated our portion size of each "H" food and reduced its volume by 50% (that means we cut the serving in half). H foods are High in saturated fats, refined carbohydrates, and sodium.

STEP 3: We made a shopping list of our "new" preferred foods and phased in their purchase one or two items at a time.

STEP 4: Now you could select a popular family dish such as lasagna. Assess the "H" ingredients, reduce by 50%, and check your preference sheet for foods to fill in for what was removed.

STEP 5: If you have diabetes or are insulin resistant, check your blood glucose two hours after you eat the modified dish. Adjust the ingredients if necessary (if your blood sugar is too high) or write it down as approved!

STEP 6: Be sure to drink enough water every day. Many people drink only sodas or coffee, when what the body really needs is water. Another thing to consider is the research on the healthy benefits of drinking tea—green tea, black tea, or red tea, it doesn't matter. All have antioxidants to keep your body healthier. And with all the teas on the market these days, you can find different tastes to please you.

Option 2: Exercise

We could say physical activity or movement, but you know what we mean.

STEP 1: Purchase a good pedometer with a strong belt clip (they tend to come off). Simply write in your journal the number of steps you take day by day for a normal week. This becomes your baseline . . . it gives you a starting point that's real.

STEP 2: Consider your whole day . . . it's got 1440 minutes and somewhere, somehow, you need to find 60 minutes (one twenty-fourth of the day) for "movement." You can cut it into two parts or three, but it should total 60 minutes every day! NOTICE: At this point, you are not doing it, you are only trying to find the time.

STEP 3: Put the time you selected to the test . . . imagine stretching, walking, and doing simple weight training within your time frame. DON'T DO IT . . . just think about it . . . you may need an alarm clock to remind you. Does it work? I need to tell you here that you may not feel strong or energetic enough . . . your back or feet may hurt . . . but since you don't have to actually do it, there is no active rejection of the idea. After one week of imagining, you are now ready to start with just one 20-minute segment, the one that seemed easiest for you to do consistently every single day.

STEP 4: Begin by walking at your most comfortable pace for 10 to 20 minutes. If you don't even walk to the end of your driveway right now, you may need to aim for 5 minutes of walking. At the end of the day check your pedometer to see the increase in your steps . . . well done!

STEP 5: Your very own daily Olympics give you a huge benefit in how you feel emotionally and physically, IF you don't try to break any records . . . especially your own! Let your body tell you and very gradually, increase in easy steps until the target 60 minutes is reached.

STEP 6: Having proven to yourself that you can actually move as consistently as you can sit, it's time to find someone to help you with stretching and simple free weights (those little dumbbells you can hold in your hands). I've done a ten-minute set of stretches every single day for years that has kept my back flexible following our major traffic accident back in 1971. Free weights are a more recent addition to my program, but I can really feel the benefit, and at 70, I've regained most of the flexibility and strength that I enjoyed in my 50s.

SPECIAL NOTE: We find that the time set apart for movement is enormously important in dealing with depression, weight control, blood sugar management, and the good (HDL) cholesterol. All this, and you'll even look better, too (if that matters to you!). Keep a record of this information in your journal, and you'll see what it can do for you.

Option 3: Sleep

Our good friend Dr. James Maas, of Cornell University, told us that the single best indicator of a long life and good health was how much sleep we had. His estimate is that nine hours is optimal and that when we get less than nine hours, we tend to sag in the mid-afternoon. Our interest in sleep began with this research, and we put it to the test. When we get 8–9 hours, there really is no sag time!

STEP 1: Record how much sleep you get at night in your journal. Also note any sag times for a full month before you make any changes. Again, this is your baseline information.

STEP 2: Buy a VCR or invest in TIVO. You will want to avoid watching TV after 9:00 p.m. With the right equipment, you can record your favorite prime time program and see it before 9:00 p.m. This is so valuable that it's well worth the expense! Again, in our lives it has been an enormous boost to our well-being. Our sleep time is now 9:00 or 10:00 p.m. to 6:00 a.m.

STEP 3: Does your sleeping pillow bend in the middle and just stay bent? If it does, consider replacing it. When folded it should unfold on its own. We are so used to ours that we travel with them!

STEP 4: Invest in the book *Power Sleep* by James B. Maas, Ph.D. It can transform your life with so many simple steps you can take!

Option 4: Stress Management

When exceeding life's speed limits.

I'm sure you must have heard about the need for appropriate stress without which, for example, a bridge would not remain standing? Treena and I have come to see our lives as another kind of bridge . . . one that floats. We have a couple of floating bridges in Seattle that span Lake Washington to the eastside cities.

When the wind blows hard from either the northwest or southeast, the lake can be whipped into angry waves that hit the bridge hard and bounce back on themselves, creating a turmoil of heaped waters raging against each other. Yet on the other side of the bridge, it's flat calm. We see our life like this . . . occasionally there is a challenging gale that beats down upon us. We have three choices:

- Try and stop the wind, waves, and confusion.
- Move away to the sheltered side until the wind drops.
- Stay on the bridge and keep moving.

Long experience has taught us to keep on doing what we do . . . to keep making gentle progress in spite of the conditions. We don't run away in search of a sheltered place, and we have certainly stopped trying to make the challenging situation go away. It has amazed us how soon the adverse "gales" tend to blow themselves out and even though we slowed down . . . we were always ahead of the game if we just kept going!

STEP 1: How short is your fuse? Really . . . I'm not kidding! When life fires a shot across your bows and somehow gets in the way of what you want to do . . . how do you react? Do you slow down, even stop and wait until the interruption goes away . . . or do you explode? It depends on the length of your fuse. Some of us get lit by adversity and go off almost immediately. This could mean that we are living with constant, unrelenting, damaging stress.

The old advice to "count to ten . . . slowly" is a proven way to lengthen your fuse. During that count there's often time to put the issue into its proper place and not fly off the handle at the unexpected. So, the goal for step one is to practice the "ten count" and during it, try to see the interruption in a different light.

STEP 2: Practice breathing. The idea is to find the odd "quiet moments" of a day and sit still. Consciously breathe in . . . filling your abdomen (just under your ribs), then let the breath out slowly, for example, to a slow count of four or a quicker count to eight. You can breathe in by mouth and out through the nose. Do slow, deep breathing several times whenever there's a small break in your day. See each breath as adding length to your fuse. This kind of breathing can do wonders for such things as blood pressure because it certainly helps to reduce stress. It lowers blood sugar, too!

STEP 3: This is where you link up with the exercise/movement option . . . a brief but active walk can be an immediate remedy to stress. For example, we always try to get in a good brisk walk at airports . . . no moving walkways, and there is less sitting around. It helps us to relieve the stress of modern travel, and it promotes good circulation that jet travel tends to decrease.

STEP 4: Is technology really helping you . . . or do you get uptight and feel that there's nowhere to hide? Every now and again we get the chance to speak out publicly about lifestyle issues. On one of those occasions, we received 1.6 million hits on our website within minutes of the broadcast! Among those hits were hundreds of emails. To attempt to answer them all was impossible. We wanted to give a personal answer, to reach out and touch each writer, but the gale of email was too much. So, we accept the reality and work within our capacity and are not tempted to overgrow ourselves with expensive technology that "sort of" answers people. To be well we have to be real and set some limits. For example, we have limited our cell phone use to family or emergency only. It's "we'll call you . . . don't call us . . . unless!"

So, for this step, review your use of technology. If you are "at work" almost all the time and have little time to reflect about what really is important outside of business . . . then try to lessen its intrusion. By all means, be of service to others . . . but by no means should you be eaten alive.

Option 5: Faith

The point is that mankind didn't make the Earth, and all our technology cannot control nature. We are part of a world, seen and unseen, that is mysterious. Sooner or later you have to wonder about who's in charge on this planet. I don't want to presume on your understanding of faith, but if you will permit me, I'd like to explore what we think about the word "faith." You can skip this and go directly to compassion if you feel that I'm in danger of intruding into your very private spiritual space. But if you're curious, let's have a go!

Faith is, for Treena and I, an opportunity to put our selves in second place. We believe there is an overwhelmingly powerful entity who is perfectly aware of our individual journey past, present, and future and who loves us intimately . . . moment by moment . . . and who wants the very best for us, including our freedom.

Now I admit that life's many defeats seem to fly in the face of this idea; but, we have been able to see the silver lining in some of the worst events and have seen awful circumstances turned into our eventual good. Certainly there is a time lag between pain and providence, but then faith is more about the unseen than the seen.

A visual might help here. Try to see this powerful yet loving entity as an absolutely constant breeze . . . always coming from one direction at exactly the same speed . . . utterly predicable. Now picture yourself (or me if you'd prefer) holding a dandelion puffball of seeds before my mouth and facing into the wind. I take a deep breath and blow the seeds directly into the wind. For a while, the power of my own breath blows the seeds toward the source. I've done my own thing (I've been given the freedom to do so) but see what happens . . . the seeds begin to slow down and then, for a moment, they stop. And then curving around softly, they are carried along on the gentle consistent breeze until they lodge and germinate somewhere other than where I had planned.

This is how I have come to see personal freedom. I can choose to do things that are destructive, and there will be consequences for my actions that may be painful. And yet, if I'm careful to see what's going on and that I can make other choices . . . my initial poor choice can become the source of great benefit for myself and others.

When you realize that the seeds are blowing back in your face, you can understand the "not my will but your will" idea. You make a conscious decision to put your own will into second place . . . to turn around and use your breath to speed the seeds (choices of life) on their way along with the consistent gentle breeze.

STEP 1: Learn more about the spiritual world. And here, our bias must surface. Our lives turned around, as previously described on pages 19–26, because of our recognition of God the Father, as made known to mankind through the life of Jesus Christ of Nazareth, God the Son, under the inspiration of God the Holy Spirit. If you are a seeker after spiritual truth, you may want to read the Biblical accounts of the life of Jesus Christ as told by Matthew, Mark, Luke, and John. They explain for some of us where the gentle breeze comes from and why it is so consistent.

STEP 2: A connection with the Divine can give you energy, focus, new goals, and peace. Having made contact with the power of God, you may find yourself overwhelmed by gratitude and begin to see how you might find another direction to face when blowing your seeds of choice—into or with the wind.

Option 6: Compassion

To me compassion means helping others by becoming a channel for God's love, so it can flow into the world. I think it works like this . . . and here again I need you to think through a word picture. Imagine, please, a compass on a boat. My willingness (and yours?) to be used to help alleviate pain and injustice in the world is to volunteer to step onto the compass of life. We find ourselves somewhere in the 360 degrees of the circle that surrounds the central post. Each degree represents a real human need in our world. Now imagine God is the central post, and His compassionate love radiates out equally to every one of these human needs.

You find yourself drawn to one particular degree on the compass. You face the need . . . be it child abuse, drug addiction, hunger, homelessness, AIDS hospice, . . . the list is endless. You stopped here because you intercepted God's compassion for a specific need. His love begins to flow through you en route to specific people in that group. Helped by that "feeling" you experience a sense of purpose quite beyond the normal feelings of sympathy or empathy. You have, in fact, been drawn by compassion and are now a direct conduit for God's love.

Over the past thirty years both Treena and I have experienced this strong connection and have marveled at how very different is its outcome compared to sympathetic emotions. You can feel sorry for people, you can be sympathetic . . . but compassion is a call to action. We feel that we begin by committing ourselves to be available (we set foot on the compass). God then directs our attention to a need, and by responding, we begin to practice consistency. Once committed to action, we continue in it. Consistency is an antidote to the hopelessness and despair experienced through fickle funding and its natural by-product, manipulative fund-raising.

Here are the steps we took to finding the degrees of need that would help to change our lives.

STEP 1. We made notes of our response to the tragic tales being told on the evening news. It was uneven. Of course we are moved by the plight of millions of refugees or of blind and otherwise physically handicapped people, but we couldn't do everything for everyone, and even to try is what we call the "Jesus Junior Syndrome." We did notice how strongly we responded to a particular need of children in Africa. So . . . step one was to discover the need that called to us.

STEP 2. We searched the Web for information about childhood hunger in Africa and found Compassion International. We found that, for $25.00 a month, we could provide the funds that would support a child's education, health care, and food . . . what an incredible bargain!

STEP 3. We had a need that "rang our bell" and had found someone with that need. We also had an amount. Now where to find the money? We decided to look for it in our own food budget. Could we reduce our consumption of foods that might harm us and convert our possible "indulgence" into the support of a child . . . or maybe more than one child?

We took our receipts from the supermarket and drew a ring around foods that might pose a health threat if we ate too much. If we bought less of these foods, then we could take the "H" out of the word *threat,* and it would become a true *treat* for us all!

We reduced the amount of meat that we ate each week by 50%, and saved $20 a week for our family of four. Of course we had to increase the amount of vegetables to take the place of the missing meat on the plate, and that cost $10 per week. So, we had $10 a week to give and that amounted to $520 for the year.

We began our support of a child in Ethiopia in the early 1990s. Because we have not increased our meat consumption since then, we continue to feel that a habit that harmed us became a resource that could heal Sadik in North Africa. We call this "The Double Benefit," and really, it's as simple as it sounds. What has been truly wonderful is that the healing went both ways. We were able to reduce the risk in our lives and in Sadik's.

He got decent food . . . and so did we . . . it really was a "Double Benefit." We've often wondered whether we would have been so consistent in his support had we not carefully found that new money from an old habit?

Option 7: Attitude

Yes, you can choose your attitude. So many issues spring to mind on attitude that another book could easily be written, however I'd like to keep this to the two attitudes that have been developed in our own lives as we've struggled with life's challenges.

The first is our degree of willingness, and we've already taken up a good deal of space on that issue (page 32).

The second is the choice to be made between criticism and contribution.

It seems to me, just by listening to the nightly news on PBS, that our world is almost submerged in critics who sit in judgment of all the wrongs about which we are well aware. Now and again there is an individual who tells about an actual contribution he or she is making and resists judging or condemning anyone. What an incredible joy to hear such a refreshing example of positive attitude!

In my case, I regret to say I've spent far too many years getting upset by indulgence and far too little time exploring outdulgence. Back in the year 2000, I was invited to speak in a university setting aboard a liner bound for Alaska. The adults had brought their children . . . over 900 of them.

I was speaking on the benefits of eating together as a family and was on the schedule for the second day of the trip. All I could see, on day one, were truly sad examples of men talking to other men at large tables and ignoring their children. Everywhere I looked I saw this obvious failure!

A well-known politician was also speaking, but under the press of so many children, he wanted to get off quickly. Would I swap my time with his? I agreed to wait until day five. This gave me more time to settle into my judgmental groove. What I'd seen on day one was endlessly repeated . . . the children were literally isolated from table discussions. I became quite depressed and that's unusual for me. Treena noticed and suggested that I should watch my critical attitude!

In something of a huff (you know what men are), I went off to hear Father Robert Spitzer S.J., the President of Gonzaga University in Spokane. He was wonderful, one of the best speakers I've ever heard anywhere. He spoke about being judgmental and used the Genesis account of Adam and Eve. He made it clear that it was not a sermon but a useful example perhaps?

His point was that before the first bite of the apple (surely not an apple . . . you can't walk around naked where apples grow well), Adam and Eve were created to be contributors. After they had eaten from the tree of the knowledge of good and evil (Genesis 3:1-7), they became judgmental and critical.

"Now" he said . . . "If you are feeling critical of anyone today," he seemed to look at me, "then don't be hard on yourself. You are hard wired from that first bite to follow along setting yourself up as a judge of others."

I felt a degree of relief at being inescapably normal. *Normal*?

"If, however, you'd like to experience what it was like before the first bite . . . then next time you feel critical or judgmental, just step back across that line and ask yourself a simple question."

By now I was sitting up straight and listening hard.

"Ask yourself . . . can I make a contribution? If you can't . . . then SHUT UP!"

It fit me like a glove and has ever since. Certainly I remain critical of others . . . especially when they knowingly harm the people they serve . . . but on every occasion, when I feel the judgment welling up, I breathe out the question: "Can I make a contribution?" So often I find I can't. (I tried to make a whole-grain [healthy] donut once . . . but it was so heavy it wouldn't rise to the surface!) And when that happens, I simply shut up.

I had an immediate opportunity to test the idea aboard that cruise ship. I went into every meal from that day on looking with new eyes . . . and all I could see everywhere were fathers in really meaningful discussions with their children.

Surely they hadn't changed, but I had. And I'm so grateful that this attitude has remained with me. Frankly, it has re-colored my perception of life, and one of the best outcomes is this book. Rather than be critical, Treena and I decided that it was time for us to be contributors.

I'm not sure that I know how to translate this personal story into steps for you to try. If you find yourself being critical, you can stop, ask yourself the question, and find a way to be a contributor. It's much more fun.

Summary of All the Steps

We've looked at diet, movement, sleep, stress, faith, compassion, and attitude. It's time now to move to the recipes. If you've hung in with us this far (for which we are so grateful, by the way), then I need to add how extremely important it is for you to see the recipes as a guide. By all means, adjust, adjust, adjust these recipes to suit your own taste preferences and most importantly, your own unique circumstances.

CHAPTER FIVE

The Recipes

This is my 26th cookbook, and I find myself writing this brief how-to-use-these recipes introduction with the usual sinking feeling that very few people will ever read it! So . . . if you've gotten this far, you are, therefore, unique, and I'd like to give you the hug of a lifetime!

My joy comes from knowing that these next words can virtually guarantee you success with everything you cook from this time forward. (A little overstated perhaps, but let's see how you do.)

In Order to Cook Well, You've Got to be Real

You are the sum of all your experiences. Nobody else has had your exposure to foods nor your experiences with eating and drinking, and nobody can tell you what to like and not like. So . . . please take the time to complete the Food Preference Sheets (FPS) found on pages 81–95. There are complete instructions included. To record your family's preferences and find the foods you all love in common, go to www.grahamkerr.com and click on Food Preference Sheet.

Exercise Your Rights as an Individual

When you have completed the FPS, you will know all the ingredients you love, those you will accept, those you don't like, and those you've never tried or even heard of. In short, you will have an MRI of your taste-buds and personal responses to food, something very few people have ever attempted to know. Now, it's time to put your preference to work within my recipes. (I really want you to do this . . . please!)

Send In Your Other Players

Flip through the recipes, scan the ingredients. Now, is there a food that you really dislike? Okay. Don't discard the whole recipe, just think about what the offending food has to offer in sensual terms . . . that is its taste, aroma, color, and texture. Does it major in one or more of these areas? For instance, many people think they dislike the anchovy, that little brown fish fillet with a biting salty taste and strong fishy aroma. It's contribution is primarily a salty taste. So, you don't like anchovies. Go to the taste listing on your FPS, find salt, and run your fingers down the list of your favorites. You may have chosen capers, gherkins, or dill pickles. Hey, why not substitute one of them for the anchovies? Out with my anchovy and in with your pickle? In one move, you have made my recipe yours. Every time you do this, you'll gain confidence, and you will own the result. I call this Indivity for individual creativity.

Now Add Your Circumstances to Your Food Preferences. I Call This Springboarding!

Springboarding is bouncing up and down on the diving board of the cooking method (how ingredients are assembled into a dish) and doing your own dive (using your preferred ingredients) into the pool (your special circumstances, especially as they relate to your own health and well being).

Your physical or nutrition counselor may have suggested that you make some changes in the way you eat and drink. It could be to reduce the amount of animal fat or refined processed carbohydrates. They may have suggested that you eat less and move more. The list goes on and on. Your health goals combine to become your own swimming pool. It's a new way of life, possibly for months or years to come. So, why not make it more appealing by using your list of the foods you love that do you no harm?

If you show your FPS to your caregiver, it becomes a wonderful tool (insight) into your world of food. It is easier to make adjustments using foods that you like, and these are more likely to be lasting favorites than recipes that are completely foreign to your experience.

Make Each Recipe Your Own

Treena and I have been through this sequence, and the recipes that follow have been and remain a valued part of our new lifestyle. Here are some unique characteristics to each recipe.

- SMALLER PORTIONS: We have both battled weight gain (it's an occupational hazard), so, the calories matter. As a result, our portion sizes tend to be smaller. Less food equals fewer calories. It helps to use a smaller plate. Ours measure 9 inches in diameter.
- LOWER SATURATED AND TRANS FATS FOR HEART DISEASE: Because of our history, the recipes we created since 1987 have been adjusted to lower the risk of another stroke or heart attack.
- LOWER CARB FOR TYPE 2 DIABETES: Our experience with diabetes came later, and so, I have used a small icon <c to show that the carbohydrates in the heart-healthy recipe *might* contribute to higher blood sugars. When the <c is used, you will find a box marked "To cut carb" below the recipe, and the new nutrient analysis numbers that show the change in carb. Other icons mean the following:

  < Less of another ingredient that isn't a carbohydrate.
  +> More of another ingredient.

- VEGETABLES AND FRUIT: These foods are high in water and high in fiber, which is very good news for any diet. I have given you plenty of new ideas here (see the back flap for a great list). May I earnestly recommend that you make full use of them; these foods have been our key to reducing LDL cholesterol and managing blood sugars. Be sure to add up the grams of carbohydrates when putting a whole meal together. You can do this by using the nutrient numbers with each recipe and when you substitute vegetables, by referring to the lists printed on the inside covers back and front.

■ NUMBER OF INGREDIENTS/LENGTH OF RECIPE: You may notice that some recipes appear long and have quite a few ingredients. This does not mean that they are "difficult" or even time consuming. Here's what it does mean:

Length: We put in enough description to help you master the recipe. Sometimes, short and "simple" recipes fail to give you enough instructions.

Ingredients: I believe in the value of multiple layers of flavor. The best way to change a recipe from "threat to treat" is to replace the risky ingredient with healthier foods that add taste, aroma, color, and texture. A long list of ingredients is often simply seasonings. When you've got ground cumin seed, for example, it doesn't take long to loosen the top and shake some in, but a cook without seasonings has to rely on the blunt instruments of salt, fat, sugar, and large pieces of meat to "satisfy."

Okay, let's try some of these and see if it's worth the trouble to be well.

The Food Preference Sheet (FPS)

My best hope is that you will make out this sheet, and then you will invest in a consultation with a Registered Dietitian (RD) who can use your completed FPS to tailor nutritional advice to you as a unique individual.

To locate a RD who lives near you call 1-800-877-1600 (or go to www.eatright.org) and ask for a list of local RDs and an estimate for the cost of 2 hours of consultation time. If you have been diagnosed with diabetes, 10 hours of diabetes and nutrition education is covered by government health insurance and most private companies, too. Education is the best way to prevent complications down the road.

If possible, take your most recent blood cholesterol and other lab reports and maybe a letter from your physician. The RD can put your health profile alongside your FPS and be able to tell, at a glance (almost), whether what you like to eat likes you or if it might be doing you harm.

After talking with you about your food choices, the RD may circle those foods you love (but don't love you) and suggest smaller portions, eating them less often, or, in some rare cases, removing that food from your meals.

The truth is that very few foods are actually "bad." It's usually the amount we eat that turns a treat into a threat. Having the treat is not the problem; the problem is the volume of it that you eat.

Now, what if you are unable to get to the RD . . . can you use the FPS yourself? The answer is yes, but a guarded yes. Guarded because I think your personal health and the wellbeing of those who love you are worth the time, effort, and money to have professional guidance.

1. Now, go through the list and mark the foods with an H that you think may be HIGH in

   - animal fats: meats, some dairy products, and poultry
   - trans fatty acids: baked goods, cookies, hard margarine, French fries
   - refined carbohydrates: baked goods, cookies, cakes, some breads, bagels, doughnuts, etc. All candy, all soda pop with sugar, some pastas, white rice, etc.

2. Write down the foods and amounts that you are eating now. Be ruthlessly honest. Next to each beloved food write the amount you eat as one serving and how often; for example, ice cream, 1 cup, 5 times a week.

You might, then, decide to reduce your serving of ice cream to 1/2 cup and still have it 5 times a week. But that's such a small portion . . . can you do that and be content? Probably not, if it's a long established habit. You'll want that sweet taste. So, now you look under the sweet sense on the FPS and run your fingers down the list. What whole fruit did you check off as one you love? How would a half-cup of orange or peach or cherries or grapes do with the ice cream?

You can now plan to add say, red grapes to the ice cream—two things you love and now together. It could be even better than 1 cup of ice cream on its own.

This is what we have done. In trading loved foods, we have reduced the H factor (foods high in fats, salt, sugars, starches) so that what was a tHreat is now a treat. In addition, we eat many more fruit and vegetables, which give us so much good stuff.

It will take you a little while to work it out, but let me promise you that every moment is well spent and reaps positive rewards almost immediately. Surely it's worth it?

Food Preference Sheet

TASTES

❧ 1 Salt

Food	Like	Don't Like	Don't Know
Anchovies			
Vegemite/Marmite			
Potato chips			
Tortilla chips			
Nuts			
Bacon			
Soy sauce (low sodium)			
Fish sauce (Asian)			
Capers			
Pickles			
Worcestershire sauce			
French fries			
Parmesan cheese			
Canadian bacon			
Ham hocks			
Prosciutto			
Smoked salmon			
Salami			
Chutneys			
Ham			
Lox			
Cheeses			
Pretzels			
Corned beef			
Rotisserie chicken			
Canned soups			
Canned sauces			
Packaged soups			
Packaged sauces			
Olives			
Smoked turkey			
Celery			

❧ 2 Sour

Food	Like	Don't Like	Don't Know
Lemon			
Vinegar, malt			
Vinegar, white wine/cider			
Vinegar, red wine			
Pickles			
Capers			
Vinegar, balsamic			
Lime			
Vinegar, rice			
Quince			
Beets, pickled			
Dijon mustard etc.			
Ketchup			
Rhubarb			
Raspberries			
Strawberries			
Pineapple			
Kiwi fruit			
Apples			
Cherries			
Tangerines			
Oranges			
Nectarines			
Peaches			
Apricots			
Blackberries			
Blueberries			
Seville marmalade			
Mayonnaise			
Cranberries (unsweetened)			
Tomatillos			

TASTES

❧ 3 Sweet

Food	Like	Don't Like	Don't Know
Honey			
White sugar			
Hard candy			
Candy bars			
Brown sugar			
Maple syrup			
Corn syrup			
Coffee/flavored syrups			
Chocolate syrup			
Chocolate			
Molasses			
Glazed ginger			
Cookies			
Glazed doughnuts			
Frosted cake			
Sweetened condensed milk			
Jams			
Jellies			
Coconut (sweetened)			
Colas			
Doughnuts			
Cake			
Cold cereal			
Raisins			
Dates			
Cranberries (sweetened)			
Dried fruits			
Preserves			
Ice cream			
Frozen yogurt			
Sorbets			
Prunes			

Food	Like	Don't Like	Don't Know
Fruit juices			
Muffins			
Hot cereal			
Pineapple			
Lychee (in syrup)			
Marmalade			
Yogurts (sweetened)			
Beets			
Teas (sweetened)			
Sweet bell peppers			
Sweet onions			
Corn			
Chutneys			
Ketchup			
Mangoes			
Parsnips			
Sweet potato/yam			
Nectarines			
Oranges			
Pears			
Plums			
Tangerines			
Peaches			
Carrots			
Bok choy			
Tomato juice			
Rutabagas			
Jicama			
Banana			
Figs			
Grapes			
Melon			

TASTES

❧ 4 Bitter

Food	Like	Don't Like	Don't Know
Citrus zest			
Nuts			
Brussels sprouts			
Ryvita			
Broccoli			
Tomato paste			
Wheat kernels			
Rhubarb			
Chutneys			
Broad beans (fava), fresh			
Kiwi fruit			
Persimmons			
Collards			
Celeriac			
Eggplant			
Asparagus			
Cabbage			
Cauliflower			
Fennel			
Salad greens			
Green onions			
Cucumbers			

❧ 5 Umani

Food	Like	Don't Like	Don't Know
Cheese, parmesan			
Fish sauce			
Dried lever seaweed			
Soy sauce			
Soy beans, fermented			
Onions			
Wakame seaweed			
Kelp seaweed			
Scallops			
Alaska king crab			
Blue crab			
Beets			
White shrimp			
Snow crab			
Apples			
Cheese, cheddar			
Eggs			
Chicken			
Beef			
Pork			
Cabbage			
Asparagus, green			
Mushrooms			
Salmon			
Avocado			
Cod			
Corn			
Green peas			
Shitake mushrooms			
Tomato			
Spinach			
Carrots			
Peppers			
Potatoes			
Grapes			
Kiwi			
Milk			

AROMAS

✤ 1 Volatiles

Food	Like	Don't Like	Don't Know
Port			
Brandy			
Sherry			
Red wine			
Balsamic Vinegar			
White wine			
Soy sauce			
Vanilla, other essence			
Almond extract			

✤ 2 Passive *Unheated aroma from fruits/vegetables*

Food	Like	Don't Like	Don't Know	Food	Like	Don't Like	Don't Know
Apples				Melons (honeydew, etc.)			
Apricots				Baked beans			
Avocados				Beets			
Bananas				Broccoli			
Raspberries				Cabbage			
Strawberries				Cauliflower			
Blueberries				Celeriac			
Blackberries				Celery			
Cherries				Corn			
Dates				Fennel			
Grapefruit				Green onions			
Grape juice (and DA wines)				Ginger			
Kiwi fruit				Marmalade			
Lemon				Leeks			
Lime				Onions			
Mangoes				Parsnips			
Nectarines				Peas			
Oranges and juices				Peppers (sweet bell)			
Papaya				Tomatoes			
Peaches				Smoked salmon			
Pears				Parmesan cheese			
Pineapple				Nutritional yeast			
Prunes				Olive oil (virgin)			
Tangerines				Sesame seed (toasted)			
Watermelon				Nut oils (avocado etc.)			

AROMAS

ℰ 3 Passive *Herbs, spices and seasonings/sauces, etc. (uncooked or heated)*

Food	Like	Don't Like	Don't Know
Bombay duck			
Sambal Oleck			
Thai fish sauce (NamPla)*			
Anchovies			
Garlic*			
Ginger (powdered)			
Ginger root*			
Curry powder*			
Allspice			
Clove			
Cumin			
Molasses			
Nutmeg*			
Kimchee			
Oyster sauce			
Lemon grass*			
Maple syrup			
Rosemary*			
Citrus zests			
Fennel*			
Anise			
Basil			
Cardamom			
Chili powder			
Oregano*			
Turmeric*			
Parmesan			
Peppercorns (fresh ground)			
Saffron*			

Food	Like	Don't Like	Don't Know
Bacon, Canadian*			
Mint			
Sage*			
Thyme			
Worcestershire sauce			
Coconut essence			
Tarragon			
Vinegars, various			
Cocoa			
Ketchup			
Vanilla			
Caraway*			
Cilantro			
Dill weed/seed			
Soy sauce*			
Sour cream			
Buttermilk			
Bayleaf*			

* = improves with heat

AROMAS

❧ 4 Oil Sack/Malliard/ Caramel Reactions

Food	Like	Don't Like	Don't Know
Garlic			
Ginger			
Green onions			
Onions			
Citrus zest			
Leeks			
Cinnamon			
Clove			
Curry powder			
Garam Masala			
Fennel			
Chili powder			
Cumin			
Canadian bacon			
Tomatoes (esp. tomato paste)			
Ketchup			
Rosemary			
Saffron			
Sage			
Sweet corn			
Parsnips			
Chiles (hot-spicy)			
Coconut essence			
Bran muffins			
Bread			
Cookies			
Cakes / Pastries			
Peppers (sweet bell)			
Pumpkins (winter squash)			
Sweet potatoes			
Tomatillos			
Bagels			
Cornmeal			
Rutabagas			
Jasmine rice			
Cassava			
Potatoes			

Malliard reaction (meats)

Food	Like	Don't Like	Don't Know
Meats			
Poultry			
Seafood			
Eggs			

COLORS

❧ Red

Food	Like	Don't Like	Don't Know
Strawberries			
Peppers, sweet bell			
Small peppers			
Peppers, red chili			
Radish			
Tomatoes			
Crabapple			
Swiss chard stalks (raw)			
Red currants			
Paprika			
Cayenne			
Persimmons			
Cranberries (dried)			
Raspberries			
Cherries (fresh and dried)			
Kidney beans			

❧ Orange

Food	Like	Don't Like	Don't Know
Oranges			
Marmalade			
Sweet potato			
Tangerines			
Carrots			
Sweet bell pepper			
Apricots			
Papaya			
Mango			
Pumpkin			
Acorn squash			
Hubbard squash			
Butternut squash			
Lentils ("red")			
Chickpeas (garbanzo beans)			

❧ Purple

Food	Like	Don't Like	Don't Know
Beets			
Eggplant			
Blood orange			
Cherries (fresh and dried)			
Blueberries (deep)			
Blackberries (deep)			
Plums			
Grapes			
Pepper (sweet bell)			
Radish			
Carrots (purple)			
Potatoes			
Onions ("red")			

❧ Yellow

Food	Like	Don't Like	Don't Know
Sweet bell peppers			
Patti Pans summer squash			
Crookneck summer squash			
Whole eggs			
Eggbeaters			
Corn			
Tomatoes			
Pineapple			
Nectarines			
Peaches			
Cornmeal			
Parsnips (pale)			
Delicata squash			
Yellow fin potatoes (pale)			
Lentils			
Bananas (pale)			
Jerusalem artichokes			
Swiss chard			

COLORS

✑ Green (leaf)

Food	Like	Don't Like	Don't Know
Collard			
Spinach			
Savory			
Beets (greens)			
Kale			
Mustard greens			
Bok choy (tops)			
Romaine			
Arugula			
Watercress			
Pea vines			
Escarole			
Cabbage (drum head)			
Butterleaf			
Chinese (Napa)			
Curly endive			
Iceberg lettuce			

✑ Green

Food	Like	Don't Like	Don't Know
Green beans			
Asparagus			
Soy beans (young)			
Peas, green			
Peas, snow			
Green onions			
Fennel tops			
Kiwi fruit			
Artichokes (globe)			
Brussels sprouts			
Cherkin			
Capers			
Avocados			
Grapes (pale)			
Tomatillos (pale)			
Lima beans			
Celery (pale)			
Fava beans			
Cucumber			

✑ Pink

Food	Like	Don't Like	Don't Know
Salmon			
Shrimp, flesh			
Cherries			
Lobster, flesh			
Crab, flesh			
Arctic char			
Watermelon			
Radish			
Swiss chard stalks			
Grapefruit			
Pickled ginger			
Rhubarb			

✑ Brown & Deeper Colors

Food	Like	Don't Like	Don't Know
Beans, black			
Chocolate			
Dates			
Coffee, instant			
Raisins			
Cocoa			
Wild rice			
Meats, surface cooked			
Nuts, various			
Balsamic vinegar			
Garam masala			
Soy sauce			
Tomato paste (malliard)			
Beans, various			
Bread			
Muffins			
Cookies			
Doughnuts			
Pastry			
Wheat kernels			
Sultanas			
Bulgur			
Brown rice (pale)			

COLORS

❧ White/Cream

Food	Like	Don't Like	Don't Know
Potato			
Bagel (inside)			
Egg white			
Scallops			
Bok choy (stalks)			
Vanilla ice cream			
Vanilla iced yogurt			
Yogurt			
Cream			
Icing sugar			
Fish (some)			
Fennel			
Milks			
Daikon (radish)			
Water chestnut			
Soy			
Rice			
Pasta			
Noodles			
Soy beans (dried)			
Endive (chicory)			
Udon			
Tofu			
Lychee			
Butterbeans			
Navy beans			
Celeriac			
Jicama			
Onions			
Eggplant (inside)			
Barley			
Couscous			
Cassava			

Food	Like	Don't Like	Don't Know
White asparagus			
Turnips			
Yam			
Quinoa			
Chicken			
Apple (inside)			
Oatmeal (darker)			
Bamboo shoots			
Gnocchi			
Turkey			
Popcorn			
Bananas			
Evaporated skim milk			
Rutabagas (deep cream)			
Taro			

TEXTURES

❧ Spicy

Food	Like	Don't Like	Don't Know
Habanero pepper (Scotch Bonnet)			
Datil pepper			
Wasabi (green 'mustard')			
Jalapeño pepper			
Cayenne (red pepper)			
Horseradish			
White peppercorn			
Black peppercorn			
Hot sauces, various			
Tabasco			
Mustards, various			
Anaheim pepper			
Radish			
Arugula (Rocket)			

❧ Mouth Round Fullness (MRF)

Food	Like	Don't Like	Don't Know
Custards			
Flan (molded custards)			
Butter			
Eggs			
Margarine, various			
Cream			
Chocolate			
Smoothies			
Bananas			
Nut butters			
Avocado			
Oatmeal			
Bagel			
Pear			
Scallops			
Arrowroot			
Root vegetables as 'velvet' (purees)			
Peas and corn as 'velvet' (purees)			
Yogurt cheese			
Ice cream			
Gelatin (Agar)			
Yogurt			
Cheese			
Hummus			
Spinach as saag (Indian cooking)			
Cornstarch			
Potato starch			
Pasta			
Cornmeal (polenta)			
Milk			
Cassava (Manioc)			

OTHER FOOD EXPERIENCES

AND NOW . . . TO COMPLETE THE FUN: Simply circle your rating on the scale of 1–10 that shows how much you value the following 'other' experiences (that don't quite fit under our ingredient list).

Sample Rating

1	2	3	4	5	⑥	7	8	9	10

Not Important   Neutral   Somewhat Important   Extremely Important

❧ Appearance

Complimentary colors on one plate

1   2   3   4   5   6   7   8   9   10

Color that clash—vivid—bold

1   2   3   4   5   6   7   8   9   10

Food that glistens – reflects light

1   2   3   4   5   6   7   8   9   10

Food with a soft matte surface

1   2   3   4   5   6   7   8   9   10

Medium to small portions

1   2   3   4   5   6   7   8   9   10

Large servings, enough to take home

1   2   3   4   5   6   7   8   9   10

Simple plate presentation (elegant?)

1   2   3   4   5   6   7   8   9   10

Highly decorated/garnished dishes

1   2   3   4   5   6   7   8   9   10

❧ Appearance

Easy to eat food

| 1 | 2 | 3 | 4 | 5 | 6 | 7 | 8 | 9 | 10 |

Foods with complex structure (i.e. in 'towers')

| 1 | 2 | 3 | 4 | 5 | 6 | 7 | 8 | 9 | 10 |

Meats etc. fully coated with sauces

| 1 | 2 | 3 | 4 | 5 | 6 | 7 | 8 | 9 | 10 |

Meats etc. partially coated or set over a sauce

| 1 | 2 | 3 | 4 | 5 | 6 | 7 | 8 | 9 | 10 |

❧ Texture

Foods that are crisp

| 1 | 2 | 3 | 4 | 5 | 6 | 7 | 8 | 9 | 10 |

Crunchy

| 1 | 2 | 3 | 4 | 5 | 6 | 7 | 8 | 9 | 10 |

Al dente (as in pasta)

| 1 | 2 | 3 | 4 | 5 | 6 | 7 | 8 | 9 | 10 |

Tender

| 1 | 2 | 3 | 4 | 5 | 6 | 7 | 8 | 9 | 10 |

Springy (as in wild salmon)

| 1 | 2 | 3 | 4 | 5 | 6 | 7 | 8 | 9 | 10 |

Moist

| 1 | 2 | 3 | 4 | 5 | 6 | 7 | 8 | 9 | 10 |

Opposites (i.e. brittle/soft as in crème Brule)

| 1 | 2 | 3 | 4 | 5 | 6 | 7 | 8 | 9 | 10 |

❧ Texture

Hot foods (temperature)
    1   2   3   4   5   6   7   8   9   10

Cold foods (temperature)
    1   2   3   4   5   6   7   8   9   10

❧ Preparation

Poach (fish/vegetables/fruits/eggs)
    1   2   3   4   5   6   7   8   9   10

Shallow fry (sauté)
    1   2   3   4   5   6   7   8   9   10

Deep fry
    1   2   3   4   5   6   7   8   9   10

Bake (pies, cakes etc.)
    1   2   3   4   5   6   7   8   9   10

Barbequed
    1   2   3   4   5   6   7   8   9   10

Spit roast
    1   2   3   4   5   6   7   8   9   10

Casserole
    1   2   3   4   5   6   7   8   9   10

Stews
    1   2   3   4   5   6   7   8   9   10

Soups
    1   2   3   4   5   6   7   8   9   10

❧ Preparation

Poele (sauté then steam/poach)

| 1 | 2 | 3 | 4 | 5 | 6 | 7 | 8 | 9 | 10 |

Steam

| 1 | 2 | 3 | 4 | 5 | 6 | 7 | 8 | 9 | 10 |

Oven roast (meat etc.)

| 1 | 2 | 3 | 4 | 5 | 6 | 7 | 8 | 9 | 10 |

Broil (grill, radiant)

| 1 | 2 | 3 | 4 | 5 | 6 | 7 | 8 | 9 | 10 |

Griddle (flat metal sheet)

| 1 | 2 | 3 | 4 | 5 | 6 | 7 | 8 | 9 | 10 |

❧ Cultural Styles of Cooking

French

| 1 | 2 | 3 | 4 | 5 | 6 | 7 | 8 | 9 | 10 |

Italian

| 1 | 2 | 3 | 4 | 5 | 6 | 7 | 8 | 9 | 10 |

Chinese (USA styled)

| 1 | 2 | 3 | 4 | 5 | 6 | 7 | 8 | 9 | 10 |

Thai

| 1 | 2 | 3 | 4 | 5 | 6 | 7 | 8 | 9 | 10 |

Mexican

| 1 | 2 | 3 | 4 | 5 | 6 | 7 | 8 | 9 | 10 |

Japanese

| 1 | 2 | 3 | 4 | 5 | 6 | 7 | 8 | 9 | 10 |

❧ Cultural Styles of Cooking

British
    1   2   3   4   5   6   7   8   9   10

Indian
    1   2   3   4   5   6   7   8   9   10

North African
    1   2   3   4   5   6   7   8   9   10

Caribbean
    1   2   3   4   5   6   7   8   9   10

Mediterranean
    1   2   3   4   5   6   7   8   9   10

❧ United States Styles of Cooking

South West (Tex/Mex)
    1   2   3   4   5   6   7   8   9   10

South Eastern (Cuban)
    1   2   3   4   5   6   7   8   9   10

East Coast (Italian/European/...)
    1   2   3   4   5   6   7   8   9   10

Pacific Northwest (seafood/Asian)
    1   2   3   4   5   6   7   8   9   10

California (fusion/fresh)
    1   2   3   4   5   6   7   8   9   10

Midwest (ranchers)
    1   2   3   4   5   6   7   8   9   10

Now you have it . . . the most complete assessment of your senses

AMBIANCE

There is still remaining the final 'A' in TACTA. The issue of what the French call "ambiance" . . . or the environmental/emotional impact of the immediate surroundings. This is so much a question of individual taste (in style). It is important because it shows that you want people to feel comfortable (at home) in your home.

Ambiance is the sum of several decisions. Here are quite a few of those that are important to consider:

- Wall colors, drapes etc. Yellow/green are OK but not when vivid.
- Lighting, watch out for ugly shadows—use a dimmer.
- Candles may look nice but can be a problem (shadows).
- Natural tabletops, use wood or tile, cloth . . . plastic can be ugly/cold.
- Seats need soft padding to encourage sitting long over a meal.
- Tables need to be about 2'6" above floor level.
- Flat wear should have smooth rounded ends for comfort.
- Table flowers should be non-aromatic—they compete with wine/food.
- Please try to do without TV whilst you eat. It can be an insult to the cook.
- Music in background is fine… if kept below conversation level.
- Dining room/areas need less small decorative items. Simple is best.
- Conversation needs to be affirming, never negative!
- Better to be understated (simplicity) than ostentatious!

Above all, have fun, enjoy one another—our times at the table build extremely fond memories for both families and good friends.

Recipes

Breakfast and Brunch

Omelet with Peppers, Mushrooms, and Spinach

SERVING SIZE: 1/2 omelet, SERVES: 2

  1 tsp extra virgin olive oil, divided
1/2 cup chopped onion
  1 clove garlic
  1 cup chopped red bell peppers
1/2 cup sliced mushrooms
  2 cups fresh spinach, trimmed and cut in strips
  4 eggs or 2 eggs and 2 egg whites or 1 cup egg substitute
1/4 tsp salt
1/4 freshly ground black pepper
  2 Roma tomatoes, seeded and chopped
  2 Tbsp chopped fresh basil, chives or parsley (or all three mixed)

1 Heat 1/2 tsp of the oil in a skillet on medium high. Cook the onion until tender but not brown, about 3 minutes. Add the garlic, bell peppers, and mushrooms and cook until soft, 3 or 4 more minutes. Stir in the spinach and remove from the heat.

2 Beat the eggs and add the salt and pepper. Heat the remaining 1/2 tsp oil in a 10-inch omelet pan (this is a fry pan with rounded, low sides) on medium high. Pour in the eggs and push gently to the center with a rubber spatula allowing the uncooked eggs to flow to the outside of the pan. When the egg is cooked, remove from the heat and top with the prepared vegetables.

3 Fold in half, cut in two, and serve on hot plates. Scatter the chopped tomatoes and herbs over the top.

Per serving (2 eggs): 246 calories, 13 g fat, 4 g saturated fat, 15% calories from saturated fat, 18 g carbohydrate, 4 g dietary fiber, 477 mg sodium
Exchanges: 2 Medium Fat Meat, 3 Vegetable, 1/2 Fat
Per serving (1 egg and 1 egg white): 187 calories, 8 g fat, 2 g saturated fat, 10% calories from saturated fat, 17 g carbohydrate, 4 g dietary fiber, 464 mg sodium
Exchanges: 1 Medium Fat Meat, 3 Vegetable, 1/2 Fat
Per serving (egg substitute): 157 calories, 3 g fat, 0 g saturated fat, 0% calories from saturated fat, 18 g carbohydrate, 4 g fiber, 551 mg sodium
Exchanges: 1 Very Lean Meat, 3 Vegetable, 1/2 Fat

Artichoke Omelet

SERVING SIZE: 1/6 of recipe, SERVES: 6

    1 Tbsp extra virgin olive oil
    1 bunch green onions
    3 cloves garlic, chopped
  1/2 cup chopped red bell pepper
    1 cup zucchini, chopped in 1/2-inch pieces
    1 cup shredded collard greens
    8 Greek olives, pitted and chopped
    1 cup frozen or canned artichoke heart quarters
    2 Roma or Viva Italia tomatoes, seeded and chopped
  1/2 tsp dried oregano
  1/2 tsp dried basil
    2 Tbsp chopped fresh parsley
  1/4 tsp freshly ground black pepper
  1/8 tsp salt
    2 Tbsp plus 1 tsp grated Parmesan cheese
1 3/4 cups egg substitute

1 Preheat the oven broiler. Heat 1 tsp of the oil in a heavy skillet on medium. Slice the white ends of the green onions and finely chop the green parts. Sauté the white parts with the garlic about 1 minute to release the flavors. Add the red pepper, zucchini, collard greens, olives, artichoke hearts, oregano, and basil and cook 8 minutes or until the vegetables are tender but still crisp and colorful.

2 Stir in the tomatoes, pepper, salt, and 1 Tbsp each of the parsley and Parmesan cheese. Pour the egg substitute into the vegetables, shaking the pan to distribute it evenly. Scatter the second Tbsp of Parmesan over the top. Cook on medium about 6 minutes or until the bottom is done and the top is still runny. Place under the broiler for 2 minutes to finish cooking. Scatter the remaining teaspoon of Parmesan and a Tbsp each of the green onion tops and chopped parsley on top. Drizzle with the remaining extra virgin olive oil. Cut into four wedges and serve. It's a great brunch.

Per serving: 170 calories, 5 g fat, 1 g saturated fat, 5% calories from saturated fat, 17 g carbohydrate, 5 g dietary fiber, 453 mg sodium
Exchanges: 1 Very Lean Meat, 3 Vegetable, 1 Fat

Frittata Primavera

SERVING SIZE: 1/2 frittata, SERVES: 2

3 tsp olive oil
1/4 cup chopped onion
1 clove garlic, finely chopped
1/2 cup fresh asparagus pieces
1/2 cup canned or frozen artichoke hearts,
chopped
1/2 cup sugar snap peas, strings pulled
and cut in 1/2-inch pieces

1/4 tsp dried basil
1/8 tsp pepper
3/4 cup egg substitute
1 Tbsp plain low-fat yogurt
1 Tbsp grated Parmesan
cheese

1 Heat 1 tsp of the oil in the skillet and cook onion 2–3 minutes or until soft.
Add the garlic and cook 1 minute more. Stir in the asparagus, artichoke
hearts, peas, basil, and pepper and cook, stirring occasionally until tender
but still slightly crisp, about 3–5 minutes. Set aside.

2 Preheat the broiler. Beat the egg substitute or eggs with the yogurt and
another pinch of pepper. Heat the remaining oil in a heavy bottom skillet.
Pour in the egg mixture and cook until just set on the bottom but still wet on
the top, about 1 minute. Scatter the vegetables over the top and set in the
oven to finish cooking, about 2 minutes. Dust the top with the Parmesan
cheese, cut into wedges, and serve.

Per serving: 125 calories, 3 g fat, 1 g saturated fat, 7% calories from saturated
fat, 11 g carbohydrate, 2 g dietary fiber, 248 mg sodium, 14 g protein
Exchanges: 2 Very Lean Meat, 2 Vegetable, 1/2 Fat

Grapefruit Sections with Mint Sauce

SERVING SIZE: 1/2 grapefruit, SERVES: 4

2 large red grapefruit
1 cup unsweetened apple juice
1/4 cup fresh mint leaves
2 tsp cornstarch or arrowroot mixed with 2 Tbsp apple juice (slurry)

1 Cut the ends off the grapefruit. Cut away the rind with the white pith and skin underneath. Hold the naked grapefruit in your hand and remove the sections by cutting the flesh away from the dividing membrane. Place the sections in the refrigerator to chill.

2 Heat the apple juice with the mint leaves and simmer a minute or two. Stir in the slurry and heat to thicken and clear. Strain and chill.

3 Divide the grapefruit among 4 bowls. Spoon the mint sauce over the grapefruit and serve.

Per serving: 76 calories, 0 g fat, 0 g saturated fat, 0% calories from saturated fat, 19 g carbohydrate, 1 g dietary fiber, 4 mg sodium
Exchanges: 1 Fruit

Asparagus Omelet

SERVING SIZE: 1/2 of recipe, SERVES: 2

8 stalks asparagus	1/2 tsp non-aromatic olive oil
pinch salt and pepper	1 cup egg substitute or 4 eggs
1 tsp grated Parmesan cheese	1 cup sliced tomatoes
1/2 tsp butter	

1 Snap the tough ends off the asparagus and discard. Cut the tender stalks in 1-inch pieces. Place in a steamer basket, season with salt and pepper and sprinkle with lemon juice. Steam or microwave 5 minutes or until tender. Set aside.

2 Heat the omelet pan and melt the butter with the oil. Pour in the eggs and cook, pushing the eggs to the center of the pan and tipping the pan to cook evenly. When the eggs are ready, scatter with Parmesan cheese and add the asparagus. Roll up, cut in half, and serve garnished with the tomatoes.

Per serving (with egg substitute): 131 calories, 4 g fat, 1 g saturated fat, 7% calories from saturated fat, 10 g carbohydrate, 3 g dietary fiber, 352 mg sodium
Exchanges: 2 Very Lean Meat, 2 Vegetable, 1/2 Fat
Per serving (with eggs): 237 calories, 5 g fat, 1 g saturated fat, 4% calories from saturated fat, 40 g carbohydrate, 6 g dietary fiber, 353 mg sodium
Exchanges: 2 Very Lean Meat, 2 Vegetable, 1/2 Fat

Waffles with Spiced Applesauce

SERVING SIZE: 2 waffles, SERVES: 4

<C 8 frozen waffles
<C 2 cups unsweetened applesauce
<C 1/4 cup brown sugar

1/4 tsp allspice
    pinch ground cloves

1 Heat waffles according to package instructions.

2 Heat the applesauce on medium heat in a saucepan. Stir in the brown sugar, allspice and cloves.

3 Lay the waffles on hot serving plates and spoon the applesauce over the top.

<C To Cut Carb

Waffles: reduce to 4 only. To increase the plate "appearance" you can add fresh berries in season
Applesauce: reduce to 1 cup.
Brown sugar: reduce to 2 Tbsp and add 2 Tbsp Splenda.

Per serving: 296 calories, 7 g fat, 2 g saturated fat, 4% calories from saturated fat, 56 g carbohydrate, 2 g dietary fiber, 442 mg sodium
Exchanges: 2 Starch, 1 Fruit, 1/2 Fat, 1 Carbohydrate

Low Carb

Per serving: 151 calories, 3 g fat, 1 g saturated fat, 5% calories from saturated fat, 29 g carbohydrate, 1 g dietary fiber, 221 mg sodium
Exchanges: 1 Starch, 1/2 Fruit, 1/2 Fat, 1/2 Carbohydrate

Breakfast Taco with Refried Beans

SERVING SIZE: 1 taco, SERVES: 4

Yogurt Guacamole

  1 avocado
  1 Tbsp freshly squeezed lime juice
1/4 cup yogurt cheese

1/4 tsp salt
    pinch cayenne pepper

Refried Beans

1/2 tsp non-aromatic olive oil
1/4 cup finely chopped onion
1 clove garlic, bashed and chopped

<C 1 cup cooked pinto beans or
   nonfat canned refried beans
1 cup bean cooking liquid

Eggs

1 Tbsp finely diced reconstituted ancho
   chili (soak in hot water to reconstitute)
2 cups egg substitute
4 oz finely diced Canadian bacon

1/4 cup thinly sliced green onions
1/8 tsp salt
4 warm flour tortillas

1 Mash the avocado with a fork. Add the lime juice, yogurt cheese, salt, and cayenne. Cover closely with plastic wrap and set aside.

2 Heat the oil in a skillet on medium high. Sauté the onion until tender then add garlic and cook 30 seconds longer. Add the beans, mashing as you fry them. Pour in cooking liquid as you need it. As a nice brown crust forms on the bottom of the pan, push it into the beans giving them more and more flavor as you continue to cook them. When they are dark and flavorful and a good spreading consistency, set aside and cover to keep warm.

3 Spread refried beans on each warm tortilla. Heat a small nonstick omelet pan on medium. Spray with pan spray and pour in 1/2 cup of the egg substitute. Push in the sides of the omelet as it cooks to a soft, still wet-looking texture. Sprinkle with 1/4 of the Canadian bacon, green onion, and a little salt. Lift and lay on a bean-covered tortilla. Repeat with the other three. Top with a dollop of yogurt guacamole and some chopped cilantro.

<C To Cut Carb

Beans: reduce to 2/3 cup of both the beans and the cooking liquid.

Per serving: 365 calories, 13 g fat, 2 g saturated fat, 5% calories from saturated fat, 37 g carbohydrate, 8 g dietary fiber, 977 mg sodium
Exchanges: 2 1/2 Starch, 3 Lean Meat, 1/2 Fat

Low Carb

Per serving: 345 calories, 13 g fat, 2 g saturated fat, 5% calories from saturated fat, 34 g carbohydrate, 6 g dietary fiber, 977 mg sodium
Exchanges: 2 Starch, 3 Lean Meat, 1/2 Fat

Blake Island Skillet Soufflé

SERVING SIZE: 1/4 of recipe, SERVES: 4

1/4 cup sun-dried tomatoes
2 green onions
4 oz salmon lox
1/2 tsp non-aromatic olive oil
1/2 cup 2% milk
1 Tbsp cornstarch
pinch nutmeg
pinch saffron

1/4 tsp freshly ground black pepper
1 egg yolk
1 tsp chopped fresh tarragon or 1/4 tsp dried
4 large egg whites
1/4 tsp cream of tartar
1 tsp butter
1 Tbsp Parmesan cheese
1 Tbsp chopped parsley

Vegetarian Option

1/2 cup roasted sweet red peppers, cut in strips
2 Tbsp capers

You can make this dish vegetarian by replacing the salmon lox with the roasted sweet red peppers and the capers.

1 Bring 1 cup water to a boil in a small saucepan, add the sun-dried tomatoes, reduce the heat, and simmer 15 minutes. Drain and chop. Slice the green onions and set aside. Lay the slices of lox on top of each other and cut into 1/2-inch pieces.

2 Heat the oil in a saucepan on medium high. Sauté the onions 1 minute to release the flavors and add the tomatoes. Combine the milk, cornstarch, nutmeg, saffron, and pepper and add to the onion mixture. Stir until thick, 30 seconds, then remove from the heat to cool. Mix in the egg yolk and tarragon and set aside.

3 Preheat the oven broiler. Beat the egg whites until foamy. Add the cream of tartar and continue beating until stiff peaks form. Stir 1/3 of the whites into the flavor base to lighten then fold in the rest gently.

4 Melt the butter in a hot 10-inch omelet pan and allow it to brown slightly. Pour in the egg white mixture, stir quickly, then smooth and cook 30 seconds on medium high. Scatter the salmon evenly over the top and sprinkle with the cheese. Cook under the preheated broiler 3 to 4 minutes or until

puffed and golden. Garnish with the parsley. Take the hot pan to the table, cut into fourths, and serve on 4 hot plates. Served with an attractive salad, this can make a wonderfully tasty light brunch or supper dish.

Per serving: 128 calories, 6 g fat, 2 g saturated fat, 14% calories from saturated fat, 6 g carbohydrates, 1 g dietary fiber, 400 mg sodium
Exchanges: 2 Very Lean Meat, 1 Vegetable, 1 Fat

Vegetarian
Per serving: 99 calories, 5 g fat, 2 g saturated fat, 18% calories from saturated fat, 7 g carbohydrates, 1 g fiber, 178 mg sodium
Exchanges: 1 Very Lean Meat, 1 Vegetable, 1 Fat

Mediterranean Omelet

SERVING SIZE: 1/6 of recipe, SERVES: 6

2 tsp extra virgin olive oil	1/2 tsp dried oregano
1 bunch green onions, sliced	1/2 tsp dried basil
3 cloves garlic, chopped	1/4 tsp freshly ground black pepper
3 cups chopped fresh spinach	1/8 tsp salt
6 Greek olives, pitted and chopped	2 Tbsp grated Parmesan cheese
2 Roma tomatoes, seeded and chopped	1 1/2 cups egg substitute

1 Preheat the oven broiler. Heat 1 tsp of the oil in a heavy skillet on medium. Sauté the onions with the garlic about 1 minute to release the flavors.

2 Add the spinach, olives, oregano, and basil and cook 3 or 4 minutes, or until the vegetables are tender but still crisp and colorful. Stir in the tomatoes, pepper, salt, and 1 Tbsp Parmesan cheese.

3 Pour the egg substitute into the vegetables, shaking the pan to distribute it evenly. Scatter the second Tbsp of Parmesan over the top. Cook on medium about 6 minutes or until the bottom is done and the top still runny. Place under the broiler for 2 minutes to finish cooking.

4 Drizzle with the remaining tsp of olive oil. Cut into four wedges and serve. It's a great brunch.

Per serving: 148 calories, 7 g fat, 2 g saturated fat, 10% calories from saturated fat, 7 g carbohydrate, 4 g dietary fiber, 392 mg sodium, 14 g protein
Exchanges: 2 Very Lean Meat, 1 Vegetable, 1 Fat

Summer Tomato-Scrambled Eggs

SERVING SIZE: 1/4 of recipe, SERVES: 4

  4 eggs or about 1 cup egg substitute
1/4 cup finely sliced sun-dried tomatoes

> Spray a non-stick pan with cooking spray and heat over medium heat.
> Whisk eggs and add tomatoes. Pour into prepared pan and stir occasionally
> until eggs are cooked through. Serve warm.

Per serving (with eggs): 84 calories, 5 g fat, 2 g saturated fat, 15% calories from
saturated fat, 213 mg sodium, 2 g carbohydrate, 0 g dietary fiber,
7 g protein
Exchanges: 1 Medium Fat Meat
Per serving (with egg substitute): 39 calories, 0 g fat, 0 g saturated fat, 0% calories from saturated fat, 3 g carbohydrate, 0 g dietary fiber, 116 mg sodium,
7 g protein
Exchanges: 1 Very Lean Meat

Blintzes with Strawberries

SERVING SIZE: 1/6 of recipe, SERVES: 6

Crepe Batter

1 whole egg
1 egg yolk
1 cup skim milk

1/2 cup all-purpose flour
  1 tsp light olive oil

Strawberry Salsa

    3 cups chopped fresh strawberries (about two pints whole berries)
    1 medium crisp apple, unpeeled, chopped (about 1 cup)
    1 small jalapeno pepper, cored, seeded, and finely chopped
<C 1 Tbsp sugar
   1/8 tsp freshly ground black pepper

Filling

3/4 cup yogurt cheese

1/4 cup chopped dried strawberries

<c 2 tsp maple syrup

1/4 tsp vanilla extract

2 tsp cornstarch

1. To prepare the crepe batter, beat the whole egg, egg yolk, and milk in a large bowl. Whisk in the flour and the oil. Let the batter rest for 30 minutes before cooking.

2. While the batter is resting, prepare the salsa. In a small bowl, combine the chopped strawberries, apples, and jalapeno. Sprinkle with the sugar and black pepper and set aside.

3. To prepare the filling, gently combine the yogurt cheese, dried strawberries, maple syrup, vanilla, and cornstarch in a small bowl. Set aside while you cook the crepes.

4. To cook the crepes, spray a medium (7-inch) crepe pan or skillet with cooking spray and warm over medium heat. It is important that the skillet be good and warm before adding the batter. Pour a scant 1/4 cup of the batter into the pan, gently tilting the pan back and forth to coat the bottom with batter. When the top dulls and bubbles form, about 35-40 seconds, flip the crepe onto a paper towel, cooked side up. The crepe will be a pale golden color on the cooked side.

5. Repeat this process with the remaining batter, spraying the skillet with cooking spray if needed to keep the crepes from sticking. You may go ahead and fill each crepe while the next one is cooking, or you may stack the finished crepes until ready to fill.

6. To fill the blintzes, spoon 2 generous Tbsp of the filling into the center of the cooked side of a crepe. Fold the edges in toward the center to make a small square envelope. Repeat with the remaining crepes. If they will not be cooked immediately, store the blintzes seam side down in a single layer in a shallow container. They will keep in the refrigerator overnight.

7. When ready to cook the blintzes, preheat the broiler. Spray a baking sheet with cooking spray and lay the filled crepes on the baking sheet, seam side down. Spray the tops with cooking spray and broil for 5 minutes, or until golden brown.

8. To serve, spread a generous 1/2 cup of the salsa on each dessert plate. Lay a hot blintz on top of the salsa.

(Continued)

Per serving: 179 calories, 3 g fat, 1 g saturated fat, 5% calories from saturated fat, 31 g carbohydrate, 3 g dietary fiber
Exchanges: 1 Starch, 1 Fruit, 1/2 Fat

Low Carb
Per serving: 170 calories, 3 g fat, 1 g saturated fat, 5% calories from saturated fat, 29 g carbohydrate, 3 g dietary fiber
Exchanges: 1 Starch, 1 Fruit, 1/2 Fat

French Toast with Blueberry-Orange Sauce

SERVING SIZE: 2 slices, SERVES: 4

Sauce

2 cups fresh or frozen blueberries

1/4 cup orange juice concentrate

French Toast

1/2 cup egg substitute
1/4 cup evaporated skim milk

1/2 tsp vanilla
<C 8 slices whole-wheat bread

1 Stir the blueberries and orange juice concentrate together in a saucepan and heat gently.

2 Preheat the oven to 250°F. Combine the egg substitute with the milk and vanilla. Heat a large heavy skillet and coat with pan spray. Dip as many slices of bread as will fit in the pan into the egg mixture and cook until brown on one side. Turn and brown the other side. Keep warm in the oven. Repeat with the rest of the bread.

3 Divide the French toast among 4 hot plates and spoon the sauce over them.

Whole-wheat bread: serve only 1 slice of bread for a lower-carb snack.

Per serving: 235 calories, 3 g fat, 1 g saturated fat, 2% calories from saturated fat, 45 g carbohydrate, 6 g dietary fiber, 377 mg sodium
Exchanges: 2 Starch, 1 Very Lean Meat, 1 Fruit

Low Carb
Per serving: 166 calories, 2 g fat, 0 g saturated fat, 0% calories from saturated fat, 32 g carbohydrate, 4 g dietary fiber, 230 mg sodium
Exchanges: 1 Starch, 1 Very Lean Meat, 1 Fruit

Broiled Grapefruit

SERVING SIZE: 1 grapefruit half, SERVES: 4

2 large pink grapefruit, cut in half
2 large fresh strawberries, cut in half lengthwise

8 tsp strawberry jam
1 Tbsp chopped fresh mint

> For a hearty but less fancy variation, substitute 1 tsp of brown sugar for the 2 tsp of jam on each half and forget the mint and strawberry halves. Watch carefully during the broiling process because the sugar will burn easily.

1 Set the oven rack in the top third of the oven and preheat the broiler. Spread the grapefruit halves with the jam and set on a broiler pan. Place under the broiler and cook until the jam darkens and bubbles, 3–5 minutes depending on your broiler.

2 Sprinkle with the chopped mint, lay a strawberry half in the middle, and serve as a brunch (or dessert) treat.

Per serving: 100 calories, 0 g fat, 0 g saturated fat, 0% calories from saturated fat, 23 g carbohydrate, 4 g dietary fiber, 26 mg sodium
Exchanges: 1/2 Fruit, 1 Carbohydrate

Poached Eggs Cartagena

SERVING SIZE: 1/6 of recipe, SERVES: 6

Salsa

  6 large Italian plum tomatoes, such as Roma
  1 Anaheim chili, cored, seeded, and finely chopped (1/4 cup)
  1 1/2 cups cooked black beans (15 oz), rinsed and drained
  3 large cloves garlic, peeled, bashed, and chopped (1 Tbsp)
3/4 cup sliced green onions
 12 small stuffed green olives, sliced
1/4 tsp freshly ground black pepper
1/4 tsp ground cumin
  1 tsp mild chili powder
1/2 tsp salt
  1 Tbsp arrowroot
  2 Tbsp water
  4 Tbsp chopped fresh cilantro, 1 Tbsp reserved for garnish

Eggs and Tortillas

  6 white corn tortillas (6-inch diameter)
  6 whole eggs or 1 1/2 cups egg substitute

Garnish

  Chopped fresh cilantro
 1 tsp dried crushed red pepper flakes

1 Preheat the oven to 350°F. Take eggs out of refrigerator so they can warm to room temperature.

To Prepare the Salsa

2 Bring a large saucepan of water to a rolling boil. Core the tomatoes and drop them into the boiling water for 1 minute. (This will loosen the skin enough to peel.) Remove the tomatoes and dip in cold water or allow them to cool on a plate. When the tomatoes are cool, peel and discard skins.

3 Dice the tomatoes and put them into a medium saucepan. Add the chopped chili, black beans, garlic, green onions, olives, pepper, cumin, chili powder, and 1/4 tsp of the salt. Cook for a few minutes over medium heat.

4 Combine the arrowroot with 2 Tbsp of water to make a slurry. Add the slurry to the tomato mixture and stir over medium heat until the salsa is glossy and thickened. Set aside until the eggs are ready, along with 3 Tbsp of the chopped cilantro, which should be added just before serving.

To Prepare the Tortillas and Eggs

5 Oil a large cookie sheet with cooking spray and cover with the tortillas. Spray the tortillas lightly with cooking spray. Warm in the preheated oven for 5 minutes.

6 Add 2 inches of water and the remaining 1/4 tsp of salt to a large, shallow skillet and bring to a simmer. Break an egg into a small dish or saucer and slide gently into the simmering (not boiling) water. Repeat with the rest of the eggs, one by one. When all the eggs have been added, give the pan a gentle "Amtrak" shake to allow the hot water to flow over the tops of the eggs and cook them lightly. (Keep the water just barely simmering.) After about 4 minutes, the whites should be firm and the yolks should be runny. Serve immediately.

7 If you choose to use egg substitute, heat a medium skillet over medium-low heat. Spray with cooking spray and pour in the egg substitute. When the eggs start to set, push gently with a spatula, moving the cooked part to the center of the pan and letting the uncooked part run to the bottom of the pan. It is important that the eggs stay soft and glossy. They can be ruined by over cooking or over stirring.

To Serve

8 Stir the 3 Tbsp of cilantro into the thickened salsa. Place a hot tortilla on each warmed salad plate and spoon a healthy dollop of the salsa into the middle of the tortilla. Top with a poached egg or a 1/4-cup scoop of the scrambled eggs. For garnish, sprinkle the chopped cilantro and red pepper flakes over the eggs. Offer more pepper flakes in a small dish for those who like it more than just hot.

Per serving (with eggs): 188 calories, 7 g fat, 2 g saturated fat, 9% calories from saturated fat, 22 g carbohydrate, 4 g dietary fiber, 9 g protein
Exchanges: 1 1/2 Starch, 1 Medium Fat Meat
Per serving (with egg substitute): 131 calories, 2 g fat, 0 g saturated fat, 0% calories from saturated fat, 22 g carbohydrate, 4 g dietary fiber, 6 g protein
Exchanges: 1 1/2 Starch, 1 Very Lean Meat

Pineapple Crêpes

SERVING SIZE: 2 crêpes, SERVES: 6

Crêpe Batter

1 whole egg
1 egg yolk
1 cup 2% milk

1/2 tsp vanilla extract
1/2 cup all-purpose flour
1 tsp light olive oil

Pineapple Sauce

1/2 tsp light oil
1 lime, zest cut into thin strips
<C 1/3 cup pineapple juice concentrate
+> 2/3 cup water
<C 3/4 cup plus 2 Tbsp fruity white wine (I prefer nonalcoholic white zinfandel)
<C 2 Tbsp chopped crystallized ginger
<C 1 Tbsp brown sugar
1 Tbsp cornstarch
1/2 cup yogurt cheese (page 475)
<C 3 slices of fresh pineapple, 1/4-inch thick, cut into quarters (reserve the best-looking leaves)

Garnish

instant coffee granules or a few ground coffee beans
reserved pineapple leaves

To Prepare the Crêpes

1. Beat the whole egg, egg yolk, milk, and vanilla in a large bowl. Whisk in the flour, then let the batter rest for 30 minutes before cooking.

2. When you are ready to cook the crêpes, warm a crêpe pan or an 8-inch non-stick frying pan with low sides over medium heat. Add the oil and swirl it around to coat the bottom of the pan, then pour the excess into the batter. It is important that the skillet be good and warm before cooking the crêpes.

3. Pour 1/4 cup of batter into the skillet and gently tilt the pan back and forth to coat the bottom. When the top dulls and turns waxy, about 30 to 45 seconds, turn the crêpe over and cook the other side for about 15 seconds. When done, slip the crêpe onto a paper towel, light side up.

4. Repeat this process with the remaining batter, spraying the pan with cooking spray if needed to keep the crêpes from sticking. When all the crêpes are cooked, wrap them in a cloth napkin, where they will keep quite well for at least six hours.

To Prepare the Sauce

5 Warm the oil in a 10-inch nonstick skillet over medium-high heat. Sauté the lime zest for about 1 minute to extract the volatile oils. Add the pineapple juice concentrate, water, and 1/2 cup of the wine. Simmer for 6 minutes.

6 Strain the sauce into a small saucepan, discarding the zest. Add the crystallized ginger and brown sugar and stir over medium heat until the sugar dissolves.

7 Combine the cornstarch with 2 Tbsp of the wine to make a slurry. Pull the pan off the heat and stir in the slurry, then return to the heat and stir until thickened and clear.

8 Spoon the yogurt cheese into a 2-cup glass measuring cup and add a small amount of the warm sauce to temper the yogurt. Whisk until completely smooth, then add the rest of the sauce.

9 Rinse the saucepan with the remaining 1/4 cup of wine and pour the liquid into the skillet. Stir in the yogurt sauce over very low heat. Place one cooked crêpe in the sauce and coat well on both sides. Using a spoon and a fork, fold the crêpe into quarters (the crêpe will be in the shape of a triangle). Move the folded crêpe to the side of the pan. Repeat the coating and folding process with the remaining crêpes.

To Serve

10 Place two crêpes per serving on warmed dessert plates.

11 Add the pineapple slices to the sauce remaining in the pan and warm them through, then spoon two pieces of pineapple alongside the crêpes. Dust with coffee granules and garnish with pineapple leaves.

<c **To Cut Carb** ════════════════════════════════

White wine: reduce to 1/2 cup.   Brown sugar: reduce to 2 tsp.
+> Water: increase to 1 cup.   Pineapple slices: reduce to 2 slices.
Ginger: reduce to 1 Tbsp.

Per serving: 176 calories, 4 g fat, 1 g saturated fat, 6% calories from saturated fat, 29 g carbohydrate, 1 g dietary fiber, 63 mg sodium, 6 g protein
Exchanges: 1/2 Fat, 2 Carbohydrate

Low Carb
Per serving: 163 calories, 4 g fat, 1 g saturated fat, 6% calories from saturated fat, 26 g carbohydrate, 0 g dietary fiber, 62 mg sodium, 6 g protein
Exchanges: 1/2 Fat, 2 Carbohydrate

Muesli

SERVING SIZE: 1/2 of recipe, SERVES: 2

    1/2 cup rolled oats
    1/4 cup dark raisins
      1 Granny Smith apple, cored and grated with peel left on
      2 Tbsp lemon juice
<C   2 Tbsp sweetened condensed nonfat milk
      2 Tbsp Graham's Seed Mix (page 138)

Special Note for People with Diabetes

During the summer, Treena has this for breakfast in place of the Kerr-Mush (see page 118). The post-prandial numbers (2 hours after the *start* of the meal) run as high as 188-210. Included in this meal are one slice of Flax toast and 2 Wasa crisp bread with marmalade. *Altogether* it goes over our normal post-prandial limit of 140–180, however its betaglucan fiber is important in our cholesterol management, so we've grown to live with it.

---

1 Soak the oats and raisins in water overnight.

2 In the morning, drain and stir in the grated apple and lemon juice. Combine with the condensed skimmed milk and stir into the oat mixture.

3 Sprinkle with Graham's Seed Mix and serve.

<C **To Cut Carb**

Sweetened condensed milk: delete and use plain, non-fat yogurt sweetened with 1 tsp Splenda.

Per serving: 289 calories, 6 g fat, 1 g saturated fat, 3% calories from saturated fat, 55 g carbohydrate, 6 g dietary fiber, 27 mg sodium, 8 g protein
Exchanges: 1 Starch, 2 Fruit, 1 Fat, 1/2 Carbohydrate

Low Carb
Per serving: 243 calories, 6 g fat, 1 g saturated fat, 4% calories from saturated fat, 44 g carbohydrate, 6 g dietary fiber, 19 mg sodium, 7 g protein
Exchanges: 1 Starch, 2 Fruit, 1 Fat

Eggs Ottawa

SERVING SIZE: 1/4 of recipe, SERVES: 4

1 tsp non-aromatic olive oil
4 jumbo mushroom caps
 (2 1/2-inch), stems removed
2 tsp lemon juice
1/2 tsp dill weed
1/8 tsp ground cayenne pepper
2 tsp light butter flavored margarine

1 1/2 cups egg substitute
2 English muffins, split and toasted
4 slices Canadian bacon (1 oz each)
8 slices low-fat mozzarella cheese
 (1 oz each)
1 Tbsp finely chopped green onions

1 Heat the oil in a chef's pan on medium high. Set the mushroom caps in the hot pan stem side up. Pour 1/2 tsp of the lemon juice in each one and season with dill weed and cayenne pepper. Cook 6 minutes or until the lemon juice starts to steam. Turn and cook 1 more minute. Remove to a warm plate and cover.

2 Wipe off the pan and melt the margarine on medium high. Pour in the egg substitute and let it start to cook on the bottom without stirring. Egg substitute needs to be handled gently. Slowly push the cooked part of the egg to the center of the pan with a flat-ended spatula. When it's ready, it will still be slightly runny on the top. Please don't over cook it!

3 Preheat the broiler. Place the toasted muffin halves on the rack on a broiler pan. Lay the Canadian bacon on the muffin. Cover each muffin with 1/4 of the cooked eggs, press down firmly to make an even mound. Set the cooked mushrooms, stem side down, on top of the eggs and push down so the egg goes up into the cavity. Top with 2 slices of overlapping mozzarella. Place under the broiler 1 1/2 minutes or until the cheese is melted and begins to brown. Sprinkle with green onions and serve.

Per serving: 292 calories, 8 g fat, 4 g saturated fat, 12% calories from saturated fat, 18 g carbohydrate, 0 g dietary fiber, 821 mg sodium, 37 g protein
Exchanges: 1 Starch, 4 Very Lean Meat, 1 Vegetable, 1 Fat

Kerr-Mush

SERVING SIZE: 1/2 recipe, SERVES: 2

<C   1 cup rolled oats
     1/4 cup dark raisins, unsweetened cranberries, and sour cherries mixed
  2 2/3 cups nonfat milk
     1/4 cup Graham's Seed and Nut Mix (see sidebar)
<C   2 tsp brown sugar

Graham's Seed and Nut Mix

Combine equal measures of sunflower seeds, unhulled sesame seeds, green pumpkin seeds, sliced almonds, walnuts, and pecan pieces, and a half measure of ground flax seeds. Make a big batch and keep it tightly covered in the refrigerator for handy use.

---

1 Simmer oats, raisins, and milk over low heat, covered until warmed through and plump.

2 Raise the heat to medium, and stir vigorously until it goes creamy-thick in texture, less than one minute.

3 Add seed and nut mix, and dust with brown sugar—not more than 1 tsp.

<C To Cut Carb

Oats: reduce to 2/3 cup.
Sugar: replace with Splenda.

Per serving: 448 calories, 13 g fat, 2 g saturated fat, 3% calories from saturated fat, 64 g carbohydrate, 7 g dietary fiber, 178 mg sodium
Exchanges: 2 Starch, 1 Fruit, 1 1/2 Fat-free Milk, 2 Fat

Low Carb

Per serving: 381 calories, 12 g fat, 2 g saturated fat, 3% calories from saturated fat, 51 g carbohydrate, 6 g fiber, 175 mg sodium
Exchanges: 1 Starch, 1 Fruit, 1 1/2 Fat-free Milk, 2 Fat

Breakfast Bonanza

SERVING SIZE: 1/2 of recipe, SERVES: 2

1/3 cup blueberries
1/3 cup cherries, halved
1/3 cup peach or nectarine slices

<C 1 cup low-fat, low-sugar cold cereal
1 cup 1% or skim milk

Combine the blueberries, cherries, and peaches and scatter over two bowls of cereal. Add milk and enjoy!

<C **To Cut Carb**

Cereal (preferably high fiber): reduce to 3/4 cup.

Per serving: 162 calories, 1 g fat, 0 g saturated fat, 0% calories from saturated fat, 35 g carbohydrate, 6 g dietary fiber, 281 mg sodium
Exchanges: 1 Starch, 1/2 Fruit, 1/2 Fat-Free Milk

Low Carb

Per serving: 143 calories, 1 g fat, 0 g saturated fat, 0% calories from saturated fat, 30 g carbohydrate, 5 g dietary fiber, 227 mg sodium
Exchanges: 1 Starch, 1/2 Fruit, 1/2 Fat-Free Milk

Appetizers

Broiled Shrimp with Chili Sauce Barra Vieja

SERVING SIZE: 1/6 of recipe, SERVES: 6

Chili Sauce

6 dried New Mexico chilis
3 ancho chilis
3 cloves garlic, peeled, bashed, and chopped
2/3 cup chopped onion
4 Italian plum tomatoes, such as Roma, quartered

1/2 tsp ground cumin
1/2 tsp dried marjoram
1/2 tsp dried oregano
1/8 tsp ground cloves
1/4 tsp salt
1 Tbsp white distilled vinegar
1 Tbsp molasses

Yogurt Mayonnaise

1/2 cup yogurt cheese (page 475)
1 Tbsp fresh lime juice

1 pinch of powdered saffron
1/4 tsp salt

Other Ingredients

24 cherry tomatoes
6 medium shrimp (about 2 ounces or 55 g each)
1 bunch watercress, thoroughly washed

Garnish

1 tsp mild chili powder
1 Tbsp chopped fresh cilantro

6 corn tortillas

Vegetarian Option

12 oz baby carrots (2 1/4 inch apiece)

Replace the shrimp with baby carrots (you could call them "garden prawns"), steamed for 6 to 8 minutes, or until tender but still crisp. Coat the carrots with 1/2 cup of the chili sauce and serve over watercress and tomatoes.

---

1 To prepare the New Mexico and ancho chilis, remove the stems and slice the chilis open lengthwise. Remove the seeds and pulp with the tip of a knife blade or a small spoon. Put the chilis in a saucepan with 1 cup of water and bring to a boil. Turn off the heat, cover, and let soak for 10 minutes.

2 While the chilis are soaking, make the yogurt mayonnaise. Whisk together the yogurt cheese, lime juice, saffron, and salt. Cover and set aside.

3 To finish the chili sauce, strain the soaked chilis, reserving the liquid. Transfer the chilis to a food processor or blender. Add the garlic, onion, tomatoes, cumin, marjoram, oregano, cloves, salt, vinegar, and molasses. Pulse, then blend until smooth, about 4 minutes. Transfer the sauce to a small saucepan. Rinse the processor bowl or blender jar with 1 cup of the pepper-soaking liquid and stir into the sauce. Bring to a boil over medium heat, then lower heat and simmer for 15 minutes.

4 Meanwhile, warm a medium frying pan over medium-high heat. Cook the cherry tomatoes until lightly browned on the outside. Transfer the tomatoes to a plate and gently mash with a fork. Remove most of the seeds.

5 Preheat the broiler.

6 Peel the shrimp, leaving the tail shell attached. Slit each shrimp lengthwise down the center, being careful not to cut all the way through. Remove the sand-filled vein and open the shrimp out flat, like a butterfly. Weave a toothpick through the thickest part of the meat, so that the two halves of the shrimp remain flat. Brush each shrimp generously on both sides with the chili sauce. Place the shrimp on a broiler pan and broil for 3 minutes on each side. Serve immediately.

7 To serve, divide the watercress among small salad plates. Arrange 3 crushed tomatoes and one shrimp on top of the watercress. Spoon a little chili sauce over each shrimp and top with a dollop of yogurt mayonnaise. Dust with mild chili powder and garnish with the chopped cilantro and hot tortillas.

Per serving: 172 calories, 2 g fat, 0 g saturated fat, 0% of calories from saturated fat, 23 g carbohydrate, 3 g dietary fiber
Exchanges: 1 Starch, 1 Very Lean Meat, 2 Vegetable

Vegetarian
Per serving: 135 calories, 1 g fat, 0 g saturated fat, 0% of calories from saturated fat, 27 g carbohydrate, 4 g dietary fiber
Exchanges: 1 Starch, 3 Vegetable

Pesto Bean Dip

SERVING SIZE: 1/2 cup, SERVES: 4

2 cups Great Northern beans (or other white beans), drained and rinsed
1 cup lightly packed fresh basil leaves
1/4 cup grated Parmesan cheese
1 tsp roasted garlic
2 Tbsp lemon juice
1/4 tsp salt
pinch pepper

1 Place the beans, basil, Parmesan cheese, garlic, lemon juice, salt, and pepper into a processor or blender and whiz until smooth. If you use a blender, you will have to add a little water to get it all moving.

2 Serve in a bowl surrounded with an assortment of raw vegetables. For an *hors d'oeuvre*, cut the tops off small cherry tomatoes and carefully clean out the pulp and seeds. Spoon the spread into a pastry bag with a plain tip and fill each tomato.

Per serving: 160 calories, 2 g fat, 1 g saturated fat, 6% calories from saturated fat, 24 g carbohydrate, 6 g dietary fiber, 239 mg sodium, 12 g protein
Exchanges: 1 1/2 Starch, 1 Very Lean Meat

Celery Peanut Butter Snacks

SERVING SIZE: 1 celery stalk, SERVES: 4

4 long celery stalks (or apples or 1 small jicama)
4 Tbsp peanut butter

1 Cut the celery on the diagonal in 3-inch long pieces. If you are using apples or jicama, cut in wedges.

2 Divide the peanut butter among the vegetable pieces, spread on them, and pack in a lunch or set on a plate to share around.

Per serving: 91 calories, 7 g fat, 1 g saturated fat, 10% calories from saturated fat, 4 g carbohydrate, 2 g dietary fiber, 36 mg sodium
Exchanges: 1 High Fat Meat

Low-Fat Ranch Dip

SERVING SIZE: 1/2 cup, SERVES: 4

1 (15 oz) can Great Northern beans, rinsed and drained
1/4 cup water
1/2 cup plain low-fat yogurt
1/2 tsp garlic powder or
    1 Tbsp roasted garlic

Pinch cayenne pepper
1/4 tsp pepper
1 Tbsp chopped fresh chives
1 Tbsp chopped fresh parsley
1/4 tsp dried tarragon

1 Blend beans and water for 2 minutes, or until silky smooth. Scrape into a medium bowl.

2 Stir in yogurt, cayenne, chives, parsley, and tarragon. Serve in a bowl surrounded by spring vegetables, such as sugar snap peas, tiny radishes, baby carrots, and lightly steamed baby new potatoes.

Per serving: 40 calories, 1 g fat, 0 g saturated fat, 0% calories from saturated fat, 8 g carbohydrate, 2 g dietary fiber, 176 mg sodium
Exchanges: 1/2 Starch

Roasted Chickpea Snacks

Servings size: 1/4 of recipe, SERVES: 4

2 tsp olive oil
  pinch turmeric
  pinch cayenne
1 Tbsp lime juice

1/2 tsp ground cumin
1/4 tsp salt
1 (15 oz) can garbanzo beans (chickpeas), rinsed and drained

1 Preheat the oven to 350°F. Combine the olive oil, turmeric, cayenne, lime juice, cumin, and salt in a bowl. Add the garbanzo beans and toss to coat.

2 Spread in a single layer on a baking sheet and bake 15 minutes in the pre-heated oven. Cool and serve.

Per serving: 148 calories, 4 g fat, 0 g saturated fat, 0% calories from saturated fat, 24 g carbohydrate, 5 g dietary fiber, 456 mg sodium, 4 g protein
Exchanges: 1 1/2 Starch, 1/2 Fat

East Indian Lentil Spread

SERVING SIZE: 1/4 of recipe, SERVES: 4

1/2 cup red or brown lentils
1/4 cup low-fat yogurt
  1 tsp non-aromatic olive oil
  1 cup chopped onions
  2 cloves garlic, peeled, bashed, and chopped

  1 Tbsp curry powder
1/4 cup currants or chopped dates
  1 Tbsp Mango Chutney (page 472)
  2 Tbsp chopped pistachio nuts

1 Cook the lentils in 2 cups of water for 30 minutes. Drain, saving any cooking liquid, and place in a blender jar. Add the yogurt and whiz in a blender until smooth. You may need some of the cooking liquid to keep the mixture moving in the jar.

2 Heat the oil in a frying pan big enough for the pureed lentils. Sauté the onions in the hot pan for 2 minutes. Add the garlic and curry powder and continue cooking until the onions are soft. Stir in the lentils, currants, and chutney and heat through. Serve in a bowl with the nuts scattered on top. Try this with toasted pita wedges or as a sandwich spread.

Per serving: 186 calories, 4 g fat, 1 g saturated fat, 5% calories from saturated fat, 30 g carbohydrate, 10 g dietary fiber, 9 g protein, 59 mg sodium
Exchanges: 1 Starch, 1 Very Lean Meat, 1 Fruit, 1/2 Fat

Texas Caviar

SERVING SIZE: 1/4 of recipe, SERVES: 4

  1 (15 oz) can black eye peas, drained and rinsed
1/2 cup chopped green onion, green and white parts
1/2 cup chopped red bell pepper
  1 clove garlic, bashed and chopped
  1 jalapeño pepper, chopped (with the seeds if you like it hot)
1/4 tsp salt
1/2 cup fat free Italian dressing

1 Combine the black eye peas, green onion, bell pepper, garlic, jalapeno pepper, salt, and dressing. Let sit for a few hours or overnight to let the flavors mellow. Serve with baked tortilla chips.

> Please notice how the tortilla chips take this great classic and push it over the top. Just 1 oz of tortilla chips nearly doubles the carbs per serving!!

Per serving: 114 calories, 0 g fat, 0 g saturated fat, 0% calories from saturated fat, 22 g carbohydrate, 6 g dietary fiber, 575 mg sodium
Exchanges: 1 1/2 Starch
Per serving (with 1 oz unsalted tortilla chips): 260 calories, 8 g fat, 1 g saturated fat, 4% calories from saturated fat, 39 g carbohydrate, 7 g dietary fiber, 643 mg sodium
Exchanges: 2 1/2 Starch, 1 1/2 Fat

Coleslaw with Color

SERVING SIZE: 1/2 cup, SERVES: 8

2 cups shredded cabbage
1 cup shredded purple cabbage
1 cup shredded carrots
2 Tbsp apple cider vinegar
2 Tbsp honey

1/4 cup nonfat cream cheese
1/2 tsp horseradish
1/4 tsp salt
1/4 tsp pepper

1 Toss cabbage, purple cabbage, and carrots together in a bowl.

2 Combine vinegar, honey, cream cheese, horseradish, salt, and pepper, mixing well.

3 Pour over salad and toss again.

Per serving: 36 calories, 0 g fat, 0 g saturated fat, 0% calories from saturated fat, 8 g carbohydrate, 1 g dietary fiber, 125 mg sodium
Exchanges: 1/2 Carbohydrate

Garlic Toast with Avocado Yogurt Cheese Spread

SERVING SIZE: 1 slice, SERVES: 6

6 slices (1/2-inch thick) of French
  baguette
1 whole clove garlic, peeled
  (optional)
1 ripe avocado

1/4 cup yogurt cheese
  (see page 475)
1/8 tsp salt
  1 tsp fresh lemon or lime juice

1 Preheat the broiler. Place the bread slices on a broiler pan and toast until lightly browned on both sides. Remove from the oven and rub one side of each slice with the garlic.

2 Peel and pit the avocado. Mash with a fork until it has the consistency of chunky guacamole. Stir in the yogurt cheese, salt, and lemon juice. If you will not be serving this immediately, lay a piece of plastic wrap directly on the surface of the spread so it won't darken, then cover with an airtight lid and refrigerate until needed.

3 To serve, spread the avocado mixture thickly on the garlic toast.

Per serving: 126 calories, 4 g fat, 1 g saturated fat, 4% calories from saturated fat, 19 g carbohydrate, 2 g dietary fiber, 257 mg sodium
Exchanges: 1 Starch, 1 Fat

Vegetable Bean Quesadillas

SERVING SIZE: 1/4 of recipe, SERVES: 4

4 large flour tortillas
1 lb can low-fat refried beans
1/2 tsp olive oil
1/2 cup chopped sweet onion
2 cloves garlic
1 cup canned or frozen corn kernels
1 cup chopped red bell pepper

1 jalapeño pepper, chopped with
  seeds if you like it hot
1/2 tsp ground cumin
1 cup grated reduced-fat
  Monterey jack cheese
1 cup low-sodium canned
  or homemade salsa

1 Lay 4 tortillas on the counter and spread with the refried beans.

2 Heat the oil in a skillet and sauté the onions 2 minutes without browning. Add the garlic, corn, red pepper, jalapeño, and cumin over medium heat until the vegetables are tender, up to 5 minutes.

3 Divide the vegetables among the tortillas and cover lightly with the cheese. Fold over and press down.

4 These can be heated several different ways. Lay on a baking sheet, cover lightly with foil, and heat 15 minutes in a 350°F oven, one at a time on top of the stove in a heavy bottom skillet (2 or 3 minutes per side), or 2 or 3 minutes in a microwave.

5 Cut in wedges and serve with the salsa.

Per serving: 352 calories, 9 g fat, 2 g saturated fat, 5% calories from saturated fat, 54 g carbohydrate, 7 g dietary fiber, 359 mg sodium
Exchanges: 1 1/2 Starch, 1 Very Lean Meat, 1 Vegetable

The Comfort of Tomatoes and Toast

SERVING SIZE: 1/4 of recipe, SERVES: 4

4 medium-sized tomatoes	2 Tbsp Parmesan cheese
1/2 tsp salt	4 slices dry toasted whole-wheat bread
1/2 tsp pepper	

1 Preheat broiler. Slice tomatoes in half and place on tray. Season with salt and pepper and broil 4 inches away from the heat for about 5 minutes. Serve on top of toast slices. Sprinkle with Parmesan cheese.

Per serving: 113 calories, 3 g fat, 1 g saturated fat, 7% calories from saturated fat, 20 g carbohydrate, 4 g dietary fiber, 474 mg sodium, 5 g protein
Exchanges: 1 Starch, 1 Vegetable, 1/2 Fat

Party Stuffed Mushrooms

SERVING SIZE: 3 mushrooms, SERVES: 4

12 large mushrooms
1/2 tsp olive oil
1 cup finely chopped onion
1 clove garlic, chopped
2 cups chopped fresh spinach or
   1 (10 oz) package frozen, thawed
   with water squeezed out

1 Tbsp chopped walnuts
2 Tbsp grated Parmesan cheese
1/2 cup unseasoned breadcrumbs
1/4 tsp salt
1/4 tsp pepper
   pinch of nutmeg
2 Tbsp finely chopped parsley

1 Clean the mushrooms with a dry cloth and remove the stems. Chop the stems finely and set aside with the whole mushroom caps.

2 Heat the oil in the large heavy skillet. Sauté the onions until very soft, about 10 to 15 minutes. Add the garlic and cook another minute. Stir in the spinach, nuts, Parmesan, breadcrumbs, salt, pepper, and nutmeg. Cook until the spinach wilts or in the case of the frozen spinach, heats through.

3 Coat the mushrooms lightly with pan spray. Stuff with the filling and bake at 350°F 15 minutes or until the mushrooms are soft and the tops light brown. Scatter parsley over the top and serve.

Per serving: 114 calories, 4 g fat, 1 g saturated fat, 8% calories from saturated fat, 16 g carbohydrate, 3 g dietary fiber, 317 mg sodium, 4 g protein
Exchanges: 1/2 Starch, 2 Vegetable, 1/2 Fat

Graham's Trail Mix

SERVING SIZE: 1 cup + 1 Tbsp, SERVES: 4

1/2 cup dried cranberries (unsweetened)
1/2 cup dried sour cherries
1/2 cup grape nuts

1/2 cup Cheerios
1/4 cup roasted almonds,
   roughly chopped

1 Combine and divide among 4 zip-top plastic bags.

Per serving: 204 calories, 4 g fat, 0 g saturated fat, 0% calories from saturated fat, 40 g carbohydrate, 4 g dietary fiber, 125 mg sodium
Exchanges: 1 Starch, 1 1/2 Fruit, 1 Fat

Garlic Herb Dip

SERVING SIZE: 1/8 of recipe, SERVES: 8

1 head garlic
1 cup yogurt cheese (see page 475)
1 Tbsp chopped parsley
1 Tbsp chopped chives
1/4 tsp coarsely ground black pepper
1/4 tsp salt

1 Preheat the oven to 375°F. Slice about 1/2-inch off the top of the garlic, wrap in aluminum foil, and bake for 1 hour or until very soft. When it is cool enough to handle, squeeze the roasted garlic from the skin. You should have a generous Tbsp.

2 Combine the yogurt cheese, roasted garlic, parsley, chives, pepper, and salt. Serve with raw vegetables or as a dressing for a baked potato.

Per serving: 33 calories, 1 g fat, 0 g saturated fat, 0% calories from saturated fat, 4 g carbohydrate, 0 g dietary fiber, 107 mg sodium
Exchanges: 1/2 Carbohydrate

Celery Slaw

SERVING SIZE: 1/4 of recipe, SERVES: 4

4 cups chopped celery
1 cup grated carrot
1/2 chopped sweet onion
1/2 cup chopped red bell pepper
1/2 cup raisins
1/4 cup mayonnaise
1/4 cup plain, nonfat yogurt
2 Tbsp cider vinegar
1 Tbsp Dijon mustard

1 Toss the celery, carrots, onions, red pepper, and raisins together in a large bowl.

2 Combine the mayonnaise, yogurt, vinegar, and mustard in a small bowl. Whisk until smooth. Pour the dressing on the vegetables, and toss to mix well.

Per serving: 209 calories, 12 g fat, 2 g saturated fat, 9% calories from saturated fat, 26 g carbohydrate, 4 g dietary fiber, 229 mg sodium
Exchanges: 2 Vegetable, 1 Fruit, 1 1/2 Fat

Matzo Dumplings

SERVING SIZE: 2 dumplings, SERVES: 4

1/2 cup matzo meal
1/4 tsp salt
1/2 tsp baking powder

1/2 cup egg substitute
1 tsp non-aromatic olive oil

1 Combine the matzo meal, salt, baking powder, egg substitute, and oil. Refrigerate 30 minutes. Form 8 dumplings using 2 dessert spoons and drop into a pan of boiling soup or stew. Reduce the heat to medium and boil gently for 15 minutes.

Per serving: 90 calories, 1 g fat, 0 g saturated fat, 1% calories from saturated fat, 15 g carbohydrate, 1 g dietary fiber, 256 mg sodium, 5 g protein
Exchanges: 1 Starch

Watercress Dipped in Vinaigrette Rolled in a Tortilla

SERVING SIZE: 1 wrap, SERVES: 4

Treena's Vinaigrette

1 clove garlic, bashed and chopped
2 Tbsp non-aromatic olive oil
1/4 cup rice vinegar

1/2 tsp dry mustard
1 tsp brown sugar
pinch cayenne pepper (optional)

Wrap

4 corn tortillas   1 bunch watercress

1 Whiz the garlic, oil, vinegar, mustard, brown sugar, and cayenne pepper in a blender until slightly thickened.

2 Wrap the tortillas in waxed paper and heat in the microwave on high 2 minutes or wrap in foil and heat at 350°F in a conventional oven for 10 minutes.

3 Wash the watercress in cold water and spin dry. Choose 2 or 3 stems per serving, dip into the vinaigrette and lay on each of the tortillas. Roll and serve alongside soup or salads. The remaining watercress will be great as part of a green salad and can be dressed with the remaining vinaigrette dressing.

Per serving: 81 calories, 2 g fat, 0 g saturated fat, 0% calories from saturated fat, 17 g carbohydrate, 1 g dietary fiber, 174 mg sodium
Exchanges: 1 Starch

Jicama and Salsa Snack

SERVING SIZE: 1/4 of recipe, SERVES: 4

2 cups jicama slices
1 Tbsp lime juice

1 cup low-sodium salsa

1 Toss the jicama slices with the lime juice. Serve on a plate alongside the salsa.

Per serving: 35 calories, 0 g fat, 0 g saturated fat, 0% calories from saturated fat, 8 g carbohydrate, 4 g dietary fiber, 142 mg sodium
Exchanges: 1 Vegetable

Tangy Bean Dip

SERVING SIZE: 1/8 of recipe, SERVES: 8

1 (15 oz) can reduced-sodium white beans
1/2 cup low-fat salad dressing

2 Tbsp chopped parsley, chives, or cilantro

1 Drain and rinse the beans and tip into your blender or processor. Pour in the salad dressing and whiz until smooth. Stir in chopped parsley. Serve as a dip with raw vegetables of your choice.

Per serving: 92 calories, 3 g fat, 0 g saturated fat, 0% calories from saturated fat, 13 g carbohydrate, 2 g dietary fiber, 150 mg sodium
Exchanges: 1 Starch, 1/2 Fat

Green Pea Dip

SERVING SIZE: 1/4 of recipe, SERVES: 4

2 cups frozen peas
2 Tbsp lemon or lime juice
1 tsp mild chili powder
1/8 tsp cayenne pepper (optional)

1 Tbsp minced onion
1 clove garlic, bashed and chopped
1/3 cup prepared salsa

1 Cook the peas in a little water until tender, about 4 minutes. Pour into a processor. Add the lemon juice, chili powder, and cayenne and pulse until almost smooth. Put into a bowl big enough to mix in the rest of the ingredients.

2 Stir in the onion, garlic, and salsa. Serve with baked tortilla or pita chips.

Per serving: 72 calories, 0 g fat, 0 g saturated fat, 0% calories from saturated fat, 14 g carbohydrate, 5 g. dietary fiber, 122 mg sodium, 4 g protein
Exchanges: 1 Starch

Bean Dip with a Kick

SERVING SIZE: 1/4 of recipe, SERVES: 4

1 (15 oz) can low-sodium Great Northern beans, rinsed and drained
1/4 cup low-fat salad dressing, any variety
1/4 tsp hot pepper flakes, or to taste
1 Tbsp chopped parsley
1 lb carrots, cut into sticks, or ready-peeled small carrots, or other cut-up veggies

1 In a blender, combine beans with salad dressing until smooth and creamy. Add hot peppers and serve as a dip alongside carrots or other cut-up vegetables.

Per serving: 176 calories, 7 g fiber, 2 g fat, 0 g sat fat, 0% sat fat, 0 mg cholesterol, 172 mg sodium, 33 g carbohydrate, 8 g protein.
Exchanges: 1 1/2 Starch, 2 Vegetable

Roasted Garlic in Yogurt Cheese

SERVING: 1/4 cup, SERVES: 4

1 cup low-fat yogurt cheese (page 475)
1 head garlic

1/4 tsp salt
1/4 tsp pepper

1 Preheat the oven to 350°F. Cut the stem end off the garlic head exposing the tops of the individual cloves. Wrap it in foil and bake 45 minutes to 1 hour in the preheated oven. It should be very soft when done. Cool, lay on the counter, and squeeze out the soft roasted garlic.

2 Combine the garlic with the yogurt cheese, salt, and pepper. Serve as a dip or potato topping.

Per serving: 95 calories, 2 g fat, 1 g saturated fat, 9% calories from saturated fat, 13 g carbohydrate, 0 g dietary fiber, 226 mg sodium, 6 g protein
Exchanges: 1 Fat-Free Milk

Hummus

SERVING SIZE: 1/4 of recipe, SERVES: 4

1 (15 1/2 oz) can reduced-sodium garbanzo beans, drained and rinsed
1 Tbsp tahini
2 Tbsp lemon juice
2 cloves chopped garlic

1/4 tsp salt
1/4–1/2 cup water
   (no more than 1/2 cup)
   pinch cayenne pepper
1/4 cup chopped parsley

1 Place beans in a processor or blender. Add tahini, lemon juice, garlic, salt, and cayenne. Blend until smooth.

2 Scrape into a bowl, and stir in parsley. Serve with fresh cut up vegetables or as a sandwich spread.

Per serving: 123 calories, 4 g fat, 0 g saturated fat, 0% calories from saturated fat, 17 g carbohydrate, 5 g dietary fiber, 261mg sodium
Exchanges: 1 Starch, 1 Fat

Classic Apples and Cheese

SERVING SIZE: 1/4 of recipe, SERVES: 4

1 apple (try a variety you've never tried before)
1 pear (look for a new variety)

4 oz low-fat cheese, cut in chunks

1 Cut the apple in quarters and core. Cut the pear in quarters and core. Arrange 2 apple quarters and 2 pear quarters on each of 4 dessert plates.

2 Divide the cheese chunks and scatter around the fruit. Serve for dessert or a snack.

Per serving: 111 calories, 3 g fat, 1 g saturated fat, 8 % calories from saturated fat, 12 g carbohydrate, 2 g dietary fiber, 50 mg sodium
Exchanges: 1 Lean Meat, 1 Fruit

Black Bean Nachos

SERVING SIZE: 1/4 of recipe, SERVES: 4

<C 2 large low-fat flour tortillas
<C 1 (15 oz) can reduced sodium black beans, rinsed and drained
    1 cup canned no-salt tomatoes
<C 1 cup frozen corn kernels
    1/2 cup sliced green onions (scallions)

    chopped garlic cloves
    2 jalapeño chilis, seeded and chopped
    1/4 teaspoon ground cumin
    1/2 cup low-fat, low-sodium Monterey jack cheese
    1/4 cup chopped cilantro

1 Preheat the oven to 375°F. Lightly coat the tortillas with pan spray and bake until crisp, about 10 minutes. Set aside.

2 While tortillas are baking, combine the beans, tomatoes, corn, green onions, garlic, green chilis, and cumin in a saucepan. Bring to a boil, reduce the heat, and simmer 5 minutes.

3 Divide the beans between the tortillas, top with cheese, and bake 5 minutes or until heated through. Scatter the cilantro over the nachos, cut in wedges, and eat.

<C **To Cut Carb**

<C Tortillas: reduce to one only.   <C Black Beans: reduce to 1/2 can
<C Corn Niblets: reduce to 1/2 cup.   (drained).

Per serving: 263 calories, 3 g fat, 2 g saturated fat, 7% calories from saturated fat, 48 g carbohydrate, 365 mg sodium, 7 g dietary fiber
Exchanges: 3 Starch, 1 Vegetable

Low Carb
Per serving: 166 calories, 3 g fat, 2 g saturated fat, 11% calories from saturated fat, 27 g carbohydrate, 246 mg sodium, 4 g dietary fiber
Exchanges: 1 1/2 Starch, 1 Vegetable, 1/2 Fat

Raw Vegetable Canapés

SERVING SIZE: 1/4 of recipe, SERVES: 4

24 slices fresh vegetable
    (such as cucumber, carrot, jicama, and/or summer squash)
1/2 cup low-fat bean dip (see page 138)
1/4 lb shrimp, roasted red pepper, tomato, or marinated artichoke heart quarters
24 small colorful strips or pieces of vegetables (such as corn kernels), olives, herbs, or edible flowers

1 A nice way to slice cucumber, carrot, jicama, or squash is in long diagonal pieces. This gives you ovals that look pretty on a plate. You can also cut jicama and carrots in fancy shapes with cookie or canapé cutters. The kids will love that!

2 Spread (or pipe from a pastry bag) the bean dip or light cream cheese on each vegetable slice. Lay a piece of shrimp, roasted red pepper, or artichoke heart on each one. Top with a bit of colorful vegetable, olive, herb, or flower.

3 Arrange the canapés on a plate and decorate with sprigs of herbs or edible flowers.

Per serving: 100 calories, 0 g fat, 0 g saturated fat, 0% calories from saturated fat, 16 g carbohydrate, 6 g dietary fiber, 267 mg sodium
Exchanges: 1/2 Starch, 2 Vegetable

Graham's Seed Mix

SERVING SIZE: 1 Tbsp, SERVINGS: 70

1/4 cup raw cashews
1/4 cup almonds
1/4 cup hazelnuts

1/4 cup sunflower seeds
1/4 cup pumpkin seeds
2 Tbsp flax seed

Combine all ingredients and store in an airtight jar in the refrigerator.

Per serving: 49 calories, 4 g fat, 1 g saturated fat, 1% calories from saturated fat, 2 g carbohydrate, 1 g dietary fiber, 2 mg sodium
Exchanges: 1 Fat

Refried Bean Dip

SERVING SIZE: 1/6 of recipe, SERVES: 6

1 cup vegetarian refried beans
1/2 cup salsa

1 Tbsp chopped cilantro

Combine the refried beans and salsa. Put in an attractive bowl and scatter cilantro over the top. Serve with raw vegetables or oven baked tortilla chips. It's especially nice with sticks of jicama.

Per serving (with jicama): 94 calories, 1 g fat, 0 g saturated fat, 0% calories from saturated fat, 18 g carbohydrate, 7 g dietary fiber, 506 mg sodium
Exchanges: 1 Starch

Soups, Salads, and Breads

Waldorf Salad

SERVING SIZE: 1/4 of recipe, SERVES: 4

     2 red-skinned crisp apples (such as Jonagold or Red Delicious), 3 cups
     2 Tbsp lemon juice
     2 ribs celery, diced (1/2 cup)
     2 Tbsp toasted, chopped walnuts
  1/4 cup low-fat mayonnaise dressing
     4 cups romaine lettuce, washed and torn into bite-size pieces
  1/4 cup raisins

1 Wash and cut the apples into quarters, core, and then dice into 3/4-inch pieces. Toss with the lemon juice. Add the celery, walnuts, and mayonnaise dressing. Mix thoroughly.

2 Place the lettuce on 4 plates or in salad bowls. Scoop the apple mixture onto each salad. Scatter raisins over the top.

Per serving: 129 calories, 4 g fat, 0 g saturated fat, 0% calories from saturated fat, 25 g carbohydrate, 4 g dietary fiber, 163 mg sodium
Exchanges: 1 Vegetable, 1 1/2 Fruit, 1/2 Fat

Warm Brussels Sprouts Salad

SERVING SIZE: 1/4 of recipe, SERVES: 4

     1 (10 oz) package frozen Brussels sprouts, or 1 lb fresh
     1 tsp extra-virgin olive oil
  1/2 tsp dried thyme
  1/4 tsp caraway seed (optional)
     2 Tbsp balsamic vinegar
  1/4 tsp salt
  1/4 tsp pepper

1 Put the Brussels sprouts in half and steam until tender, about 5 minutes.

2 Warm the oil in a skillet on medium heat. Add the thyme, caraway, and vinegar. Drop in the cooked Brussels sprouts, season with salt and pepper, and toss. Serve immediately while they are still bright green.

Per serving: 61 calories, 2 g fat, 0 g saturated fat, 0% calories from saturated fat, 10 g carbohydrate, 2 g dietary fiber, 169 mg sodium
Exchanges: 2 Vegetable, 1/2 Fat

Matzo Ball Soup with Vegetables

SERVING SIZE: 1 cup, SERVES: 6

Matzo Balls:

3 Tbsp vegetable oil
1 cup egg substitute
1 cup unsalted matzo meal
1 tsp salt
1/2 cup minced fresh dill
1/4 cup water
2 cups finely diced carrot

1 cup finely diced celery
1/2 cup finely diced fennel (optional: to simplify, you could replace fennel with more celery)
2 (32 oz) boxes low-sodium chicken broth, or
8 cups no-salt-added homemade chicken broth
1/4 cup minced scallion
1/2 tsp black pepper

1 Whisk together oil and egg substitute with a fork or small whisk. Add matzo meal, salt, dill, and water and mix until a sticky dough forms. Cover and place in refrigerator for 10 to 15 minutes to stiffen.

2 Bring 3 quarts of water to a boil in a large pot. Meanwhile, remove matzo mixture from refrigerator and form into small balls, about an inch in diameter. Wet hands to prevent sticking. Drop balls into boiling water. Reduce heat to medium and cover. Boil matzo balls gently for 30 to 40 minutes, until cooked throughout (cut one open to check).

3 Wash each of the vegetables. In a medium pot, place carrots, celery, and fennel, and add broth. Bring to a boil, lower heat, and gently boil until vegetables are soft, about 15 minutes. Stir in scallions, black pepper, and cooked matzo balls and serve.

Per serving: 171 calories, 5 g fat, 1.7 g saturated fat, 9% calories from saturated fat, 21 g carbohydrate, 2 g dietary fiber, 422 mg sodium, 8 g protein, 0 mg cholesterol
Exchanges: 1 Starch, 2 Vegetable, 1 Fat

Refreshing Carrot Salad

SERVING SIZE: 1/4 of recipe, SERVES: 4

    1 1/4 lb carrots, peeled and coarsely grated   1 Tbsp chopped fresh mint
       1 orange, peeled and chopped   juice and zest of 1 lime
<C   1/2 cup raisins

> Combine the carrots, oranges, raisins, mint, lime juice, and zest. Chill for an hour or 2 to let the flavors mingle.

<C **To Cut Carb**
<C Raisins: reduce to 1/4 cup.

Per serving: 127 calories, 0 g fat, 0 g saturated fat, 0% calories from saturated fat, 32 g carbohydrate, 6 g dietary fiber, 47 mg sodium
Exchanges: 2 Vegetable, 1 1/2 Fruit

Low Carb
Per serving: 100 calories, 0 g fat, 0 g saturated fat, 0% calories from saturated fat, 25 g carbohydrate, 5 g dietary fiber, 46 mg sodium
Exchanges: 2 Vegetable, 1 Fruit

Rainbow Salad

SERVING SIZE: 1/2 cup, SERVES: 20

2 cups shredded purple (or red) cabbage
2 cups thawed petit peas
2 cups grated carrots
2 cups corn kernels

2 cups seeded and chopped Roma tomatoes
1/2 cup sliced olives
1 cup low-fat salad dressing of your choice

> Layer the cabbage, peas, carrots, corn, and tomatoes in a straight-sided glass bowl. Scatter the olives over the top and pour in the dressing. If you would like a bigger salad, just add equal amounts to each of the vegetables. If there is a vegetable in there you don't like, substitute another or just skip it—it's your rainbow!

Per serving: 60 calories, 2 g fat, 0 g saturated fat, 0% calories from saturated fat, 10 g carbohydrate, 2 g dietary fiber, 173 mg sodium
Exchanges: 1/2 Starch, 1 Vegetable

Romaine Salad

SERVING SIZE: 1/4 of recipe, SERVES: 4

1 head romaine lettuce	1/4 tsp pepper
1 cup orange segments	1 Tbsp olive oil
1/4 cup chopped green onions	1 Tbsp rice vinegar
1/4 tsp salt	

1 Remove and discard the battered outside leaves of the romaine. Pull off the leaves and wash carefully. Dry in a salad spinner or colander and cut into bite size pieces. You will need about 4 cups for this salad. The rest can be put in the refrigerator for another salad tomorrow.

2 Place the lettuce in a large bowl with the orange segments, green onions, salt, pepper, oil, and vinegar. Toss well and serve.

Per serving: 65 calories, 4 g fat, 0 g saturated fat, 0% calories from saturated fat, 8 g carbohydrate, 3 g dietary fiber, 148 mg sodium
Exchanges: 1/2 Fruit, 1 Fat

Manhattan Clam Chowder

SERVING SIZE: 1/6 of recipe, SERVES: 6

   1 tsp non-aromatic olive oil
2 oz Canadian bacon, cut in 1/4-inch cubes
   1 large sweet onion, chopped (2 cups)
   4 carrots, peeled and chopped (1 1/2 cups)
   2 ribs celery, chopped (3/4 cup)
   3 cups Yellow Finn or Yukon Gold potatoes, peeled and cut in 3/4-inch cubes
   2 (10 oz) cans small whole clams, drained, juice reserved
   1 (8 oz) bottle clam juice
1/4 tsp freshly ground black pepper
1/2 tsp dried thyme
   1 bay leaf
   2 lb Roma tomatoes, peeled, seeded, and cut in 3/4-inch cubes
   2 Tbsp chopped parsley

1 Heat the oil in a Dutch oven on medium high. Drop in the bacon to fry 1 minute then the onions to cook 2 or 3 minutes more. Add the carrots, celery, and potatoes, stir and sauté 3 minutes. Pour in the reserved clam nectar and clam juice. Season with the pepper, thyme, and bay leaf. Bring to a boil then simmer 10 minutes or until the potatoes and carrots are tender.

2 Stir in the tomatoes and parsley and bring to a boil again. Cook 2 to 3 minutes to let the tomatoes cook down a little. Add the clams and serve. The chowder will be thick and stew like.

Per serving: 192 calories, 3 g fat, 1 g saturated fat, 5% calories from saturated fat, 31 g carbohydrate, 5 g dietary fiber, 706 mg sodium, 10 g protein
Exchanges: 1 Starch, 1 Very Lean Meat, 3 Vegetable

Plum and Red Cabbage Salad

SERVING SIZE: 1/8 of recipe, SERVES: 8

Salad

```
  1  small head red cabbage, shredded (4 cups)
  8  yellow, purple, or green sweet plums, pitted and sliced
1/4  cup chopped parsley
```

Dressing

```
1 Tbsp non-aromatic olive oil          1/4  tsp salt
3 Tbsp balsamic or rice vinegar        1/4  tsp pepper
```

1 Combine the shredded cabbage, plums, and parsley. Whisk the oil, vinegar, salt, and pepper together and toss with the prepared vegetables.

Per serving: 49 calories, 2 g fat, 0 g saturated fat, 0% calories from saturated fat, 9 g carbohydrate, 1 g dietary fiber, 78 mg sodium
Exchanges: 1/2 Fruit, 1/2 Fat

Chinese Mustard Green Soup

SERVING SIZE: 1/4 recipe, SERVES: 4

4 cups low-sodium chicken stock
(page 463)
1 Tbsp grated ginger root
2 cups sliced mushrooms
4 cups sliced mustard greens or
1 package frozen

1 Tbsp light soy sauce
1/4 tsp salt
1/2 tsp toasted sesame oil
2 cups cooked long-grain
white rice, hot

1 Bring stock and ginger to a boil in a large saucepan. Add mushrooms and greens, and cook 3 minutes.

2 Stir in soy sauce, salt, and sesame oil. Place 1/2 cup rice in each of 4 bowls. Ladle soup over the top and enjoy!

Per serving: 137 calories, 1 g fat, 0 g saturated fat, 0% calories from saturated fat, 25 g carbohydrate, 2 g dietary fiber, 342 mg sodium
Exchanges: 1 1/2 Starch, 1 Vegetable

Italian Bread with Olives and Rosemary

SERVING SLICE: 1 wedge, SERVES: 12

1 cup warm water
1 tsp dry yeast
1/4 tsp salt
1/2 tsp dried oregano
1/2 tsp dried basil

1 1/2 tsp dried rosemary
2 to 2 3/4 cups all purpose flour
1/2 cup chopped Italian black olives
1 tsp olive oil
1/4 tsp kosher or ground sea salt

1 Sprinkle the yeast over the warm water in a large bowl and let set until creamy, about 10 minutes. Stir in the salt, oregano, basil, and 1 tsp of the rosemary. Add 2 cups of the flour and mix thoroughly, adding more flour until you have a nice medium-firm dough. Turn out onto a floured surface and knead until the dough is smooth and springy, at least 5 minutes. Place the dough in an oiled bowl, cover, and allow to rise until doubled in size, 1 1/2 to 2 hours.

2 Preheat the oven to 425°F. Pat the dough into a large rectangle, scatter on the olives, and fold over the sides. Knead into the dough making sure they are well dispersed. Spray a skillet or pie pan with pan spray. Pat the dough out to fit the pan, cover, and let rise for 30 minutes.

3 Make deep dimples into the slightly risen dough with your fingertips. Drizzle the oil over the top and scatter on a pinch of kosher salt. Bake in the preheated oven for 30 minutes or until golden brown. Cool on a rack for 10 minutes before cutting into wedges.

Per serving: 104 calories, 2 g fat, 0 g saturated fat, 0% calories from saturated fat, 20 g carbohydrate, 1 g dietary fiber, 138 mg sodium
Exchanges: 1 1/2 Starch

Jeweled Watermelon Soup

SERVING SIZE: 1/4 of recipe, SERVES: 4

1 pink grapefruit
1 pomegranate
6 cups 1-inch cubes watermelon, seeded

Juice of 1 lime
2 tsp confectioners' sugar

1 Peel grapefruit. Slice horizontally into thin, attractive slices. Discard (or eat) end pieces. Set aside. Seed pomegranate and discard peel and membrane. Set aside.

2 Place watermelon, lime juice and sugar in a blender or food processor and puree until very smooth. Pour into shallow bowls and garnish with a grapefruit slice or two and a sprinkle of pomegranate seeds. Serve chilled.

Per serving: 129 calories, 1 g fat, 0 g saturated fat, 0% calories from saturated fat, 31 g carbohydrate, 2 g dietary fiber, 6 mg sodium, 2 g protein, 0 mg cholesterol
Exchanges: 2 Fruit

Asparagus Salad

SERVING SIZE: 1/4 of recipe, SERVES: 4

2 pounds fresh asparagus (3 cups)
1 tsp extra virgin olive oil
1 Tbsp red wine vinegar

1/4 tsp salt
1/4 tsp freshly ground black pepper
2 Tbsp chopped fresh dill

1 Wash and snap the ends off the asparagus. Steam over boiling water 3 to 5 minutes or until tender but still crisp. Plunge into cold water to stop the asparagus from further cooking. Drain and cut on the diagonal in 1-inch pieces. Place in a bowl.

2 Drizzle oil and vinegar and scatter salt, pepper, and herbs over the top. Toss gently and let sit for 1/2 hour. Serve at room temperature or chilled.

Per serving: 32 calories, 1 g fat, 0 g saturated fat, 0% calories from saturated fat, 4 g carbohydrate, 1 g dietary fiber, 150 mg sodium
Exchanges: 1 Vegetable

Greek Vegetable Salad

SERVING SIZE: 1/4 of recipe, SERVES: 4

Salad

1/2 cup red bell pepper strips
1 cup cucumber
1 cup seeded, chopped tomatoes

8 Greek olives, pitted and halved
2 Tbsp crumbled feta cheese

Dressing

1 Tbsp extra virgin olive oil
1 Tbsp vinegar
2 Tbsp tomato juice

1/2 tsp dried oregano
1/4 tsp freshly ground black pepper

1 Combine ingredients for salad and then drizzle with dressing.

Per serving: 89 calories, 7 g fat, 2 g saturated fat, 20% calories from saturated fat, 5 g carbohydrate, 1 g dietary fiber, 242 mg sodium
Exchanges: 1 Vegetable, 1 1/2 Fat

Summer Berry Salad

SERVING SIZE: 1/4 of recipe, SERVES: 4

1/3 cup apple juice
2 Tbsp lemon juice
1/4 tsp freshly ground black pepper
1 tsp cornstarch or arrowroot
1 cup blueberries

1 cup quartered strawberries
1 cup raspberries or blackberries
4 leaves butter lettuce
3 cups (1 bunch) watercress

1 Stir the apple juice, lemon juice, pepper, and cornstarch together in a small saucepan. Heat to thicken then refrigerate to chill.

2 Combine the blueberries, strawberries, and raspberries in a large bowl. Pour on the dressing and toss gently.

3 Divide the lettuce leaves among 4 salad plates, lay the watercress on the lettuce, and spoon the berries on top.

Per serving: 64 calories, 1 g fat, 0 g saturated fat, 0% calories from saturated fat, 15 g carbohydrate, 4 g dietary fiber, 12 mg sodium
Exchanges: 1 Fruit

Wilted Winter Salad

SERVING SIZE: 1/4 of recipe, SERVES: 4

1 bunch Swiss chard
1 tsp olive oil
1/2 cup roasted red peppers, cut in strips

1/2 cup water chestnuts, cut in quarters
2 Tbsp balsamic vinegar

1 Wash chard and remove stems. Chop the stems in 1/2-inch pieces. Cut the leaves in bite-size pieces. Heat the oil in a large pan on medium-high. Sauté the stems until crisp-tender, about 3 minutes. Add the leaves and cook until just wilted, 2 or 3 minutes.

2 Toss with the red peppers, water chestnuts, and balsamic vinegar. Serve warm.

Per serving: 54 calories, 1 g fat, 0 g saturated fat, 0% calories from saturated fat, 11 g carbohydrate, 2 g dietary fiber, 211 mg sodium
Exchanges: 2 Vegetable

Creamy Vegetable Soup

SERVING SIZE: 1/4 of recipe, SERVES: 4

1 large (1/2 lb) russet potato, peeled
  and cut in eighths
  (or 2 peeled and chopped parsnips)
1 small onion, peeled and sliced
3 cups low-sodium chicken or
  vegetable broth (pages 463, 473)

3/4 cup chopped carrots
3/4 cup chopped mushrooms
3/4 cup frozen peas, thawed
  2 Tbsp chopped parsley
1/4 tsp salt
1/4 tsp pepper

1 Preheat oven to 400°F. Roast potatoes and onions 30 minutes or until tender. Blend with enough broth to cover. Pour pureed vegetables and remaining broth into a large saucepan, and bring to a boil.

2 Add carrots and cook 15 minutes or until tender. Stir in mushrooms, peas, and parsley, and heat through. Season with salt and pepper, and serve. A wonderful lunch with a slice of crusty bread and a salad.

Per serving: 134 calories, 2 g fat, 1 g saturated fat, 7% calories from saturated fat, 24 g carbohydrate, 4 g dietary fiber, 307 mg sodium
Exchanges: 1 Starch, 2 Vegetable

Bulgur Nut Salad

SERVING SIZE: 1/4 of recipe, SERVES: 4

<C 1 cup dry bulgur wheat
    2 cups boiling water
    1 tsp olive oil
<C 1 1/2 cups chopped sweet onion
    1/2 cup tomato puree
    1 Tbsp dried mint or
      1 tsp fresh

1 tsp ground cumin
1/2 tsp ground allspice
1/4 cup chopped toasted walnuts
1/4 cup lemon juice
  2 cups fine chopped fresh vegetables
    such as tomatoes, cucumbers, and/or
    sweet peppers; it's your choice.

1 Pour the boiling water over the bulgur and let sit 30 minutes or until soft. Drain and squeeze dry.

2 Heat the oil in a skillet and sauté the onion until soft but not brown, 3 to 5 minutes. Add the tomato puree, mint, cumin, and allspice.

3 Stir in the bulgur and walnuts. Add the lemon juice and mix thoroughly. Let sit at least 30 minutes to blend the flavors. Add chopped fresh vegetables like cucumber, tomatoes, and/or sweet peppers just before serving.

<C **To Cut Carb**
<C Bulgar wheat: either reduce to 1/2 cup or substitute Quinoa.
<C Onions: reduce to 1/2 cup.

Per serving: 234 calories, 7 g fat, 0 g saturated fat, 0% calories from saturated fat, 41 g carbohydrate, 10 g dietary fiber, 141 mg sodium
Exchanges: 2 Starch, 2 Vegetable, 1 Fat

Low Carb
Per serving: 159 calories, 6 g fat, 0 g saturated fat, 0% calories from saturated fat, 24 g carbohydrate, 6 g dietary fiber, 137 mg sodium
Exchanges: 1 Starch, 2 Vegetable, 1 Fat

Corn and Tomato Salad

SERVING SIZE: 1/6 recipe, SERVES: 6

1/4 cup unsweetened apple juice	3 large tomatoes	
2 Tbsp balsamic vinegar	9 large basil leaves	
1/2 tsp arrowroot or cornstarch	6 small basil sprigs	
1 1/2 cups fresh or frozen corn kernels		

1 Preheat oven to 425°F. Combine apple juice, vinegar, and arrowroot or cornstarch in a small saucepan. Stir over medium-high heat until clear and thickened. Set aside to cool.

2 Spread corn on a baking sheet in a single layer. Lightly coat with olive oil pan spray. Roast in oven 5 minutes or until it begins to turn brown.

3 Slice the tomatoes and arrange on 6 salad plates. Scatter corn over tomatoes, and drizzle sauce around vegetables. Stack basil leaves, roll, and slice into thin strips. Sprinkle over top and lay a basil sprig on each plate.

Per serving: 56 calories, 0 g fat, 0 g saturated fat, 0% calories from saturated fat, 14 g carbohydrate, 2 g dietary fiber, 9 mg sodium
Exchanges: 1/2 Starch, 1 Vegetable

Celeriac Apple Salad

SERVING SIZE: 1/4 of recipe, SERVES: 4

1 small celeriac or celery root, peeled and sliced (1 1/2 cups)
2 small (or 1 large) red-skinned apples, cored and chopped (1 1/2 cups)
2 Tbsp rice vinegar
4 butter lettuce leaves

1 Tbsp non-aromatic olive oil
1 tsp Dijon mustard
1/2 tsp dried tarragon
1/4 tsp salt
1/4 tsp pepper

1 Drop the celeriac slices into boiling water. Bring back to a boil, and cook 3 minutes. Drain, and run under cold water to cool. Cut into strips. Mix with the chopped apples.

2 Combine the rice vinegar, oil, mustard, tarragon, salt, and pepper. Pour over the celeriac and apples, and toss to coat. Spoon onto the lettuce leaves and serve.

Per serving: 84 calories, 4 g fat, 1/2 g saturated fat, 5% calories from saturated fat, 13 g carbohydrate, 2 g dietary fiber, 234 mg sodium
Exchanges: 1 Vegetable, 1/2 Fruit, 1 Fat

Green and Yellow Bean Salad

SERVING SIZE: 1/4 of recipe, SERVES: 4

Salad

1 1/2 cups green beans, stem end cut off, cut in 3-inch lengths
1 1/2 cups yellow (wax) beans, stem end cut off, cut in 3-inch lengths
1 cup canned reduced sodium garbanzo beans, rinsed and drained
1/4 red onion, cut in strips
3 Roma tomatoes, seeded and cut in strips

Dressing

2 Tbsp balsamic vinegar
1 Tbsp extra virgin olive oil
1 tsp chopped garlic
2 Tbsp chopped fresh basil

2 Tbsp chopped fresh parsley
1/4 tsp salt
1/4 tsp pepper

1 Steam the green and yellow beans 6 minutes, remove from heat and plunge into cold water to stop cooking. Drain and transfer to a large bowl. Add garbanzo beans, onion, and tomato and toss.

2 Combine vinegar, oil, garlic, basil, parsley, salt, and pepper. Pour over the vegetables and mix to coat. Let sit for 30 minutes to allow the flavors to mingle.

Per serving: 150 calories, 5 g fat, 0 g saturated fat, 0% calories from saturated fat, 23 g carbohydrate, 7 g dietary fiber, 156 mg sodium
Exchanges: 1 Starch, 2 Vegetable, 1/2 Fat

Tossed Mixed Greens

SERVING SIZE: 1/4 of recipe, SERVES: 4

2 cups collard greens	1/2 cup chopped parsley
2 cups Swiss chard	1/4 cup chopped cilantro
4 cups spinach	2 tsp ground cumin
1 Tbsp extra virgin olive oil	juice of 1 lemon (1/4 cup)
4 cloves garlic, bashed and chopped	1/4 tsp salt

1 Place the collards in a large steamer over boiling water. Steam 2 minutes, add the Swiss chard, and steam 2 minutes more. Now add the spinach and steam 4 minutes longer. Turn out into a sieve when tender and squeeze out the excess liquid with the back of a wooden spoon. Chop roughly.

2 Combine the olive oil, garlic, parsley, cilantro, cumin, and lemon juice in a large skillet. Warm, add the chopped greens and salt, and mix thoroughly. Serve immediately while the greens are still bright and beautiful.

Per serving: 69 calories, 4 g fat, 0 g saturated fat, 0% calories from saturated fat, 5 g carbohydrate, 5 g dietary fiber, 235 mg sodium, 3 g protein
Exchanges: 1 Vegetable, 1 Fat

Turnberry Isle Red Pepper Soup with Floating Avocado Toast

SERVING SIZE: 1/6 of recipe, SERVES: 6

Soup

4 large red bell peppers
4 fresh Italian plum tomatoes, such as Roma
1/2 tsp light olive oil
1/2 cup finely diced onion
2 cloves garlic, peeled, bashed, and minced

4 cups low-sodium chicken stock (page 463)
1/8 tsp salt
1/8 tsp freshly ground black pepper
1 tsp balsamic vinegar
6 fresh basil stems

Floating Avocado Toast

6 slices (1/2-inch thick) of French baguette
1 whole clove garlic, peeled (optional)
1 ripe avocado

1/4 cup yogurt cheese (see page 475)
1/8 tsp salt
1 tsp fresh lime juice

Toast Garnish

6 fresh basil leaves

Vegetarian Option

Use 4 cups vegetable stock instead of chicken stock in step 7.

 Preheat the broiler.

2 Cut both ends off the peppers and remove the seeds and pulp. Slice each pepper twice from top to bottom to make three rectangular sections. Press the pieces flat with the palm of your hand. Remove the stems from the caps and press the caps flat.

3 Place the pepper pieces, skin side up, on a broiler pan and broil until the skins blacken and blister.

4   Transfer the peppers to a paper or plastic bag, seal the bag, and set aside for at least 10 minutes to steam. When the peppers are cool enough to handle, peel and discard the charred skins. Chop the remaining flesh and set aside.

5   Bring a large saucepan of water to a rolling boil. Drop the tomatoes into the boiling water for 1 minute (this will loosen the skin enough to peel). Transfer the tomatoes to a basin of cold water or allow them to cool on a plate. When the tomatoes are cool enough to handle, peel and discard the loose skins.

6   Quarter each tomato lengthwise and scoop the seeds into a strainer set over a bowl. Discard the seeds and reserve the juice. Dice the tomatoes and set aside.

7   Warm the oil in a large saucepan over medium heat. Sauté the onion until soft but not browned, about 2 minutes. Add the garlic and cook an additional 3 minutes. Stir in the peppers, tomatoes, reserved tomato juice, stock, salt, pepper, and vinegar. Bruise the basil stems and tie them in a bundle with string, or enclose in a mesh herb ball. Drop the stems into the stock, cover, and bring to a boil. Reduce the heat and simmer for 10 minutes. Remove the basil stems.

8   Transfer half of the soup to a blender or food processor and purée until smooth. Return the purée to the pan and stir well. Reheat the soup before serving.

To Prepare Toast

9   Place the bread slices on a broiler pan and toast until lightly browned on both sides. Remove from the oven and rub one side of each slice with the garlic.

10 To prepare the spread, peel and pit the avocado. Mash the avocado with a fork until it has the consistency of chunky guacamole. Stir in the yogurt cheese, salt, and lime juice. If you will not be serving this immediately, lay a piece of plastic wrap directly on the surface of the spread so it won't darken, then cover with an airtight lid and refrigerate until needed.

11 To serve, slice the basil leaves into thin slivers. Spread the avocado mixture thickly on the garlic toast. Spoon the hot soup into warmed bowls, float an "avocado island" in the center of each bowl, and sprinkle with basil.

Per serving: 126 calories, 4 g fat, 1 g saturated fat, 7% calories from saturated fat, 20 g carbohydrate, 2 g dietary fiber, 2 g protein
Exchanges: 1 Starch, 1 Vegetable, 1/2 Fat

Union Square Summer Salad

(aka, Tomato and Sweet Corn with Balsamic Sauce)

SERVING SIZE: 1/6 of recipe, SERVES: 6

Salad

2–3 ears fresh corn, shucked   3 large ripe tomatoes

Balsamic sauce

1/4 cup unsweetened apple juice   3/4 tsp arrowroot
  2 Tbsp balsamic vinegar

Garnish

9 large basil leaves   6 fresh basil sprigs

To Prepare the Salad

1 Drop the ears of corn into a pot of rapidly boiling water and cook for 5 minutes. Remove from the heat and immediately immerse in ice water to chill. When cool enough to handle, cut the kernels from the cobs. Discard the cobs and refrigerate the kernels.

2 Core the tomatoes by cutting a shallow cone around the stem. Cut each tomato in half lengthwise, top to bottom and lay the tomato halves, cut side down, on a cutting board. With a sharp knife held parallel to the cutting board, cut thin slices across the tomato from the blossom end toward the stem end, stopping just before you cut all the way through. Make about six slices, discarding the top slice, which is completely covered with skin. Repeat with all six tomato halves and set aside until ready to serve.

To Prepare the Sauce

3 Combine the apple juice, vinegar, and arrowroot in a small saucepan. Stir over medium-high heat until the sauce thickens and turns glossy. Set aside to cool.

To Serve

4 Scatter the corn on individual salad plates. Lay a tomato half in the center of each plate and press down gently to fan out the slices. Drizzle about

1 Tbsp of the sauce over each tomato. Slice the basil leaves into thin strips and sprinkle over the corn and tomato. Lay a sprig of basil at the base of the tomato fan.

Per serving: 67 calories, 0 g fat, 0 g saturated fat, 0% calories from saturated fat, 16 g carbohydrate, 2 g dietary fiber, 10 mg sodium
Exchanges: 1/2 Starch, 1 Vegetable

Winter Sunshine Carrot-Orange Soup

SERVING SIZE: 1/4 of recipe, SERVES: 4

1 lb carrots, peeled, washed, and cut into 1/4-inch pieces
2 cloves garlic, crushed
1 (14 oz) can low-sodium chicken broth
1 (14 oz) can nonfat evaporated milk

Juice and zest of 1 orange
1 1/4 tsp pumpkin pie spice
1 tsp black pepper
1/2 tsp grated fresh ginger
1/2 tsp salt
1 Granny Smith apple, chilled

1 Preheat oven to 350°F. Coat carrots and garlic lightly with vegetable cooking spray and roast, covered, until carrots are soft, about 1 hour. Transfer carrots and garlic to a blender, add chicken broth, and puree until smooth. Transfer puree to a medium pot, whisk in milk, juice, zest, and seasonings. Heat on low until warm throughout and no sharp garlic taste remains. Add water or milk to thin, if necessary.

2 To serve, slice pre-washed apple into matchstick-shaped slivers and divide among four bowls. Ladle the hot soup over the chilled apple, and serve immediately.

Per serving: 171 calories, 1 g fat, 0 g saturated fat, 0% calories from saturated fat, 31 g carbohydrate, 1 g dietary fiber, 468 mg sodium, 9 g protein, 3 mg cholesterol
Exchanges: 2 Vegetable, 1/2 Fruit, 1 Fat-Free Milk

Thai Chicken and Shrimp Soup

SERVING SIZE: 1/4 of recipe, SERVES: 4

  5 cups low-sodium chicken stock (page 463)
  1 lb raw chicken, equal parts dark and light meat, cut in 1/2-inch pieces
  1 tsp olive oil
  1 Tbsp finely sliced lemon grass
1-inch ginger root, chopped fine
  1 clove garlic, bashed and chopped
  4 green onions, white parts cut in 1-inch lengths, greens cut in 1/2-inch rings
  1 (5 1/2 oz) can baby corn, drained
  1 (8 oz) can bamboo shoots with juice
  8 medium mushrooms, cut in quarters
  2 red jalapeño (Fresno) peppers, seeded and chopped
  1 tsp cilantro stems, chopped fine
  3 Tbsp lime juice
  1 Tbsp Thai fish sauce (nam pla), or light soy sauce
  1 tsp chopped cilantro
1/4 cup onion greens
  4 cups sliced Chinese (Napa) cabbage
1/2 cup small cooked shrimp

Vegetarian Option

  5 cups low-sodium vegetable stock (page 473)
  2 chayote squash, cut in 1/2-inch dice
     handful baby carrots
  1 Tbsp light soy sauce

To make a vegetarian version of this recipe, start at step 2. Fry the lemon grass, ginger, garlic, and onion tops for a minute. Pour in the vegetable stock and add the corn, bamboo shoots, mushrooms, chiles, cilantro stems, lime juice, and chayote squash in place of the chicken. You can add a handful of baby carrots to add color since you won't be using the baby shrimp. Season with the soy sauce. Bring to a boil, reduce the heat, and simmer until the vegetables are tender, 5 to 10 minutes. Now add the cilantro, green onion tops, and cabbage and simmer 1 more minute. Proceed with step 3.

1 Bring 2 cups of the chicken stock to a boil in a large saucepan. Drop in the dark meat and simmer 1 minute. Add the white meat and simmer 4 minutes more. Remove the chicken to a small bowl and cover. Strain the stock into a bowl and set aside.

2 Reheat the pan and add the oil. Toss in the lemon grass, ginger, garlic, and onion whites and sauté for just a minute to release the flavorful oils. Pour in the strained stock and add the corn, bamboo shoots, mushrooms, chilis, cilantro stems, lime juice, remaining 3 cups stock, and fish sauce. Bring to a boil, reduce the heat, and simmer 5 minutes. Add the cilantro, green onion tops, cabbage, and shrimp and simmer 1 more minute to heat through. This dish can be served as a soup or stew.

3 To finish as a stew, drain the liquid into a measuring cup or bowl. Thicken 1 cup of liquid by stirring in a slurry made of 1 Tbsp arrowroot mixed with 2 Tbsp water and return it to the drained ingredients. Spoon the stew on each plate with some rice on the side and the extra liquid in a glass to sip. As a soup, it can be ladled into a bowl over a scoop of rice. For those who like more flavor, pass Thai chili paste, lime wedges, chopped cilantro, and the rest of the onion greens.

Per serving: 230 calories, 6 g fat, 2 g saturated fat, 7% calories from saturated fat, 10 g carbohydrate, 3 g dietary fiber, 615 mg sodium, 34 g protein
Exchanges: 3 Lean Meat, 2 Vegetable

Vegetarian
Per serving: 184 calories, 3 g fat, 0 g saturated fat, 2% calories from saturated fat, 32 g carbohydrate, 3 g dietary fiber, 729 mg sodium
Exchanges: 1 1/2 Starch, 2 Vegetable, 1/2 Fat

Chilled Pumpkin Soup

SERVING SIZE: 1/4 of recipe, SERVES: 4

1 (16 oz) can pumpkin
1 (12 oz) can evaporated skim milk

2 green onions, finely diced
1/4 tsp red pepper flakes

1 Blend pumpkin and milk until smooth. Stir in onions and pepper flakes and chill. Serve cold on a hot summer's day.

Per serving: 115 calories, 1 g fat, 0 g saturated fat, 0% calories from saturated fat, 20 g carbohydrate, 3 g dietary fiber, 115 mg sodium
Exchanges: 1 Starch, 1/2 Fat-free Milk

Pea Salad with Curry and Almonds

SERVING SIZE: 1/4 of recipe, SERVES: 4

2 cups thawed petit peas
1 cup peeled and chopped jicama
1 heaping tsp roughly chopped
  toasted almonds
2 Tbsp roughly chopped
  toasted almonds

1/4 cup light mayonnaise
1/4 cup nonfat plain yogurt
1 tsp mild curry powder
  pinch cayenne
1/4 tsp salt
1/4 tsp pepper

1 Place the peas, jicama, and almonds in a bowl.

2 Combine the mayonnaise, yogurt, curry powder, cayenne, salt, and pepper. Add to the vegetables and mix well.

Per serving: 118 calories, 3 g fat, 0 g saturated fat, 0% calories from saturated fat, 18 g carbohydrate, 7 g dietary fiber, 161 mg sodium, 5 g protein
Exchanges: 1 Starch, 1/2 Fat

Mediterranean Lentil Salad

SERVING SIZE : 1/4 of recipe, SERVES: 4

Lentils

1 cup dried brown or green lentils
1 small onion, peeled and chopped (1/2 cup)

2 cloves garlic, peeled
1 bay leaf

Salad

1/4 cup pitted and chopped
  Greek olives
1 cup chopped celery
1 cup chopped red bell pepper
2 Tbsp chopped parsley
1/4 cup lemon juice

2 Tbsp extra virgin olive oil
2 cloves garlic, crushed
2 tsp fresh or 1/2 tsp dried thyme
  leaves
1/4 tsp salt
1/4 tsp pepper

1. Wash the lentils, picking out any small stones. Place in a pan with the onion, garlic, bay leaf, and 3 cups water. Bring to a boil, reduce the heat, and simmer 15 to 20 minutes or until tender but not mushy. Drain, discard the onion, garlic cloves, and bay leaf, and chill under cold water.

2. Place the lentils in a bowl with the olives, celery, red pepper, parsley, lemon juice, oil, thyme, salt, and pepper. Toss and serve warm or cold over mixed bitter greens.

Per serving: 253 calories, 8 g fat, 1 g saturated fat, 4% calories from saturated fat, 33 g carbohydrate, 16 g dietary fiber, 255 mg sodium
Exchanges: 1 1/2 Starch, 1 Very Lean Meat, 2 Vegetable, 1 Fat

Roasted Red Pepper Soup

SERVING SIZE: 1/6 of recipe, SERVES: 6

4 large red bell peppers	4 cups low-sodium chicken or vegetable broth
1 tsp olive oil	
1/2 cup diced sweet onions	1/4 tsp salt
2 cloves garlic	1/4 tsp pepper
1 (15 oz) can diced tomatoes in juice	1 Tbsp balsamic vinegar (optional)

1. Preheat the broiler. Cut the tops off the peppers and remove the stems from the tops and the core from the bodies. Cut through the bodies so you can flatten them. Place the long bodies and the round tops on a large baking sheet, skin side up. Broil 4 inches to 6 inches from the heat source 10 minutes or until the skin is thoroughly blackened. Place in a plastic bag to cool 20 minutes. Remove the skin and chop.

2. Heat the oil in a large saucepan on medium high. Sauté the onions 2 minutes then add the garlic and fry 1 minute more. Add the tomatoes and broth and bring to a boil. Reduce the heat and simmer 10 minutes.

3. Whiz half the soup in a blender then pour back into the rest. Season with salt, pepper, and balsamic vinegar. Divide among 6 hot soup bowls.

Per serving: 48 calories, 1 g fat, 0 g saturated fat, 0% calories from saturated fat, 8 g carbohydrate, 1 g dietary fiber, 361 mg sodium, 2 g protein
Exchanges: 2 Vegetable

Senate Bean Soup

SERVING SIZE: 1/6 of recipe, SERVES: 6

     1 lb smoky ham hock
     1 bay leaf
     3 whole cloves
<C 1 lb navy beans, rinsed, picked over, and soaked overnight
    1/2 tsp non-aromatic olive oil
<C 1 large sweet onion, chopped (1 1/2 cups)
     4 cloves garlic, bashed and chopped
<C 2 carrots, peeled and cut in 1/4-inch dice (1 1/2 cups)
+> 2 ribs celery, cut in 1/4-inch dice (1 cup)
<C 1 medium russet potato, peeled and chopped (1 1/2 cups)
    1/2 tsp cumin
    1/4 tsp summer savory
     2 Tbsp chopped parsley
    1/2 tsp salt
    1/4 tsp pepper

1 Cover the ham hock with 8 cups water in a large kettle. Toss in the bay and cloves and bring to a boil over high heat. Reduce the heat and simmer 1 1/2 hours or until the meat is tender. You can do this step in a pressure cooker with the same ingredients and cooked for 30 minutes. Strain the resulting stock into a fat strainer to remove the fat. Pour the defatted liquid back into the soup kettle, adding water to make 7 cups. Add the beans, bring to a boil, reduce the heat and simmer another 1 1/2 hours or until the beans are tender but not mushy. This too can be accomplished in a pressure cooker. Check the manufacturer's instructions for time. Cut the meat from the ham hock to put into the soup later and discard the fat, skin, and bone.

2 Heat the oil in a chef's pan or skillet on medium high. Sauté the onion for 2 minutes and then add the garlic, carrots, celery, and potato. Cook for 3 more minutes before adding to the cooked beans. Stir in the cumin and savory and simmer 20 minutes or until the vegetables are tender.

3 Pour about 1/3 of the bean mixture into a blender and whiz until smooth. Return it to the rest of the beans and stir in the reserved meat, parsley, salt, and pepper. Serve with more chopped parsley.

<c Navy beans: reduce to 2/3 lb (12 oz).   <c Celery: increase to 2 cups.

<c Sweet onion: reduce to 1 cup.   <c Potatoes: reduce to 1 cup.

<c Carrots: reduce to 1 cup.

Per serving: 344 calories, 2 g fat, 0 g saturated fat, 0% calories from saturated fat, 64 g carbohydrate, 15 g dietary fiber, 322 mg sodium
Exchanges: 3 1/2 Starch, 1 Very Lean Meat, 2 Vegetable

Low Carb
Per serving: 244 calories, 2 g fat, 0 g saturated fat, 0% calories from saturated fat, 44 g carbohydrate, 10 g dietary fiber, 335 mg sodium
Exchanges: 2 1/2 Starch, 1 Vegetable

Spinach Salad with Marinated Vegetables

SERVING SIZE: 1/4 of recipe, SERVES: 4

  1 cup small, bite-sized cauliflower pieces (use fresh or thawed frozen)
  1 cup sliced button mushrooms
  8 stalks fresh asparagus, sliced on the diagonal into bite-sized pieces (about 1 cup)
  1 (14 oz) can quartered artichoke hearts in water, drained
1/2 cup reduced-fat red wine vinaigrette or Italian dressing, divided
  4 slices white or sourdough bread (crust removed and bread sliced into bite-sized cubes)
  5 cups tightly packed spinach leaves (about 6 oz, sliced into bite-sized pieces)

1 Preheat oven to 350°F. Steam or microwave cauliflower, mushrooms, and asparagus until asparagus is tender-crisp. Place in a medium bowl with artichoke hearts and toss with 3 Tbsp dressing. Cover and refrigerate.

2 Spread bread cubes in a shallow glass pan and toss with 2 Tbsp vinaigrette. Bake 10 minutes, until golden brown. Let cool. Toss spinach leaves with remaining dressing and croutons in a large serving bowl. Top with marinated vegetables and serve.

Per serving: 166 calories, 6 g fat, 1 g saturated fat, 3% calories from saturated fat, 25 g carbohydrate, 9 g dietary fiber, 448 mg sodium, 9 g protein
Exchanges: 1 Starch, 2 Vegetable, 1 Fat

Creamy Clam Chowder

SERVING SIZE: 1/6 of recipe, SERVES: 6

    4 1/2 lb small live clams
        2 cups water
     1/2 tsp non-aromatic olive oil
        4 oz Canadian bacon or smoked salmon
<C   1 large sweet onion, chopped (2 cups)
<C 1 1/2 lb medium red potatoes, peeled and cut in 3/4-inch dice (4 cups)
        1 bay leaf
     1/2 tsp dried thyme
     1/4 tsp freshly ground black pepper
        3 cups 1% milk
<C   1/3 cup cornstarch mixed with 2/3 cup water (slurry)
        1 (12 oz) can nonfat evaporated milk

1   Rinse clams, scrub if need be. Bring water to a boil in a large skillet. Add clams, cover, and bring back to the boil. Cook 5 minutes or until clams open. Discard unopened ones. When they cool, drain, saving the liquid, and pick out the meats. Strain the liquid through cheesecloth if you see any sand. You should have 2 cups clams and 3 cups juice. Add water to make 3 cups if you are short.

2   Heat oil in a Dutch oven. Sauté bacon (skip this if you are using smoked salmon) 1 to 2 minutes. Add onions and cook 3 minutes or until translucent. Stir in potatoes, bay leaf, thyme, and pepper. Pour in reserved clam juice and milk, and bring to a boil. Reduce heat and simmer, uncovered, 10 minutes or until potatoes are tender.

3   Stir in the slurry, and boil 30 seconds to thicken. Add evaporated milk and clams, and heat. The smoked salmon may be flaked and added at this time. Light water crackers aren't necessary with nearly 50 grams of carbohydrate in the chowder. Serve in warm soup bowls.

<C **To Cut Carb**

<C Onion: reduce to 1 cup (chopped).
<C Potatoes: reduce to 1 lb, about 3 cups (chopped).
<C Cornstarch: reduce to 1/4 cup.

Per serving: 339 calories, 4 g fat, 1 g saturated fat, 3% calories from saturated fat, 45 g carbohydrate, 3 g dietary fiber, 578 mg sodium
Exchanges: 2 Starch, 2 Very Lean Meat, 1 Vegetable, 1 Fat-free Milk

Low Carb
Per serving: 303 calories, 4 g fat, 1 g saturated fat, 3% calories from saturated fat, 37 g carbohydrate, 2 g dietary fiber, 575 mg sodium
Exchanges: 1 1/2 Starch, 2 Very Lean Meat, 1 Vegetable, 1 Fat-free Milk

Summer Corn Chowder

SERVING SIZE: 1/4 of recipe, SERVES: 4

<C 4 cups fresh or frozen/thawed corn kernels, divided
<C 1 (12 oz) can evaporated skim milk
1 tsp non-aromatic olive oil
2 green onions, sliced thin

2 oz Canadian bacon, cut in slivers
+> 1 cup zucchini, cut in matchsticks
1/2 tsp salt
1/4 tsp pepper
1/4 tsp pepper
2 Roma tomatoes, seeded and diced

1 Puree 3 cups of the corn in a blender or processor using just enough evaporated milk to keep it moving. Whiz 2 minutes to get it really smooth.

2 Heat the oil in a large saucepan on medium high. Fry the onions and Canadian bacon 1 minute. Add the zucchini and cook 1 minute more.

3 Pour the pureed corn through a sieve into the saucepan. Press with the back of a spoon or spatula to get all the liquid. Add the remaining evaporated milk, corn, salt, and pepper and heat through. Stir in the tomatoes just before serving.

<C **To Cut Carb**

<C Corn: reduce to 3 cups. Use only 2 cups in step 1.
<C Evaporated milk: reduce to 1 cup (8 oz) or replace with chicken stock.
+> Zucchini: increase by 1 cup.

Per serving: 254 calories, 3 g fat, 1 g saturated fat, 4% calories from saturated fat, 46 g carbohydrate, 5 g dietary fiber, 642 mg sodium
Exchanges: 2 Starch, 1 Fat-Free Milk, 1/2 Fat

Low Carb
Per serving: 201 calories, 3 g fat, 1 g saturated fat, 3% calories from saturated fat, 35 g carbohydrate, 4 g dietary fiber, 601 mg sodium
Exchanges: 1 1/2 Starch, 1 Vegetable, 1/2 Fat-Free Milk, 1/2 Fat

Sumptuous Summer Salad

SERVING SIZE: 1/6 of recipe, SERVES: 6

1 cup chopped zucchini
1 cup fresh, canned or frozen
  corn kernels
1 cup chopped seeded
  tomatoes
1 cup fresh or frozen peas
1/4 cup sliced green onions

2 cup cooked rice, quinoa,
  bulgar, or millet
1/4 cup chopped fresh basil
1/3 cup low-fat vinaigrette
  salad dressing
6 large butter of leaf lettuce leaves

1 Combine the zucchini, corn, tomatoes, peas, onion, rice, basil, and salad dressing in a large bowl. Mix well and let sit for at least 1/2 hour.

2 Serve on lettuce leaves with a good slice of crusty whole-wheat bread.

Per serving: 164 calories, 5 g fat, 1 g saturated fat, 5% calories from saturated fat, 26 g carbohydrate, 4 g dietary fiber, 118 mg sodium, 2 g protein
Exchanges: 1 Starch, 1 Vegetable, 1 Fat

Winter Fruit Salad

SERVING SIZE: 1/6 of recipe, SERVES: 6

1/2 cup sliced canned peaches in
  light syrup, drained
1/2 cup sliced canned pears in
  light syrup, drained
1/2 cup pineapple chunks in light syrup,
  drained

1/2 cup fresh orange sections
1/2 cup diced fresh apple
1/2 cup orange juice
1 tsp honey
1 Tbsp lime juice

1 Place the peaches, pears, pineapple, oranges, and apples in a bowl.

2 Combine the orange juice, honey, and lime juice and pour over. Chill for an hour and serve.

Per serving: 64 calories, 0 g fat, 0 g saturated fat, 0% calories from saturated fat, 17 g carbohydrate, 2 g dietary fiber, 3 mg sodium
Exchanges: 1 Fruit

Butternut and Ginger Soup

SERVING SIZE: 1/6 of recipe, SERVES: 6

1 tsp non-aromatic olive oil	<C 1/2 lb potatoes, peeled and chopped
1 1/2 cups chopped onion	<C 1/2 lb potatoes, peeled and chopped
3 cloves garlic, bashed and chopped	1 cup unsweetened apple juice
2 tsp chopped fresh ginger	3 cups water or vegetable broth
1 1/2 lb peeled raw butternut or other winter squash	1/2 cup nonfat milk or soy milk
	1/2 tsp salt

Garnish

1/2 Granny Smith apple, chopped
 2 Tbsp chopped parsley

1 Heat the oil in a high-sided skillet or large saucepan on medium high. Sauté the onion 3 minutes or until it starts to wilt. Add the garlic and ginger and cook 1 minute longer.

2 Add the squash, potatoes, apple juice, and water or broth. Bring to a boil, reduce the heat and simmer 35 to 40 minutes or until very soft.

3 Whiz in a blender or processor, in batches, until smooth. Pour back into the pan and stir in the milk and salt. Reheat and serve topped with shopped apple and parsley.

<C **To Cut Carb**

<C Potatoes: remove entirely.

Per serving: 135 calories, 1 g fat, 0g saturated fat, 0% calories from saturated fat, 31 g carbohydrate, 4 g dietary fiber, 214 mg sodium
Exchanges: 1 1/2 Starch, 1/2 Fruit

Low Carb
Per serving: 110 calories, 1 g fat, 0 g saturated fat. 0% calories from saturated fat, 25 g carbohydrate, 3 g dietary fiber, 213 mg sodium
Exchanges: 1 Starch, 1/2 Fruit

Quick Smoky Vegetarian Bean Soup

SERVING SIZE: 1/6 of recipe, SERVES: 6

  1/2 tsp non-aromatic olive oil
     1 large sweet onion, chopped
     4 garlic cloves, bashed and chopped
<C 2 carrots, peeled and cut in 1/4-inch dice (1 1/2 cups)
     2 ribs celery, cut in 1/4-inch dice (1 cup)
<C 1 medium russet potato, peeled and chopped (1 1/2 cups)
     8 cups vegetable broth
<C 6 cups canned navy beans
  1/2 tsp cumin
  1/4 tsp summer savory
     2 Tbsp chopped parsley
  1/2 tsp salt (optional)
     3 tsp rinsed, seeded, and chopped canned chipotle chili or chipotle sauce
        to taste

1 Heat the oil in a soup kettle on medium high. Sauté the onion for 2 minutes and then add the garlic, carrots, celery, and potato. Cook for 3 more minutes. Pour in the vegetable stock and canned beans. Stir in the cumin and savory and bring to a boil. Reduce the heat and simmer 20 minutes or until the vegetables are tender.

2 Pour about 1/3 of the bean mixture into a blender and whiz until smooth. Return it to the rest of the beans and stir in the parsley and chipotle. Taste before adding salt as the canned beans and vegetable stock may be quite salty. Serve with more chopped parsley.

<C To Cut Carb

<C Carrots: reduce to 3/4 cup.

<C Potatoes: reduce to just 1/2 cup (it is now a garnish).

<C Navy beans: reduce to 4 cups and add 2 cups of your favorite non-root vegetable which you cut in 1/4-inch pieces and add at step 1.

Per serving: 385 calories, 2 g fat, 0 g saturated fat, 0% calories from saturated fat, 70 g carbohydrate, 16 g fiber, 1255 mg sodium
Exchanges: 4 Starch, 1 Very Lean Meat, 2 Vegetable

Low Carb
Per serving: 267 calories, 2 g fat, 0 g saturated fat, 0% calories from saturated fat, 48 g carbohydrate, 12 g dietary fiber, 863 mg sodium
Exchanges: 2 1/2 Starch, 1 Very Lean Meat, 2 Vegetable

Southwest Kidney Bean Pasta Salad

SERVING SIZE: 1/6 of recipe, SERVES: 6

<C 10 oz dry bow tie or other small pasta shape
<C 1 (15 oz) can kidney beans, rinsed and drained
<C 1 (15 1/4 oz) can corn niblets, rinsed and drained
<C 1 1/2 cups prepared chunky salsa, divided
   4 green onions, sliced
   1/2 tsp ground cumin
   1/4 cup chopped cilantro (optional)
   3 Tbsp olive oil

1 Cook pasta according to package instructions. Drain and rinse with cold water to stop cooking.

2 Combine the beans, corn, pasta, onions, cumin, 1 cup of the salsa, and cilantro. Let sit in the refrigerator for at least an hour. Before serving, stir in the remaining salsa and the olive oil.

<C **To Cut Carb**

<C Pasta: reduce to 3 cups cooked (5 oz raw).
<C Kidney beans: reduce to 12 oz (1 cup).
<C Corn niblets: reduce to 12 oz (1 cup).
<C Salsa: reduce to 1 cup.

Per serving: 352 calories, 8 g fat, 1 g saturated fat, 3% calories from saturated fat, 59 g carbohydrate, 4 g dietary fiber, 485 mg sodium
Exchanges: 3 1/2 Starch, 1 Vegetable, 1 Fat

Low Carb
Per serving: 221 calories, 8 g fat, 1 g saturated fat, 4% calories from saturated fat, 32 g carbohydrate, 4 g dietary fiber, 223 mg sodium
Exchanges: 2 Starch, 1 1/2 Fat

Island Greens Salad with Papaya Seed Dressing

SERVING SIZE: 1/6 of recipe, SERVES: 6

Salad

- 1 head napa cabbage, washed and cored
- 1/3 English cucumber
- 6 green onions cut diagonally into 1/2-inch pieces
- 1 cup loosely packed mung bean sprouts, rinsed
- 4 cups washed and stemmed spinach
- 30 small cilantro leaves, very finely sliced
- 1 lime, peeled, sectioned, and chopped, juice reserved
- 2 Tbsp pumpkin seeds
- 1 large, ripe papaya, peeled and cut into 1/2-inch cubes or scooped into balls with a melon baller (reserve the seeds)

Papaya Seed Dressing

- 4 thin slices of peeled ginger root, about 1/4-inch thick
- 2 cloves garlic, peeled and thinly sliced
- 1 tsp mustard powder

- 1 Tbsp papaya seeds (optional)
- 1/2 cup rice vinegar
- 1/4 cup light olive oil
- 1 Tbsp brown sugar
- 1 Tbsp low-sodium tamari

To Prepare the Salad

1. Pick out six of the nicest, largest cabbage leaves and refrigerate the rest for another use. Cut out the white stems and slice them crosswise into strips. You should have about 1 cup. Wrap the leaves loosely in a towel and refrigerate.

2. Peel the cucumber and trim the sides flat so that it forms a long rectangle, then cut into a 1/2-inch dice.

3. Put the cabbage stems, cucumber, onions, sprouts, spinach, cilantro, lime, lime juice, and pumpkin seeds in a large salad spinner. Add the papaya and toss gently. Refrigerate the ingredients in the salad spinner until ready to serve.

To Prepare the Dressing

4. Process the ginger, garlic, mustard, papaya seeds, rice vinegar, oil, brown sugar, and tamari in a blender at high speed for about 1 minute.

To Serve

5 Pour the dressing over the greens in the salad spinner. Give the spinner a few good turns to allow the extra dressing to spin off. Collect the dressing from the bottom of the spinner and sprinkle 2 Tbsp over the top of the greens. The leftover dressing will keep in the refrigerator for several days. (I often use this technique for dressing green salads. The spinner distributes the dressing evenly over the greens, and the excess doesn't collect on the leaves near the bottom, as often happens in a salad bowl.)

6 Place a chilled cabbage leaf on each salad plate and arrange a portion of the salad on top.

Per serving: 88 calories, 4 g fat, 1 g saturated fat, 10% calories from saturated fat, 11 g carbohydrate, 4 g dietary fiber, 2 g protein
Exchanges: 1 Vegetable, 1/2 Fruit, 1 Fat

Szechuan Cucumber Salad

SERVING SIZE: 1/4 of recipe, SERVES: 4

1 lb cucumbers, peeled, seeded and cut into 2-inch strips	1/2 tsp toasted sesame oil
3 green onions, sliced	1 tsp rice vinegar
1 tsp chopped garlic	1/4 tsp granulated sugar
1 1/2 Tbsp light soy sauce	1/8 tsp ground allspice
	1/4 tsp hot pepper flakes

1 Combine the cucumbers, onions, and garlic in a glass bowl.

2 Whisk together the soy sauce, sesame oil, rice vinegar, sugar, allspice, and hot pepper flakes.

3 Pour the dressing over the vegetables, toss, and let sit for 10 minutes before servings.

Per serving: 28 calories, 1 g fat, 0 g saturated fat, 0% calories from saturated fat, 5 g carbohydrate, 1 g dietary fiber, 79 mg sodium
Exchanges: 1 Vegetable

Southern Japanese Miso and Sweet Potato Soup

SERVING SIZE: 1/4 of recipe, SERVES: 4

<C   8 oz soba (Japanese buckwheat) noodles or whole-wheat spaghetti
6 cups low-sodium chicken stock (page 463)
3 dried shitake mushrooms, stems removed and discarded
6 green onions, white parts cut on the diagonal in 1/2-inch slices, greens cut in 1/4-inch rings
2 carrots, cut on the diagonal in 1/2-inch slices
<C   1 medium sweet potato, cut in 1/2-inch pieces (1 1/2 cups)
1 medium turnip, cut in 1/2-inch strips
1/4 cup white miso
1/4 tsp cayenne pepper
2 (5 oz) boneless, skinless chicken breasts, cut in half lengthwise then across in 1/2-inch strips
1 bunch Swiss chard, stems removed, cut in 1/2-inch strips

Vegetarian Option

10 oz light tofu, cut in 1-inch cubes
6 cups low-sodium vegetable stock

For a lovely vegetarian miso soup, simply leave out the chicken and replace it with the firm, silken tofu. Use low-sodium vegetable stock instead of chicken broth.

---

1 Place the noodles into a large pan of vigorously boiling water and cook for 10 minutes or until tender but not soft. Drain, rinse in cold water to stop the cooking, and set the colander over a pan of hot water to reheat.

2 Whilst the noodles are cooking, bring the stock to a boil in a large saucepan. Add the dried shitakes and soak for 10 minutes off the heat. Remove, cut in thin strips, and set aside.

3 Bring the stock back to a simmer on medium heat. Place the white parts of the onion and the carrots into the simmering broth and cook gently for 5 minutes. Add the sweet potato, turnip, and mushroom strips and simmer 10 more minutes until the vegetables are tender but still firm.

4 Dissolve the miso paste in hot stock, add cayenne, and stir it into the soup. Scatter the pieces of chicken and chard onto the surface, stirring until well mixed. Simmer 3 minutes, being careful not to overcook the chicken.

5 Divide the noodles among four pre-heated bowls and ladle the soup on the top. Scatter the green onion rings over all. Please serve everything very hot, the rising cloud of aroma is a treat in itself.

<C **To Cut Carb**

<C Soba (whole-wheat noodles): replace with finely cut bok choy stalk.
<C Sweet potato: reduce by half.

Per serving: 453 calories, 7 g fat, 1 g saturated fat, 3% calories from saturated fat, 67 g carbohydrate, 9 g dietary fiber, 1436 mg sodium
Exchanges: 3 1/2 Starch, 3 Very Lean Meat, 2 Vegetable, 1/2 Fat

Low Carb
Per serving: 273 calories, 6 g fat, 1 g saturated fat, 4% calories from saturated fat, 31 g carbohydrate, 7 g dietary fiber, 950 mg sodium
Exchanges: 1 Starch, 3 Very Lean Meat, 3 Vegetable, 1/2 Fat

Vegetarian
Per serving: 371 calories, 3 g fat, 0 g saturated fat, 0% calories from saturated fat, 70 g carbohydrate, 9 g dietary fiber, 1819 mg sodium
Exchanges: 3 1/2 Starch, 3 Vegetable, 1/2 Fat

Summer Salad with Jicama and Strawberries

SERVING SIZE: 1/4 of recipe, SERVES: 4

4 cups mixed salad greens
1 cup jicama peeled and cut in 1/2-inch pieces

1 cup quartered strawberries
1/4 cup low-fat vinaigrette salad dressing (page 132)

| Combine the salad greens, jicama, and strawberries in a large salad bowl. Pour in the dressing and toss.

Per serving: 80 calories, 5 g fat, 1 g saturated fat, 11% calories from saturated fat, 9 g carbohydrate, 4 g dietary fiber, 102 mg sodium
Exchanges: 1 Vegetable, 1 Fat

Quick Tomato Soup

SERVING SIZE: 1/4 of recipe, SERVES: 4

1/2 tsp olive oil
1 cup chopped onion
2 cloves garlic, bashed and chopped
1 (28 oz) can diced tomatoes in juice

1 cup water
1 tsp dried basil
1 tsp dried oregano
1/4 tsp salt

1 Heat the oil in a large saucepan on medium-high. Sauté the onion 2 or 3 minutes or until the onion starts to wilt. Add the garlic and cook 1 minute, being careful not to let it brown.

2 Pour in the tomatoes and water. Crush the basil and oregano and add. Bring to a boil, reduce the heat, and simmer 15 minutes. Season with salt and serve.

Per serving: 65 calories, 1 g fat, 0 g saturated fat, 0% calories from saturated fat, 11 g carbohydrate, 3 g dietary fiber, 453 mg sodium, 3 g protein
Exchanges: 2 Vegetable

Creamy Carrot Soup

SERVING SIZE: 1/4 of recipe, SERVES: 4

1 tsp non-aromatic olive oil
1 tsp butter
<C 1 cup chopped onions
<C 1 lb carrots, peeled and chopped
4 cups low-sodium chicken broth

<C 1/2 cup uncooked white rice
<C 1/2 cup evaporated fat-free milk
1/4 cup plain nonfat yogurt
1 Tbsp chopped chives

1 Heat oil and butter in a skillet on medium high. Add onions, and cook 3 minutes or until wilted. Add carrots, and cook 3 minutes longer.

2 Pour in broth and rice. Cover, bring to a boil, and cook 20 minutes or until rice is soft. Blend in batches, being careful not to fill the jar more than half full of hot liquid. Return to pan, and stir in evaporated milk. Reheat.

3 Serve in 4 bowls swirled with yogurt. Scatter chives over the top.

<C **To Cut Carb**

<C Onions: reduce to 1/2 cup.
<C Carrots: reduce to 12 oz.
<C Evaporated milk: reduce to 1/4 cup.

<C Rice: delete white rice, use 1/4 cup brown rice.

Per serving: 227 calories, 4 g fat, 1 g saturated fat, 4% calories from saturated fat, 39 g carbohydrate, 4 g dietary fiber, 213 mg sodium
Exchanges: 1 1/2 Starch, 3 Vegetable, 1/2 Fat

Low Carb
Per serving: 158 calories, 4 g fat, 1 g saturated fat, 6% calories from saturated fat, 24 g carbohydrate, 3 g dietary fiber, 187 mg sodium
Exchanges: 1 Starch, 2 Vegetable, 1/2 Fat

Cream of Lettuce Soup

SERVING SIZE: 1/4 of recipe, SERVES: 4

  4 slices dill rye bread
  1 lb Romaine lettuce
  1 tsp non-aromatic olive oil
1 1/2 cups finely sliced onion
  2 cloves garlic, peeled, bashed, and chopped
  2 cups low-sodium chicken stock

  2 cups 1% milk
1/2 tsp salt
1/4 tsp white pepper
1/2 tsp dried dill weed
  2 Tbsp cornstarch mixed with
  4 Tbsp 1% milk (slurry)

1 Remove crusts from bread, and cut into 1-inch squares. Bake on ungreased cookie sheet at 350°F for 10 minutes. Wash lettuce leaves. Place in a large saucepan, cover, and cook over medium heat 6 minutes. Stir to make sure all lettuce is wilted, and cook for 2 more minutes if need be. Place the cooked lettuce in a blender and set aside.

2 Reheat the saucepan, and add oil. Sauté onions for 2 minutes, add garlic, and continue cooking until soft. Add to the lettuce, and blend for 2 minutes or until smooth. If too dry, add up to 1/4 cup chicken stock.

3 Pour stock and milk into the saucepan to heat. Add blended lettuce and onions to the warm liquid. Add salt, pepper and dill weed, cover, and simmer 7 minutes. Stir in the slurry, and heat to thicken.

4 Serve in warm soup bowls with a dollop of yogurt and dill weed. Pass the croutons.

Per serving: 211 calories, 3 g fat, 1 g saturated fat, 4% calories from saturated fat, 38 g carbohydrate, 4 g dietary fiber, 300 mg sodium
Exchanges: 1 Starch, 2 Vegetables, 1/2 Fat-free Milk, 1/2 Fat

Misosoba

SERVING SIZE: 1/4 of recipe, SERVES: 4

    1 lb daikon (large Japanese radish), peeled and cut into 1-inch chunks
    1 medium turnip, peeled and cut into eighths
<C 2 medium waxy potatoes, peeled and cut into eighths
    1 small winter squash (I prefer delicata), peeled, seeded, and cut into
      1-inch chunks
  12 oz low-fat extra firm tofu, cut into 1-inch cubes
   8 cups low-sodium chicken stock (page 463)
1/4 cup light soy sauce
<C 1/4 cup packed light brown sugar
    1 (10 oz) jar gefilte fish with juice
    2 Tbsp mustard powder
    2 Tbsp arrowroot
1/2 cup water
    2 hard-boiled eggs, shelled
    2 Tbsp chopped parsley

Vegetarian Option

1 lb fennel bulb, trimmed and cut lengthwise into fourths
4 oz low-fat extra firm tofu, cut into 1-inch cubes
8 cups low-sodium vegetable stock (page 473)

Add the fennel bulb to the vegetables. Increase the tofu to 1 lb and leave out the fish. Replace the chicken stock with low-sodium vegetable stock. Hard-boiled eggs are optional.

---

1 Bring a quart of water to a boil in a large saucepan. Drop in the daikon, cover, and cook for 10 minutes. Now add the turnip, potatoes, and squash and cook 12 minutes more. Drain, discarding the water, and set aside. This precooking will ensure a clear broth and good texture for the vegetables.

2 Pour boiling water over the tofu and let it soak while you do the next step.

3 Combine the chicken stock, soy sauce, and sugar in a heavy Dutch oven and bring to a boil. Drop in the vegetables, drained tofu, and gefilte fish. Turn the heat down as low as possible and simmer, uncovered, for 90 minutes. The liquid should be reduced by a little more than half, about 3 cups. Combine the mustard flour, arrowroot, and water to make a slurry. Pour into the stew, stirring while it thickens.

4 Divide among 4 warm bowls, set half a hard-boiled egg, yolk side up, in each and scatter chopped parsley over the top. Sprinkle the optional garnish over all.

<C **To Cut Carb**

<C Potatoes: reduce to zero.
<C Brown sugar: replace with Splenda.

Per serving: 403 calories, 14 g fat, 4 g saturated fat, 8% calories from saturated fat, 45 g carbohydrate, 6 g dietary fiber, 1251 mg sodium
Exchanges: 1 1/2 Starch, 3 Lean Meat, 1 Vegetable, 1/2 Fat, 1 Carbohydrate

Low Carb
Per serving: 306 calories, 14 g fat, 4 g saturated fat, 10% calories from saturated fat, 21 g carbohydrate, 5 g dietary fiber, 1243 mg sodium
Exchanges: 1 Starch, 3 Lean Meat, 1 Vegetable, 1 Fat

Vegetarian
Per serving: 292 calories, 6 g fat, 1 g saturated fat, 3% calories from saturated fat, 48 g carbohydrate, 8 g dietary fiber, 742 mg sodium
Exchanges: 1 1/2 Starch, 1 Lean Meat, 2 Vegetable, 1 Carbohydrate

Salad Greens with Kale Croutons

SERVING SIZE: 1/4 of recipe, SERVES: 4

2 cups sliced kale stems
2 Tbsp lemon juice

1/2 tsp freshly ground black pepper
4 cups fresh salad greens

Toss the kale with the lemon juice and black pepper. Refrigerate for two hours. Toss with fresh salad greens and serve.

Per serving: 29 calories, 0 g fat, 0 g saturated fat, 0% calories from saturated fat, 6 g carbohydrate, 1 g dietary fiber, 29 mg sodium
Exchanges: 1 Vegetable

Corn Chowder

SERVING SIZE: 1/6 of recipe, SERVES: 6

	1/2	tsp light olive oil
<C	2	cups finely chopped onion
<C	6	fresh ears corn, kernels shaved off the cob (about 3 1/2 cups)
	1/2	tsp dried thyme
	1	tsp finely diced parsley stalks
	1/4	tsp salt
	1/8	tsp freshly ground black pepper
<C	1	(12 oz) can evaporated skim milk
	2	cups soy milk
	2	Tbsp cornstarch
	4	Tbsp dry white wine (or nonalcoholic chardonnay)
	1/3	cup finely diced Canadian bacon
	1/3	cup finely diced red bell pepper
	1	Tbsp chopped parsley

Vegetarian Option

Omit the Canadian bacon.

1 Warm oil in large saucepan. Sauté onion and 1/2 cup corn until very soft, 12 to 15 minutes. Stir occasionally so the onion doesn't brown. Add thyme, parsley stalks, salt, and pepper.

2 Place onion mixture in a blender and add 1/2 cup evaporated milk. Purée for 2 minutes. Add remaining evaporated milk, and blend another 3 minutes, or until silky smooth. Return to saucepan with the remaining corn.

3 Rinse the blender with soy milk to pick up any flavorful bits and add to the saucepan with the corn. Bring to a boil, then reduce heat, and simmer for 10 minutes.

4 Combine cornstarch with wine to make a slurry. Remove soup from the heat and stir in the slurry. If not serving right away, set aside, and allow to cool. A few minutes before you are ready to serve, return the soup to the heat and stir occasionally until warm and slightly thickened.

5 Warm small frying pan over medium-high heat. Sauté Canadian bacon, pepper, and parsley for 3 minutes. Remove from heat and set aside.

6 Serve the chowder in warm bowls, topping each with 1 heaping Tbsp of Canadian bacon mixture.

<C **To Cut Carb**
<C Onions: reduce to 1 cup and add 1 cup diced celery.
<C Corn: reduce to 5 ears (about 2 1/2 cups).
<C Evaporated skim milk: reduce to 1 cup.

Per serving: 213 calories, 3 g fat, 0 g saturated fat, 0% calories from saturated fat, 40 g carbohydrate, 3 g dietary fiber, 9 mg sodium
Exchanges: 1 1/2 Starch, 1 Vegetable, 1 Fat-free Milk

Low Carb
Per serving: 177 calories, 3 g fat, 0 g saturated fat, 0% calories from saturated fat, 31 g carbohydrate, 3 g dietary fiber, 281 mg sodium
Exchanges: 1 Starch, 1 Vegetable, 1/2 Low-fat Milk

Vegetarian
Per serving: 217 calories, 3 g fat, 0 g saturated fat, 0% calories from saturated fat, 41 g carbohydrate, 4 g dietary fiber, 218 mg sodium
Exchanges: 1 1/2 Starch, 1 Vegetable, 1 Fat-free Milk

Risi Bisi

SERVING SIZE: 1/4 of recipe, SERVES: 4

2/3 cup arborio or pearl rice	1/4 tsp salt
1 1/3 cups low-sodium chicken or vegetable stock (page 473)	1/4 tsp pepper
2 cups frozen petit peas, thawed	2 Tbsp grated Parmesan cheese

1 Bring the rice and stock to a boil in a covered saucepan. Reduce the heat as low as possible and cook, covered, 15 minutes or until the rice is tender.

2 Stir in the peas, salt, pepper, and Parmesan cheese.

Per serving: 101 calories, 2 g fat, 1 g saturated fat, 9% calories from saturated fat, 15 g carbohydrate, 4 g dietary fiber, 323 mg sodium, 6 g protein
Exchanges: 1 Starch, 1/2 Fat

Chinese New Year Fresh Fish & Vegetable Soup

SERVING SIZE: 1/8 of recipe, SERVES: 8

<C   1 lb box rice noodles or flat noodles, like fettuccine
        1 4-oz piece fresh ginger, peeled and slivered
        2 (32 oz) boxes low-sodium vegetable broth
        1 tsp rice vinegar (optional)
        1 tsp sesame oil (optional)
        1 tsp light soy sauce
  1 1/2 lbs firm white fish, such as halibut, orange roughy, or red snapper
+>   1 cup chopped green cabbage
        2 cups fresh snow peas
    1/2 cup shredded carrots
        1 cup sliced baby bok choy
    1/2 cup fresh bean sprouts
    1/4 cup roasted chopped peanuts or sesame seeds

1 Cook noodles according to package directions.

2 Steep ginger in vegetable broth in large pot on medium heat. Add vinegar, sesame oil, and soy sauce. Bring broth to a simmer, and add fish. Simmer and poach fish, covered, until done. Cook for about 9 minutes per inch of thickness. Remove fish to a cutting board or plate.

3 Wash all the fresh vegetables. Add cabbage, snow peas, and carrots to broth, cover, and cook 7 minutes. Meanwhile, use a fork and knife to flake fish into small pieces. Set fish aside. Add bok choy and bean sprouts to other vegetables, cover, and cook 3 more minutes. Gently stir fish into soup.

4 Serve soup over noodles, and garnish with peanuts or sesame seeds.

<C **To Cut Carb**

<C Rice noodles: reduce to 4 oz.
+> Cabbage: increase by 1 cup.

Per serving: 361 calories, 5 g fat, 0.6 g saturated fat, 0% calories from saturated fat, 55 g carbohydrate, 2 g dietary fiber, 575 mg sodium
Exchanges: 3 Starch, 2 Very Lean Meat, 2 Vegetable

Low Carb

Per serving: 208 calories, 4 g fat, 0.5 g saturated fat, 0% calories from saturated fat, 20 g carbohydrate, 12 g dietary fiber, 499 mg sodium
Exchanges: 1/2 Starch, 2 Very Lean Meat, 2 Vegetable

Mesclun Salad with Fruit

SERVING SIZE: 1/6 of recipe, SERVES: 6

Dressing

1/2 tsp arrowroot
1/4 cup dry white wine
  (I prefer nonalcoholic chardonnay)

1/4 cup fresh orange juice
1 tsp rice wine vinegar

Salad

3 oranges, peeled and segmented, reserving any juice for the dressing
6 plums, quartered, pitted, and sliced

1/4 cup thinly sliced red onion
3 Tbsp slivered cilantro
3 cups mesclun (mixed salad greens)

To Prepare the Dressing

1 Combine the arrowroot with the wine in a small saucepan and stir over medium heat until clear and slightly thickened. Stir in the orange juice and vinegar. Set aside to cool.

To Prepare the Salad

2 Place the oranges, plums, onion, and cilantro in a large salad bowl. When the dressing has cooled, pour it over the fruit and toss to mix well. Set-aside until ready to serve.

3 To serve, toss mixed greens and dressed fruit.

Per serving: 68 calories, 0 g fat, 0 g saturated fat, 0% of calories from saturated fat, 17 g carbohydrate, 6 g dietary fiber
Exchanges: 1 Vegetable, 1 Fruit

Asian Pasta Salad

SERVING SIZE: 1/6 of recipe, SERVES: 6

Dressing

1/4 cup rice vinegar
2 Tbsp toasted sesame oil
1 Tbsp reduced-sodium soy sauce
1 tsp finely chopped garlic

1 tsp grated ginger
1/2 tsp crushed Chile peppers
1/4 tsp salt

Salad

2 cups cooked thin noodles
1 cup red grape halves
1 cup fresh or frozen Chinese pea pods, strings removed
1 cup mung bean sprouts
1/2 cup sliced green onions
2 cups salad shrimp or chicken breast pieces
4 large red leaf lettuce leaves

1 Combine the vinegar, oil, soy sauce, garlic, ginger, Chile peppers, and salt in a blender or small bowl and set aside.

2 Toss together the noodles, grapes, pea pods, bean sprouts, green onion, and shrimp or chicken. Pour the dressing over and mix well. Let sit 30 minutes for the flavors to mingle. Serve on beds of red leaf lettuce leaves.

Per serving: 190 calories, 6 g fat, 1 g saturated fat, 5% calories from saturated fat, 21 g carbohydrate, 2 g dietary fiber, 219 mg sodium
Exchanges: 1 Starch, 1 Very Lean Meat, 1 Vegetable, 1 Fat

Leek, Bean, and Spinach Soup

SERVING SIZE: 1/4 recipe, SERVES: 4

3 medium leeks
3 cups low-sodium canned or
   homemade vegetable stock
1 (15 oz) can navy beans (or white beans),
   rinsed and drained

1 tsp dried thyme or 1 Tbsp fresh
1 tsp dried basil or 1 Tbsp fresh
1 cup chopped fresh spinach
2 Tbsp toasted pine nuts

1 Chop white parts of leeks, saving green parts for stock. Add to vegetable broth and bring to a boil. Reduce heat and simmer 10 minutes or until leeks are tender.

2 Pour soup through a strainer. Return liquid to the saucepan and save 1/4 cup leeks for later. Blend the rest with all but 1/2 cup beans using enough soup liquid to cover.

3 Add pureed vegetables, thyme, and basil to the liquid. Bring to a boil and stir in spinach. Add pine nuts, reserved leeks, and beans. Serve immediately while spinach is still nice and green.

Per serving: 199 calories, 4 g fat, 0 g saturated fat, 0% calories from saturated fat, 32 g carbohydrate, 7 g dietary fiber, 389 mg sodium
Exchanges: 1 1/2 Starch, 2 Vegetables, 1/2 Fat

Creamy Pea Soup

SERVING SIZE: 1/4 of recipe, SERVES: 4

1 tsp non-aromatic olive oil	2 cups low-sodium vegetable broth
1/2 cup chopped onion	1/4 tsp salt
1 clove garlic, bashed, and chopped	1/4 tsp white pepper
2 cups frozen peas, thawed	1 (12 oz) can evaporated skim milk
(or corn or broccoli)	1 Tbsp chopped fresh parsley

1 Heat oil in large saucepan. Cook onions, until soft and transparent, 5 to 8 minutes. Add garlic, and cook 1 more minute. Add peas and broth, and bring to a boil. Reduce heat, and cook 3 minutes. Remove from heat.

2 Take a cup of peas out of the broth, and place in a blender. Cover with broth, and puree until smooth. For velvety soup, push the puree through a sieve; otherwise, pour it back into the broth.

3 Season with salt and pepper, and pour in evaporated milk. Heat and serve immediately while still a gorgeous green! Scatter parsley over each bowl, and serve with good whole-wheat bread.

Per serving: 166 calories, 2 g fat, 0 g saturated fat, 0% calories from saturated fat, 26 g carbohydrate, 5 g dietary fiber, 321 mg sodium
Exchanges: 1 Starch, 1 Fat-free Milk

Mixed Greens Salad with Berries

SERVING SIZE: 1/4 of recipe, SERVES: 4

Salad

    4 cups mixed salad greens
1 1/3 cup strawberries, blackberries, blueberries, or raspberries
   1/4 cup roughly chopped toasted walnuts

Dressing

1/4 cup berry vinegar (page 473)   1/4 tsp salt
  2 Tbsp olive oil   1/4 tsp freshly ground black pepper

1 Place the greens, berries, and nuts in a large bowl.

2 Combine the vinegar, oil, salt, and pepper in a small bowl. Pour over the salad and toss well.

Per serving: 89 calories, 6 g fat, 6 g saturated fat, 10% calories from saturated fat, 9 g carbohydrate, 4 g dietary fiber, 146 mg sodium
Exchanges: 1 Vegetable, 1/2 Fruit, 1 Fat

Papaya Salad Bowls with Asian Green Salad

SERVING SIZE: 1 salad bowl, SERVES: 4

Salad

2 ripe papayas   1/4 cup sliced green onions
4 cups mixed salad greens   1/2 cup alfalfa sprouts

Dressing

2 Tbsp rice vinegar   1 Tbsp light soy sauce
1 tsp toasted sesame oil   1/4 tsp grated ginger
2 Tbsp chicken broth

1 Cut the papayas in half lengthwise, remove the seeds, and peel. Place each half on a salad plate.

2 Toss the salad greens, green onions, and alfalfa sprouts together in a bowl.

3 Whisk together the vinegar, sesame oil, chicken broth, soy sauce, and ginger. Pour over the greens and toss to coat well.

4 Top each papaya half with the salad letting it spill over on the sides with the ends of the papaya peeking out.

Per serving: 87 calories, 1 g fat, 0 g saturated fat, 0% calories from saturated fat, 18 g carbohydrate, 4 g dietary fiber, 172 mg sodium
Exchanges: 1 Vegetable, 1 Fruit

Spiced Squash Soup

SERVING SIZE: 1/8 of recipe, SERVES: 8

2 Tbsp butter
2 medium onions, chopped
2 medium carrots, chopped
2 cloves garlic, chopped
1 cup tomato puree
2 fresh, hot chilis, seeded and chopped

2 1/2 lb butternut squash, chopped
5 cups low-sodium, chicken broth (remove fat)
Pepper to taste
Very small amount of salt (optional)
Lime wedges

1 In a large, non-aluminum saucepan, warm the butter over medium heat. Stir in the onions, carrots, and garlic. Cook for 3 minutes then cover the pan. Lower heat and cook for 3 or 4 more minutes, until the vegetables are very tender. Stir in the tomato puree, chilis, butternut squash, and chicken broth. Bring the soup to a simmer and cook for 30 minutes.

2 Mash the squash pieces with a potato masher or the back of the spoon (the soup does not need to be completely smooth), season to taste (optional) and serve. Pass lime wedges to be squeezed into each bowl of soup.

Per serving: 126 calories, 4 g fat, 2 g saturated fat, 14% calories from saturated fat, 23 g carbohydrate, 5 g dietary fiber, 207 mg sodium, 4 g protein, 8 mg cholesterol
Exchanges: 1 Starch, 1 Vegetable, 1/2 Fat

Carrot and Orange Soup

SERVING SIZE: 1/4 of recipe, SERVES: 4

1 Tbsp butter or butter-flavored
  margarine
2 cups copped onions
4 cups peeled and chopped carrots
4 cups low-sodium chicken broth

1 cup orange juice
1/4 tsp salt
1/4 tsp pepper
1 tsp grated orange zest
  (orange part of the peel)

1 Melt the butter, add the onions, cover, and cook over very low heat, stirring often, until very soft, about 25 minutes. Add the carrots and broth, and bring to a boil. Reduce the heat and simmer 30 minutes or until very tender.

2 Puree in batches in a blender. Be very careful to cover the blender with a towel to prevent the hot liquid from overflowing the top. Return to the pan, add the orange juice, salt, pepper, and orange zest, then reheat.

3 Serve immediately.

Per serving: 169 calories, 5 g fat, 2 g saturated fat, 9% calories from saturated fat, 28 g carbohydrate, 5 g dietary fiber, 333 mg sodium
Exchanges: 4 Vegetable, 1/2 Fruit, 1 Fat

Broccoli Endive Salad

SERVING SIZE: 1/6 of recipe, SERVES: 6

1 (1 lb) package broccoli spears
3/4 cup low fat French or Italian salad dressing, divided
1 lb Belgium endive (6 cups)
2 red bell peppers, cut in strips or 2 cup tiny tomatoes
1 Tbsp toasted pine nuts

1 Tip the broccoli into a pot of boiling water for 1 minute. Pour into a colander and run under cold water to stop cooking. Drain thoroughly in the colander then toss with 1/4 cup of the salad dressing.

2 Cut the cone shaped core out of the bottom of each endive. The leaves should separate. Toss gently with another 1/4 cup of the dressing.

3 To compose the salad on a platter or on individual plates, lay the endive leaves around the sides. Set the pepper strips on the leaves. Place the marinated broccoli in the middle and top with the pine nuts. Drizzle the remaining 1/4 cup dressing over all.

Per serving: 96 calories, 3 g fat, 0 g saturated fat, 0% calories from saturated fat, 17 g carbohydrate, 5 g dietary fiber, 272 mg sodium
Exchanges: 2 Vegetable, 1/2 Fat, 1/2 Carbohydrate

Boston Brown Bread

(*Adapted from Fanny Farmer's* Boston School Cooking Cook Book)

SERVING SIZE: 2 slices 1/2-inch thick, SERVES: 24

1 cup rye
1 cup corn meal
1 cup whole-wheat flour
2 tsp baking soda
1 tsp salt

1/2 cup molasses
1 cup plain nonfat yogurt
1 cup 2% milk
1 cup raisins

1 Combine the rye flour, whole-wheat flour, corn meal, soda, and salt in a medium mixing bowl. Stir in the molasses, yogurt, and milk until smooth. Add the raisins.

2 Wash 6 4 1/2-inch-tall tin cans and coat with pan spray. Fill half full with the batter, cover with aluminum foil, and tie with a string. Set a trivet in the bottom of a large pan. Set the cans on the trivet, fill with water half way up the cans, cover and bring to a boil. Reduce the heat and steam 1 1/2 to 2 hours or until a wooden skewer plunged into the middle comes out clean.

3 Take out of the water and cool on a rack. When cool enough to handle, loosen and shake out. Slice each into 8 slices. If you have too much, the bread can be wrapped tightly and frozen for up to 6 months. Serve with Boston Baked Beans (page 370).

Per serving: 94 calories, 1 g fat, 0.3 g saturated fat, 3% calories from saturated fat, 19 g carbohydrate, 1 g dietary fiber, 220 mg sodium
Exchanges: 1 Starch

Gazpacho

SERVING SIZE: 1/4 of recipe, SERVES: 4

3 cups fresh or canned tomatoes
1 cup peeled and seeded cucumber
1 stalk celery roughly chopped
1 cup roughly chopped red or
   yellow bell pepper
2 Tbsp chopped sweet onion
2 Tbsp chopped parsley

2 Tbsp lemon juice
1 clove garlic, finely chopped
1 Tbsp red wine vinegar
1/4 tsp salt
1/4 tsp pepper
1/4 tsp ground cumin
   Tabasco to taste

1 Place the tomatoes, cucumber, celery, and yellow pepper in a processor. Pulse to chop but not puree. Pour into a large bowl and stir in onion, parsley, lemon juice, garlic, vinegar, salt, pepper, cumin, and Tabasco. Thin with tomato juice if need be.

2 Chill 2 hours and serve.

Per serving: 73 calories, 1 g fat, 0 g saturated fat, 0% calories from saturated fat, 16 g carbohydrate, 3 g dietary fiber, 171 mg sodium
Exchanges: 3 Vegetable

Pohole or Sunflower Sprout Salad

SERVING SIZE: 1/6 of recipe, SERVES: 6

Salad

1 lb pohole or 9 oz sunflower sprouts
1 bunch green onions
1/2 cup fresh pomegranate seeds or dried cranberries

Dressing

1 Tbsp tamari
2 Tbsp rice vinegar

1/8 tsp Shanghai Ethmix (page 477)

1 Remove the heavy stalks from the bottom of the pohole and discard. Break the remaining fronds into 1-inch pieces. If you are using sunflower sprouts, wash and cut off any brown parts.

2 Cut off the white parts of the onions and set aside for another use. Wash the green parts, then slice into 1-inch pieces. Combine the pohole or sprouts with the sliced onion greens in a salad bowl.

3 Combine the tamari, rice vinegar, and Shanghai Ethmix and toss with the greens. Sprinkle the pomegranate seeds or dried cranberries over the top.

4 Serve on chilled salad plates.

Per serving: 47 calories, 0 g fat, 0 g saturated fat, 0% calories from saturated fat, 8 g carbohydrate, 0 g dietary fiber, 4 g protein
Exchanges: 2 Vegetable

Fava Bean Soup

SERVING SIZE: 1/6 of recipe, SERVES: 6

1 tsp non-aromatic olive oil	2 cups tightly packed stemmed mustard greens, finely chopped
1/2 lb sweet onions, chopped	1 lb plum tomatoes, peeled, seeded and chopped
2 cloves garlic, bashed and sliced	
1 cup chopped fennel bulb or celery	1/4 tsp black pepper
1 (10 3/4 oz) can tomato puree	1/2 tsp salt
1 quart water	
bouquet garni (page 467)	
1 (19 oz) can fava beans or	
1 lb frozen baby lima beans	

1 Heat the oil in a high-sided skillet on medium high and sauté the onion and garlic 3 minutes. Add the fennel, tomato puree, and water. Bring to a boil, drop in the bouquet garni and beans and simmer 5 minutes.

2 Add the mustard greens and tomatoes, pepper, and salt. Simmer 4 more minutes. Remove the bouquet garni and serve. Chop 1 Tbsp of the tender fennel tops ("feathers") and scatter over the top if you have used the fennel. When celery is used try some finely chopped leaves as a garnish.

Per serving: 167 calories, 2 g fat, 0 g saturated fat, 1 % calories from saturated fat, 32 g carbohydrate, 8 g dietary fiber, 243 mg sodium
Exchanges: 1 Starch, 3 Vegetable, 1/2 Fat

Colorful Fruit-and-Greens Salad

SERVING SIZE: 1/4 of recipe, SERVES: 4

3/4 cup fresh orange juice
  2 Tbsp white wine (or champagne) vinegar
  1 tsp olive oil
1/4 tsp black pepper
    pinch salt
  4 cups mixed salad greens, such as mesclun
  1 orange, peeled and sliced
1/2 fresh fennel, diced
1/2 cup strawberries, sliced
  1 Golden Delicious apple or Bartlett pear, cored and chopped

In large salad bowl, whisk together vinaigrette ingredients. Add salad greens and toss. Arrange fruit and fennel on top of greens and serve.

Per serving: 95 calories, 1 g fat, 0 g saturated fat, 0% calories from saturated fat, 17 g carbohydrate, 4 g dietary fiber, 74 mg sodium
Exchanges: 1 Vegetable, 1 Fruit

Mulligatawny Soup

SERVING SIZE: 1/6 of recipe, SERVES: 6

  4 cups low-sodium chicken
    stock (page 463)
  4 chicken thighs (1/4 lb)
  1 tsp non-aromatic olive oil
  1 medium onion, thinly sliced
  2 cloves garlic, bashed and chopped
1 1/2 cups chopped parsnips (1 large)
  4 tsp curry powder
1/2 cup dried red or brown lentils

  1 bay leaf
  1 lb broccoli, florets removed, stems peeled and chopped
1/4 tsp salt
<C 1 cup cooked long-grain white rice
3/4 cup Graham's coconut cream (page 465)

Place the thighs in a high-sided skillet and pour the stock over them. Cover, bring to a boil, reduce the heat, and simmer 35 minutes. Remove the thighs to a plate and pour the stock into a fat strainer. Set aside to use in step 2.

2 Heat the oil in the same skillet on medium high. Sauté the onion for 1 minute, add the garlic and curry and cook 2 more minutes. Stir in the parsnips, lentils, and bay leaf. Defat the stock and add enough water to make 4 cups. Pour into the pan, cover, bring to a boil, reduce the heat and simmer 15 minutes or until the parsnips are soft. Add the broccoli florets and stems and simmer 5 more minutes.

3 Remove the skin and bones from the thighs and add the meat to the soup. Stir in the rice and 1/2 cup of the coconut cream. Heat to serving temperature and ladle into bowls. Top each with a dollop of the remaining coconut cream.

<C **To Cut Carb**
<C Rice: reduce to 2/3 cup and substitute long-grain brown rice.

Per serving: 281 calories, 9 g fat, 3 g saturated fat, 9% calories from saturated fat, 31 g carbohydrate, 8 g dietary fiber, 239 mg sodium
Exchanges: 1 1/2 Starch, 2 Lean Meat, 1 Vegetable, 1/2 Fat

Low Carb
Per serving: 271 calories, 9 g fat, 3 g saturated fat, 10% calories from saturated fat, 29 g carbohydrate, 8 g dietary fiber, 239 mg sodium
Exchanges: 1 1/2 Starch, 2 Lean Meat, 1 Vegetable, 1/2 Fat

Cold Asparagus Salad

SERVING SIZE: 3/4 cup, SERVES: 4

2 lb fresh asparagus
1 tsp extra virgin olive oil
1 Tbsp red wine vinegar

1/4 tsp salt
1/4 tsp freshly ground black pepper
2 Tbsp chopped fresh dill

1 Wash and snap ends off the asparagus. Cut diagonally in 1-inch pieces. Steam over boiling water 3–5 minutes, until tender but crisp. Plunge into cold water to stop cooking. Drain and lay on a platter.

2 Drizzle oil and vinegar and scatter salt, pepper, and dill over the top. Toss gently and let sit for 1/2 hour. Serve at room temperature or chilled.

Per serving: 32 calories, 1 g fat, 0 g saturated fat, 0% calories from saturated fat, 4 g carbohydrate, 1 g dietary fiber, 150 mg sodium
Exchanges: 1 Vegetable

Cucumber Raita Salad

SERVING SIZE: 1/4 recipe, SERVES: 4

1 English cucumber	1 Tbsp lime juice
3 green onions, finely chopped	1/2 tsp ground cumin
1 Tbsp chopped cilantro	1/2 tsp ground coriander
1 Tbsp chopped spearmint	1/4 tsp salt
1/2 cup plain low-fat yogurt	1/4 tsp pepper

1 Wash the cucumber, and peel leaving alternating stripes of green skin and white flesh. Cut lengthwise into long thin slices, then across into matchsticks. Combine with green onion, cilantro, and mint in a large bowl.

2 Whisk yogurt, lime juice, cumin, coriander, salt, and pepper together to make dressing. Toss with vegetables, and let sit for 10 minutes to marinate. Serve with a hot dish to cool your burning mouth!

Per serving: 38 calories, 1 g fat, 0 g saturated fat, 0% calories from saturated fat, 6 g carbohydrate, 1 g dietary fiber, 166 mg sodium
Exchanges: 1 Vegetable

String Wing Bean Salad

SERVING SIZE: 1 cup, SERVES: 4

Salad

 1 lb green beans or wing beans, tipped, tailed, and cut in half
1/4 tsp salt
1/4 tsp freshly ground black pepper
1/8 tsp ground allspice
 4 fresh Italian plum tomatoes, such as Roma, cut lengthwise into eighths
1/4 cup roughly chopped stuffed green olives
 6 fresh basil leaves, finely sliced (1 Tbsp)
 2 green onions, sliced into 1/4-inch pieces (1/4 cup)

Glaze

1/4 cup balsamic or red wine vinegar   1/2 tsp water
1/4 tsp arrowroot

To Prepare the Salad

1 Place the beans in a large vegetable steamer and sprinkle with the salt, pepper, and allspice. Cover and steam for 5 minutes.

2 Combine the tomatoes, olives, basil, and onions in a large serving bowl and set aside.

To Prepare the Glaze

3 Combine the arrowroot with 1/2 tsp of water to make a slurry. Pour the vinegar into a small saucepan and add the slurry. Stir over medium heat until clear, glossy, and slightly thickened.

To Serve

4 Add the cooked beans to the salad bowl and toss with the warm vinegar glaze. Serve immediately.

Per serving: 49 calories, 1 g fat, 0 g saturated fat, 0% calories from saturated fat, 9 g carbohydrate, 4 g dietary fiber, 1 g protein
Exchanges: 2 Vegetable

Kale and Apple Soup

SERVING SIZE: 1/4 of recipe, SERVES: 4

2 cups low-sodium vegetable broth
1 lb kale, carefully washed and
    stems removed (4 cups)
1/4 tsp salt
1/4 tsp ground cumin

1 tsp brown sugar
1 small Granny Smith apple,
    cored and chopped (1 cup)
1/2 cup low-fat plain yogurt

1 Bring broth to a boil in a large saucepan. Add kale, cover, and simmer 8 minutes. Blend cooked kale with a little of the liquid until smooth. Return to the pan with the rest of the liquid.

2 Season with salt, cumin, and brown sugar. Stir in chopped apple, and simmer another 8 minutes. Remove from heat, and stir in the yogurt.

Per serving: 77 calories, 1 g fat, 0 g saturated fat, 0% calories from saturated fat, 15 g carbohydrate, 2 g dietary fiber, 370 mg sodium
Exchanges: 1 Carbohydrate

Spinach Salad for Spring and Summer

SERVING SIZE: 2 cups, SERVES: 2

  - 3 cups baby spinach leaves, well washed and dried
  - 1 cup seasonal fresh vegetables or fruit of your choice (raw sugar snap peas, strawberry halves, blueberries, or peach slices)
  - 3 Tbsp low-fat vinaigrette salad dressing
- 1/4 tsp black pepper

Place the spinach and seasonal fruit or vegetable in a large bowl. The more colors you add to your diet, the more cancer fighting nutrients you'll get. Toss with the dressing and serve.

Per serving (with strawberries): 59 calories, 2 g fat, 0 g saturated fat, 0% calories from saturated fat, 10 g carbohydrate, 6 g dietary fiber, 250 mg sodium
Exchanges: 2 Vegetable, 1/2 Fat

East African Peanut Soup

SERVING SIZE: 1/6 of recipe, SERVES: 6

- 1/2 tsp non-aromatic olive oil
- 1 onion, roughly chopped
- 1 red bell pepper, finely chopped
- 2 carrots, peeled and thinly sliced
- <C 3/4 cup long-grain white rice
- 2 cloves garlic, peeled, bashed and chopped
- 1 generous Tbsp finely chopped ginger root
- 5 cups water
- 1/2 cup dry roasted, low-sodium or unsalted peanuts
- 1 (6 oz) can tomato paste
- 1/2 tsp crushed red chilis
- 1/2 tsp salt
- 2 Tbsp chopped parsley

Heat the oil in a high-sided skillet or large saucepan on medium. Fry the onion 1 minute. Add the peppers and carrots and cook for 10 minutes more. Stir in the rice, garlic, and ginger and cook for 1 minute to release the flavors and turn the rice a chalky color. Pour in the water and cook until the carrots and rice are tender, about 15 minutes.

2 Add the peanuts, tomato paste, crushed chilis and salt. Stir with a whisk to dissolve the tomato paste. Bring to a boil, reduce the heat and simmer 3 minutes. Pour into a blender (in two batches if need be) and whiz 1 to 2 minutes or until the soup is smooth, thick, and a medium orange in color. Return to the pan and reheat.

3 Serve in preheated bowls with the chopped parsley scattered over the top.

<C **To Cut Carb**

<C Rice: reduce to 1/2 cup of brown rice and cook for 35 minutes. In step 1 you may need to add an extra cup of water.

Per serving: 213 calories, 7 g fat, 1 g saturated fat, 5% calories from saturated fat, 34 g carbohydrate, 4 g dietary fiber, 226 mg sodium
Exchanges: 1 1/2 Starch, 2 Vegetable, 1 Fat

Low Carb

Per serving: 186 calories, 7 g fat, 1 g saturated fat, 6% calories from saturated fat, 27 g carbohydrate, 5 g dietary fiber, 226 mg sodium
Exchanges: 1 Starch, 2 Vegetable, 1 1/2 Fat

Vegetable Pasta Salad

SERVING SIZE: 1/4 of recipe, SERVES: 4

1 cup cooked orzo pasta	1 cup chopped fresh spinach
1 cup lightly steamed asparagus, cut the same size as the pasta, or peas	1 cup small cherry tomatoes (optional)
1/2 cup chopped red bell pepper or carrots	1/4 cup low-fat vinaigrette dressing (page 132)
1/2 cup sliced green onions	2 Tbsp grated Parmesan cheese
1/2 cup chopped yellow summer squash	

1 Combine the pasta, asparagus, peppers, onions, squash, spinach, tomatoes, dressing, and Parmesan in a large bow. Toss to coat with the dressing. Serve with grilled chicken or fish at a barbecue or picnic.

Per serving: 114 calories, 2 g fat, 1 g saturated fat, 8% calories from saturated fat, 20 g carbohydrate, 3 g dietary fiber, 204 mg sodium
Exchanges: 1/2 Starch, 2 Vegetable, 1/2 Fat

Curried Butternut Soup

SERVING SIZE: 1/4 of recipe, SERVES: 4

```
  1  tsp non-aromatic olive oil
1/2  cup chopped onion
  1  Tbsp mild curry powder
  1  apple, peeled, cored, and grated
  2  cups roasted butternut squash (or other winter squash or pumpkin)
  2  cups low-sodium chicken or vegetable stock (pages 463, 473)
1/4  tsp salt
```

1 Heat oil in large saucepan. Fry onion and curry powder until onion is soft but not brown, about 5 minutes. Stir in apple and squash.

2 Pour in stock, bring to a boil, reduce heat, and simmer 15 minutes. Season with salt. If you like creamy soup, pour into a blender and purée. (When blending hot liquids, be sure to cover the top with a towel.)

Per serving: 83 calories, 2 g fat, 1 g saturated fat, 10% calories from saturated fat, 14 g carbohydrate, 4 g dietary fiber, 215 mg sodium
Exchanges: 1 Carbohydrate

Gold Medal Curry Soup

SERVING SIZE: 1/4 of recipe, SERVES: 4

```
  1  small white or yellow onion, chopped      1  cup nonfat plain yogurt
1 1/2  tsp curry powder                        1  (14 oz) can vegetable broth
  1  lb frozen or fresh cauliflower florets  3/4  tsp black pepper
1/2  cup water                                1/2  tsp salt
```

Cilantro puree

```
1/3  cup tightly packed cilantro leaves and stems
     Juice of one lemon
  1  tsp extra-virgin olive oil
     (Or garnish soup instead with 1/4 cup slivered dried apricots and
     fresh pomegranate seeds)
```

1 Spray bottom and sides of a medium pot with vegetable cooking spray. Place onion and curry powder in pot and cover. Sweat on low heat for 6–7 minutes, softening onion and releasing curry powders aroma. Add cauliflower and water, and cook on medium heat until cauliflower is done, about 10–12 minutes for frozen and less time for fresh. Transfer pot contents to a blender and puree until very smooth.

2 Place yogurt in the pot and slowly whisk in vegetable broth until a smooth emulsion forms. Slowly whisk in cauliflower puree and black pepper, blending well. Heat on low until warm enough to serve, but do not bring to a boil, as yogurt may separate.

3 To make cilantro puree, blend all ingredients until smooth in a blender or small food processor.

4 Divide soup among four bowls and drizzle with cilantro puree. Or, instead of cilantro puree, place dried apricots and fresh pomegranate seeds on the bottom of each bowl, and pour the soup over them.

Per serving: 90 calories, 2 g fat, 1 g saturated fat, 4% calories from saturated fat, 15 g carbohydrate, 2 g dietary fiber, 452 mg sodium, 6 g protein, 1 mg cholesterol
Exchanges: 3 Vegetable

Chilled Watermelon Soup

SERVING SIZE: 1/4 of recipe, SERVES: 4

4 cups watermelon pieces
1 cup orange juice

1 Tbsp lime juice
1 tsp lime zest or chopped fresh mint

1 Blend or process watermelon pieces until smooth. Stir in orange juice, lime juice, and lime zest. Chill thoroughly and serve or keep cold in an insulated cup to eat later.

Per serving: 80 calories, 1 g fat, 0 g saturated fat, 0% calories from saturated fat, 19 g carbohydrate, 1 g dietary fiber, 3 mg sodium
Exchanges: 1 1/2 Fruit

Lima Bean Soup with Carrots

SERVING SIZE: 1/4 of recipe, SERVES: 4

1 tsp non-aromatic olive oil
1 cup chopped onions
1/4 lb Canadian bacon, cut
   in 1/2-inch dice
1 cup sliced carrots
2 cups fresh or frozen baby lima beans

3 cups low-sodium chicken or
   vegetable broth
2 cups chopped fresh or
   1/2 package frozen spinach
1/4 tsp salt
1/4 tsp pepper

1 Heat oil in large saucepan. Sauté onions 2 minutes. Add bacon and continue
cooking until it browns a little. Stir in carrots and lima beans.
Pour in broth, bring to a boil, reduce heat, and simmer 20 minutes.

2 Add spinach, salt, and pepper, and simmer 5 minutes longer.

Per serving: 224 calories, 3 g fat, 1 g saturated fat, 4% calories from saturated
fat, 31 g carbohydrate, 11 g dietary fiber, 619 mg sodium
Exchanges: 1 1/2 Starch, 1 Lean Meat, 2 Vegetable

Italian Bread with
Roasted Vegetables

SERVING SIZE: 1 slice, SERVES: 12

1 cup water
1 tsp dry yeast
1 tsp olive oil
1/2 tsp dried oregano
1/2 tsp dried basil
1/2 tsp salt

2 to 2 3/4 cups all purpose flour
1 sweet onion, cut in 1-inch pieces
1 red bell pepper, cut in 1-inch pieces
2 cloves garlic, peel on
6 sun-dried tomato halves, cut in strips
1/16 tsp kosher or ground sea salt

1 Sprinkle the yeast over the warm water in a large bowl and let set until
creamy, about 10 minutes. Stir in the oregano, basil, and salt. Add 2 cups of
the flour and mix thoroughly, adding more flour until you have a nice
medium-firm dough. Turn out onto a floured surface and knead until the

dough is smooth and springy, at least 5 minutes. Place the dough in an oiled bowl, cover, and allow to rise until doubled in volume, about 1 1/2 to 2 hours.

2 Preheat the oven to 425°F. Toss the onions, peppers, and the unpeeled garlic with 1/2 tsp of the oil in a baking dish. Sprinkle with 1/8 tsp of the salt. Bake 25 minutes or until the vegetables are tender and the garlic is soft. Cool before using. Peel the garlic and cut into small pieces.

3 Preheat the oven to 400°F. Spread the dough into a large rectangle. Scatter the vegetable mixture evenly over the top. Add the sun-dried tomato pieces and fold in the sides. Knead the vegetables into the dough until they are well distributed throughout. Pat the dough to a greased 10-inch skillet or pie pan. Allow it to rise about 30 minutes.

4 Make deep dimples in the dough with your fingertips. Drizzle the remaining 1/2 tsp oil over the top and sprinkle with the kosher salt. Bake 30 minutes or until golden brown. Cool on a rack before cutting.

Per wedge: 116 calories, 1 g fat, 0 g saturated fat, 0 % calories from saturated fat, 24 g carbohydrate, 2 g dietary fiber, 91 mg sodium, 3 g protein
Exchanges: 1 1/2 Starch

Arugula Salad with Yogurt Goat Cheese Dressing

SERVING SIZE: 1/4 of recipe, SERVES: 4

4 cups washed and trimmed arugula   1 oz soft goat cheese
8 oz low-fat plain yogurt

1 Mound the arugula on each of 4 salad plates. Combine the yogurt and goat cheese. Divide the dressing among the arugula salads.

Per serving: 60 calories, 3 g fat, 2 g saturated fat, 30% calories from saturated fat, 5 g carbohydrate, 0 g dietary fiber, 71 mg sodium
Exchanges: 1/2 Fat, 1/2 Carbohydrate

Make Ahead Salad

SERVING SIZE: 1/4 of recipe, SERVES: 4

1 (15 oz) can navy or other
   white beans
2 tsp chopped fresh chives

2 Tbsp low-fat vinaigrette
   salad dressing
4 cups salad greens

1 Drain and rinse the beans. Combine them with the chives and salad dressing and store in the refrigerator.

2 Spoon over the salad greens for a quick, flavorful, nutritious salad.

Per serving: 119 calories, 1 g fat, 0 g saturated fat, 0% calories from saturated fat, 22 g carbohydrate, 6 g dietary fiber, 75 mg sodium, 6 g protein
Exchanges: 1 Starch, 1 Vegetable

Soba and Vegetable Salad

SERVING SIZE: 1/6 of recipe, SERVES: 6

Salad

<C 8 oz dry soba noodles
   1 (1 lb) package frozen broccoli florets, steamed and cooled
<C 1 cup thawed peas
   6 green onions, trimmed and cut in 1/4-inch slices (1/2 cup)

Dressing

1 Tbsp lime juice
2 Tbsp rice vinegar
2 Tbsp toasted sesame oil

1 Tbsp light soy sauce
2 tsp grated or finely chopped ginger root

Garnish

  2 Tbsp toasted sesame seeds
1/4 cup chopped cilantro

1 Cook the noodles until tender but still firm. Drain and cool quickly in ice water then drain again. Combine the noodles with the broccoli, peas, and green onions.

2 Stir together the lime juice, vinegar, oil, soy sauce, and ginger. Pour over the noodles and vegetables and toss to mix thoroughly. Chill for at least 30 minutes.

3 Serve topped with the sesame seeds and cilantro.

<c **To Cut Carb**

<c Soba noodles: reduce to 6 oz dry weight and use recipe as a side dish.
<c Peas: reduce to 3/4 cup.

Per serving: 236 calories, 6 g fat, 1 g saturated fat, 4% calories from saturated fat, 34 g carbohydrate, 6 g dietary fiber, 445 mg sodium
Exchanges: 2 Starch, 1 Vegetable, 1 Fat

Low Carb
Per serving: 193 calories, 7 g fat, 1 g saturated fat, 5% calories from saturated fat, 27 g carbohydrate, 5 g dietary fiber, 377 mg sodium
Exchanges: 1 1/2 Starch, 1 Vegetable, 1 Fat

Make-You-Feel-Better Tomato Soup

SERVING SIZE: 1/4 of recipe, SERVES: 4

1 tsp olive oil	1 (28 oz) can no-salt-added diced
1/2 large yellow onion, chopped	tomatoes
1 clover garlic, crushed	1 cup water
1 tsp dried basil	1/4 tsp salt
1 tsp oregano	

1 In a medium saucepan, heat the oil. Sauté the onions, garlic, basil, and oregano for 5 minutes. Add tomatoes, water, and salt. Bring to a boil, reduce heat, and simmer for 15 minutes.

Per serving: 63 calories, 1 g fat, 0 g saturated fat, 0% calories from saturated fat, 9 g carbohydrate, 2 g dietary fiber, 181 mg sodium, 2 g protein, 0 mg cholesterol
Exchanges: 2 Vegetable

Caraway Cabbage Soup

SERVING SIZE: 1/4 of recipe, SERVES: 4

1 tsp non-aromatic olive oil
1 cup chopped onions
1 russet potato, peeled and cut
 in 1/2-inch dice
4 cups shredded cabbage

1 tsp caraway seeds
4 cups low-sodium vegetable or
 chicken broth
1/4 tsp salt
1/4 tsp pepper

1 Heat the oil in a large saucepan on medium high. Cook the onion until it begins to wilt, 2 minutes. Add the potatoes, cabbage, and caraway seeds, and stir fry 1 minute.

2 Pour in the broth and season with salt and pepper. Bring to a boil, reduce the heat and simmer 1 hour. Serve with a piece of crusty rye bread.

Per serving: 103 calories, 2 g fat, 0 g saturated fat, 0% calories from saturated fat, 19 g carbohydrate, 3 g dietary fiber, 222 mg sodium
Exchanges: 1/2 Starch, 2 Vegetable

Red Grapefruit Salad

SERVING SIZE: 1/4 of recipe, SERVES: 4

2 whole red grapefruit (2 cups)
1 cup fresh or canned orange segments

1 cup peeled kiwi wedges
1/4 cup chopped chives

1 Cut the red grapefruit in half. Remove the fruit from the shell whole by cutting around the outside of the fruit with a spoon. Separate the segments and cut each in half. You should have 2 cups.

2 Combine the red grapefruit with the orange segments and kiwi wedges. Spoon into the shells and top with a crossed sprig of chives or a chive flower. Serve with pork or chicken.

Per serving: 112 calories, 1 g fat, 0 g saturated fat, 0% calories from saturated fat, 26 g carbohydrate, 5 g dietary fiber, 2 mg sodium
Exchanges: 2 Fruit

Cucumber Salad with Tomatoes

SERVING SIZE: 1/4 of recipe, SERVES: 4

2 cups diced cucumber
1 cup seeded and diced tomatoes
1/4 cup chopped sweet onions

2 tsp chopped fresh dill weed
    or 1/2 tsp dried
1/2 cup low-fat vinaigrette salad dressing

1 | Toss together cucumbers, tomatoes, onions, dill, and salad dressing. Chill 1 hour and serve.

Per serving: 65 calories, 5 g fat, 1 g saturated fat, 14% calories from saturated fat, 6 g carbohydrate, 1 g dietary fiber, 103 mg sodium
Exchanges: 1 Vegetable, 1 Fat

Caesar Salad with a Difference

SERVING SIZE: 1/4 of recipe, SERVES: 4

Croutons

2 cups whole-wheat bread cubes

Olive oil cooking spray

Dressing

1/2 cup plain low-fat yogurt
  2 tsp Dijon mustard
1 1/2 Tbsp balsamic vinegar

3 cloves garlic, chopped
2 anchovy fillets, chopped (optional)

Salad

8 cups torn romaine lettuce
1/4 cup grated Parmesan cheese
1 lb chicken breasts, cooked, and sliced (optional)

1 | Preheat oven to 350°F. Scatter bread cubes in a single layer on a baking sheet. Coat lightly with olive oil spray and bake 15 minutes.

2 | Whisk together yogurt, mustard, vinegar, garlic, and anchovies if you use them. Pour over the romaine lettuce and toss. Scatter the cheese on top. Divide among 4 plates and serve or lay chicken slices on top to make a full meal.

Per serving (with chicken breast, no anchovies): 277 calories, 6g fat, 2 g saturated fat, 6% calories from saturated fat, 22 g carbohydrate, 4 g dietary fiber, 384 mg sodium
Exchanges: 1 Starch, 4 Very Lean Meat, 1 Vegetable, 1/2 Fat

Side Dishes

Black Beans with Corn and Garlic

SERVING SIZE: 1/4 of recipe, SERVES: 4

1 (15 oz) can reduced sodium black beans, drained
2 cloves garlic, bashed and chopped
1 cup frozen corn
2 Roma tomatoes, chopped

1 jalapeno chili, chopped with seeds if you like it hot, without, if not
1/8 tsp cayenne pepper
1/2 tsp ground cumin
1 tsp mild chili powder
1/4 cup chopped cilantro

1 Rinse the beans and whiz half in a blender with the garlic. Add a little water to get them going.

2 Pour into a saucepan and add the remaining beans, corn, tomatoes, jalapeno, cayenne pepper, cumin, and chili powder. Heat on medium, stirring occasionally to keep from sticking. Stir in the cilantro.

3 Serve as a side dish or on hot tortillas with a salad for lunch or light dinner.

Per serving: 91 calories, 0 g fat, 0 g saturated fat, 0% calories from saturated fat, 21 g carbohydrates, 6 g dietary fiber, 203 mg sodium
Exchanges: 1 Starch, 1 Vegetable

Steamed Broccoli Sprouts

SERVING SIZE: 1/4 of recipe, SERVES: 4

4 cups broccoli sprouts
1/4 tsp salt

1 Tbsp lemon or lime juice

1 Spread the sprouts in a large steamer and season with salt. Sprinkle lemon juice over the top and steam, covered, 2 or 3 minutes or until they just begin to wilt.

Per serving: 17 calories, 0 g fat, 0 g saturated fat, 0% calories from saturated fat, 3 g carbohydrate, 1 g dietary fiber, 149 mg sodium
Exchanges: 1 Vegetable

Cauliflower and Carrots with Fennel Seeds

SERVING SIZE: 1/6 recipe, SERVES: 6

2 heads cauliflower, broken or cut into florets (6 cups)
1 tsp fennel seeds
1/4 tsp salt
6 medium carrots, peeled and cut on the diagonal into 1/4-inch slices (2 cups)

1 Place the cauliflower florets on the bottom platform of a two-tiered steamer. Sprinkle fennel seeds and salt over the top. Place the carrots in the second platform and stack it on top. Put steamer racks over the boiling water, cover, and steam 8 minutes for crisp-tender vegetables or 12 minutes if you like them softer. If you do not have a two-tiered steamer, steam the vegetables in two batches, keeping the cauliflower warm while the carrots cook.

2 Combine the cauliflower and carrots and serve.

Per serving: 66 calories, 1 g fat, 0 g saturated fat, 9% of calories from fat, 14 g carbohydrate, 6 g dietary fiber
Exchanges: 3 Vegetable

Grilled Pineapple

SERVING SIZE: 2 slices, SERVES: 4

2 Tbsp light soy sauce   8 1/2-inch slices fresh or canned pineapple
1/2 tsp toasted sesame oil

1 Preheat the barbecue or broiler. Stir the soy sauce and sesame oil together and brush lightly on the pineapple slices.

2 Grill about 2 or 3 minutes per side or until brown and bubbly. Serve with barbecued pork or chicken or cut in chunks as an appetizer.

Per serving: 66 calories, 1 g fat, 0 g saturated fat, 0% calories from saturated fat, 15 g carbohydrate, 1 g dietary fiber, 286 mg sodium
Exchanges: 1 Fruit

Artichokes, Asparagus and Peas with Tarragon

SERVING SIZE: 1/4 of recipe, SERVES: 4

1/2 cup low-sodium chicken or
    vegetable broth (pages 463, 473)
1 (8 oz) package frozen artichoke
    hearts
1 cup asparagus pieces
1 cup fresh or frozen peas

1 tsp dried tarragon
1/4 tsp salt
1/4 tsp pepper
1/2 tsp arrowroot or cornstarch mixed
    with 1 Tbsp broth (slurry)
2 Tbsp Parmesan cheese

1 Heat the broth in a large skillet. Cook the artichoke hearts 5 minutes. Add the asparagus and peas; cook 3 minutes more or until the vegetables are tender.

2 Season with the tarragon, salt, and pepper and stir in the slurry. Heat until thickened and glossy. Scatter Parmesan over the top and serve.

Per serving: 89 calories, 1 g fat, 1 g saturated fat, 10% calories from saturated fat, 14 g carbohydrate, 6 g dietary fiber, 306 mg sodium
Exchanges: 1/2 Starch, 2 Vegetable

Pureed Roasted Turnips

SERVING SIZE: 1/4 of recipe, SERVES: 4

6 medium turnips, peeled and cut in quarters

1 Preheat the oven to 375°F. Set the wedges in a baking pan and coat lightly with olive oil cooking spray. Roast 30 minutes or until soft.

2 Puree the turnips in a processor until smooth. Refrigerate or freeze until needed.

Per serving: 33 calories, 0 g fat, 0 g saturated fat, 0% calories from saturated fat, 8 g carbohydrate, 2 g dietary fiber, 78 mg sodium
Exchanges: 1 Vegetable

Buttermilk Mashed Potatoes with a Butterlike Sauce

SERVING SIZE: 1/4 of recipe, SERVES: 4

Mashed Potatoes

<C   4 medium russet potatoes, peeled and quartered
<C 1/2 to 3/4 cup buttermilk

1/4 tsp salt
1/4 tsp white pepper
1/8 tsp nutmeg

Sauce

<C   2 cups low sodium chicken broth (page 463)
     pinch saffron or turmeric
<C 1/4 tsp salt
    1 Tbsp arrowroot or cornstarch mixed with 2 Tbsp low sodium chicken broth (slurry)
    pinch chopped fresh chives (optional)

1 Cook the potatoes in boiling water until very soft, 20 to 30 minutes. Drain, return the potatoes to the pot, put a towel over the top, and let them sit on very low heat for 15 minutes to dry out.

2 Transfer to an ovenproof bowl, add 1/2 cup of the buttermilk, salt, pepper, and nutmeg and mash by hand or with an electric mixer until smooth. Add more buttermilk if they are too dry. Keep warm in the oven.

3 Boil the stock in an open pan until reduced by half, about 10 minutes. Add the saffron and salt. Remove from the heat and stir in the slurry. Return to the heat to thicken and clear.

4 Divide the potatoes among 4 hot plates. Make a well in the middle and fill with the sauce, allowing it to spill over just a little. Scatter fresh chives over the top and serve with a nice piece of fish or chicken.

<C To Cut Carb

<C Potatoes: reduce to 2 medium.
<C Buttermilk: reduce to 1/4 cup.
<C Chicken broth: reduce to 1 cup.

<C Salt: reduce to 1/8 tsp.
<C Cornstarch: reduce to 2 tsp and 1 water.

Per serving: 136 calories, 1 g fat, 0 g saturated fat, 0% calories from saturated fat, 29 g carbohydrate, 2 g dietary fiber, 347 mg sodium
Exchanges: 2 Starch

Low Carb

Per serving: 67 calories, 0 g fat. 0 g saturated fat, 0% calories from saturated fat, 14 g carbohydrate, 1 g dietary fiber, 239 mg sodium
Exchanges: 1 Starch

Parsnips Mashed with Carrots and Sesame Seeds

SERVING SIZE: 1/4 of recipe, SERVES: 4

<C   1 lb parsnips
<C   1 lb carrots
    1/4 tsp salt
1/4 tsp pepper
  3 Tbsp sesame seeds

1   Preheat the oven to 350°F. Peel and slice the carrots and parsnips. Steam over boiling water for 15 minutes or until very tender. Mash roughly and stir in the salt and pepper.

2   Place into a small baking dish, scatter the sesame seeds over the top and bake until the seeds are golden and the vegetables are hot clear through, about 20 minutes.

<C **To Cut Carb**

<C Portions: Clearly this vegetable "pie" adds up to about 32 oz or 8 oz per portion. As such, it should be served with a nice portion of fish or poultry and some other very low carbohydrate vegetable. Or the portion could simply be halved.

<C Carrots: reduce to 8 oz.

<C Parsnips: reduce to 8 oz.

Per serving: 158 calories, 4 g fat, 1 g saturated fat, 5% calories from saturated fat, 30 g carbohydrate, 9 g dietary fiber, 216 mg sodium
Exchanges: 1 Starch, 2 Vegetable, 1/2 Fat

Low Carb

Per serving: 99 calories, 4 g fat, 1 g saturated fat, 9% calories from saturated fat, 16 g carbohydrate, 4 g dietary fiber, 181 mg sodium
Exchanges: 1 Starch, 2 Vegetable, 1/2 Fat

Tofu and Mushrooms in a Spicy Miso Sauce

SERVING SIZE: 1/6 of recipe, SERVES: 6

1 1/2 tsp light olive oil
 1 large clove garlic, peeled, bashed, and chopped
 1/2 onion, thinly sliced
1 1/2 cups plus 2 Tbsp dashi broth (see attached note)
 1/4 tsp dried basil
 2 tsp hatcho miso, mixed with 1 Tbsp water
 1/4 tsp Shanghai Ethmix (page 477)
10 1/2 oz extra-firm light tofu, cut into 1-inch cubes
 1/4 lb fresh shiitake mushrooms, stemmed and halved
 1/2 lb large white mushrooms, cut into 3 thick slices top to bottom
 1/4 tsp salt
 1/4 tsp freshly ground black pepper
 1 Tbsp fresh lemon juice
 1 Tbsp chopped fresh parsley
 4 tsp arrowroot

1 Warm 1/2 tsp of the oil in a medium saucepan over medium-high heat. Sauté the garlic and onion for 5 minutes, or until the onion is soft but not browned. Stir in 1 1/2 cups of the dashi broth and the basil. Simmer for 3 minutes.

2 Strain the mixture and return the liquid to the saucepan, discarding the onion. Add the thinned miso, Shanghai Ethmix, and tofu. Set aside.

3 Warm the remaining tsp of oil in a large frying pan over medium-high heat. Add the shiitake and white mushrooms, sprinkle with the salt and pepper, and cook for 2 minutes. Sprinkle the lemon juice over the top and cook for an additional 2 minutes. Stir in the parsley then add the tofu and dashi broth mixture.

4 Combine the arrowroot with the remaining 2 Tbsp of dashi broth to make a slurry. Remove the frying pan from the heat and add the slurry, then return to the heat and stir until thickened and glossy.

5 Serve on a warmed plate with 2 taro and chili cakes, a portion of bok choy, and a wedge of kabocha squash.

Per serving: 67 calories, 2 g fat, 0 g saturated fat, 0% calories from saturated fat, 8 g carbohydrate, 1 g dietary fiber, 4 g protein
Exchanges: 2 Vegetable, 1/2 Fat

Couscous with Peppers

SERVING SIZE: 1/6 of recipe, Servers 6

3 cups low-sodium chicken or vegetable stock (pages 463, 473)
1/4 tsp almond extract
1 cup large-grain couscous
3 Tbsp finely diced red bell pepper
3 Tbsp finely diced yellow bell pepper
3 Tbsp finely diced red onion
2 Tbsp lime juice (1 lime)

1/2 tsp finely chopped cilantro stems
1 tsp arrowroot
2 tsp water
1/8 tsp salt
1 Tbsp finely sliced cilantro leaves
1/2 cup fruity white wine (I prefer nonalcoholic blanc)

1 Combine stock and almond extract in large saucepan, and bring to a boil. Toss in any vegetable or fish trimmings left over from preparing the main course. Simmer 10 minutes or so. Strain, discard the trimmings, and return stock to the pan.

2 Stir couscous into stock, and simmer 20 minutes, or until fluffy and dry. If the couscous is runny, drain excess liquid. If the couscous is too dry, add up to 1/2 cup of water or dealcoholized wine. (If you only have alcoholic wine, boil off the alcohol before adding it or the dish will be bitter.)

3 While the couscous is cooking, combine peppers and onion in a bowl. Add lime juice and cilantro stems and mix.

4 In another small bowl, mix arrowroot with 2 tsp water to make a slurry.

5 When couscous is done, stir in the slurry. (Add the slurry while the couscous is still very hot.) Add the pepper mixture and salt, and turn off the heat, and cover the pan tightly to keep warm.

6 To serve, stir cilantro and wine into the couscous.

Per serving: 144 calories, 2 g fat, 1 g saturated fat, 6% of calories from saturated fat, 26 g carbohydrate, 2 g dietary fiber
Exchanges: 1 Starch, 2 Vegetable, 1/2 Fat

Braised Celery Hearts

SERVING SIZE: 1 celery heart, SERVES: 4

1 tsp olive oil
2 cups chopped sweet onion
3 Tbsp tomato paste
1/2 tsp dried oregano

2 cups low sodium vegetable broth
1/4 tsp salt
1/4 tsp pepper
2 heads celery or 4 celery hearts

1 Preheat oven to 350°F. Heat the oil in a skillet on medium high. Sauté the onion until golden then add the tomato paste. Continue cooking until the tomato paste darkens. Add the oregano, vegetable broth, salt, and pepper. Simmer while you prepare the celery.

2 Cut the bottom 5-inch or 6-inch off the bottom of each head of celery. Cut in half, lengthwise. Remove the outer ribs until you get to the tender, lighter colored heart. Save the tops and trim for salads and stocks.

3 Lay the hearts in a baking dish in one layer and pour the tomato onion sauce over them. Cover and bake 35 to 40 minutes or until tender. Serve the hearts whole on each of 4 hot dinner plates, and spoon the sauce over them.

Per serving: 79 calories, 2 g fat, 0 g saturated fat, 0% calories from saturated fat, 15 g carbohydrate, 444 mg sodium, 4 g dietary fiber
Exchanges: 3 Vegetable

Splendid Spinach

SERVING SIZE: 1/4 of recipe, SERVES: 4

12 cups spinach leaves
1/8 tsp salt

1/8 tsp pepper
1/8 tsp nutmeg

1 Trim the heavy stalk end of the spinach leaves and wash 3 times in plenty of water. Drain in a colander or on a clean dish rack. Season lightly with salt, pepper, and nutmeg to evenly coat. Steam for 3 to 4 minutes to wilt and serve.

Per serving: 22 calories, 0 g fat, 0 g saturated fat, 0% calories from saturated fat, 3 g carbohydrate, 2 g dietary fiber, 142 mg sodium, 3 g protein
Exchanges: 1 Vegetable

Cauliflower East Indian Style

SERVING SIZE: 1/4 of recipe, SERVES: 4

1 head cauliflower
1 tsp non-aromatic olive oil
1/2 cup chopped sweet onion
1 Tbsp grated ginger
1 Tbsp mild curry powder
2 Tbsp lemon juice

1/2 cup low-sodium chicken or vegetable broth
1/4 tsp salt
1 tsp cornstarch mixed with 1 Tbsp broth (slurry)

1 Prepare the cauliflower by cutting from the bottom into small florets. Discard large pieces of stem. Rinse and allow to drain in a colander.

2 Heat the oil in a high-sided skillet on medium-high. Sauté the onion, ginger, and curry powder 2 minutes. Stir in the broth; then add the prepared cauliflower and salt. Cook, covered, about 10 minutes or until tender.

3 Push the cauliflower aside and stir in the slurry. Heat to thicken and gloss. Sprinkle with lemon juice and serve.

Per serving: 66 calories, 2 g fat, 0 g saturated fat, 0% calories from saturated fat, 10 g carbohydrate, 6 g dietary fiber, 263 mg sodium
Exchanges: 2 Vegetable, 1/2 Fat

Steamed Mustard Greens

SERVING SIZE: 1/4 of recipe, SERVES: 4

1 lb mustard greens
1 Tbsp lemon juice

1 Wash mustard greens in lots of cold water. Remove the stems and chop.

2 Steam over boiling water for 5 to 7 minutes. Sprinkle with lemon juice and serve. They are wonderful with black-eyed peas and rice, or with ham and cornbread.

Per serving: 30 calories, 0 g fat, 0 g saturated fat, 0% calories from saturated fat, 6 g carbohydrate, 4 g dietary fiber, 28 mg sodium, 1 g protein
Exchanges: 1 Vegetable

Sautéed Kohlrabi

SERVING SIZE: 1 cup, SERVES: 4

8 small kohlrabi bulbs (enough to make 4 cups)
1 tsp olive oil
1/4 tsp salt
1/4 tsp pepper
2 Tbsp lemon juice

1 Trim the stems and leaves from the kohlrabi. Remove the stems from the leaves, discard, and save the leaves for soups, pasta sauces, or stews. Peel the bulbs with a potato peeler and grate coarsely by hand or in your processor.

2 Heat the oil in a high-sided skillet, add the shredded kohlrabi and cook, stirring often, 3 or 4 minutes or until tender. Season with salt and pepper and toss with the lemon juice. This makes a wonderful nest for grilled fish and is a deliciously light side dish for summer barbecues and winter roasts.

Per serving: 48 calories, 1 g fat, 0 g saturated fat, 0% calories from saturated fat, 9 g carbohydrate, 5 g dietary fiber, 166 mg sodium
Exchanges: 2 Vegetable

Creamy Garlic Mashed Potatoes

SERVING SIZE: 1/4 of recipe, SERVES: 4

2 large russet potatoes, peeled
4 cloves peeled garlic
1/4 tsp salt
1/4 tsp freshly ground white pepper
1/2 cup low-fat buttermilk

1 Cut potatoes into 1/2-inch slices. Place in large saucepan with garlic, cover with water, and bring to a boil. Cook on medium heat for 15 minutes or until potatoes are soft. Pour off water. Put a clean dish towel into the pan to cover the potatoes, and set over low heat for 5 minutes to dry out.

2 When potatoes have a floury appearance on top, add salt and pepper, and mash, making sure garlic also gets mashed and spread through the potatoes. Stir in buttermilk, and serve immediately.

Per serving: 116 calories, 0 g fat, 0 g saturated fat, 0% calories from saturated fat, 25 g carbohydrate, 2 g dietary fiber, 177 mg sodium
Exchanges: 2 Starch

Sautéed Mushrooms and Peas

SERVING SIZE: 1/4 of recipe, SERVES: 4

2 Tbsp lemon juice
12 medium mushrooms, quartered
2 cups frozen (thawed) peas
1/4 cup chopped roasted red peppers
  or pimentos

1/4 tsp salt
1/4 tsp pepper
2 Tbsp grated Parmesan cheese
4 medium tomatoes or
  4 pre-baked squash halves

1 Heat a skillet and add the lemon juice and mushrooms. Fry them on high for 2 or 3 minutes or until they start to brown. Stir in the peas, red peppers, salt, and pepper.

2 Fill 4 medium hollowed out tomatoes or 4 pre-baked squash halves. Scatter Parmesan over the top and bake until heated through, about 10 minutes.

Per serving (stuffing only): 93 calories, 1 g fat, 1 g saturated fat, 10% calories from saturated fat, 15 g carbohydrate, 5 g dietary fiber, 282 mg sodium
Exchanges: 1 Starch

Roasted Brussels Sprouts

SERVING SIZE: 8 sprouts, SERVES: 4

32 small Brussels sprouts
2 cloves garlic, peeled and crushed
1 tsp olive oil
1/4 tsp salt

1/4 tsp pepper
2 (3-inch) sprigs rosemary or
  1/2 tsp dried, finely chopped

1 Preheat the oven to 350°F. Peel away any discolored leaves and trim the stalks of the Brussels sprouts. Cut a deep cross into the stalk ends. Combine the oil, garlic, salt, and pepper and toss with the prepared Brussels sprouts. Place in a baking dish in a single layer.

2 Lay the rosemary sprigs on top and roast 20 minutes or until tender.

Per serving: 50 calories, 1 g fat, 0 g saturated fat, 0 % calories from saturated fat, 8 g carbohydrate, 3 g dietary fiber, 162 mg sodium, 2 g protein
Exchanges: 2 Vegetable

Broiled Summer Squash with Sweet Onions and Tomatoes

SERVING SIZE: 1/4 of recipe, SERVES: 4

    2 small (not baby) zucchini squash, cut in half lengthwise
    2 small (not baby) yellow zucchini or crookneck, cut in half lengthwise
    1 sweet onion, cut in 1/2-inch slices
    4 plum tomatoes, cut in half lengthwise
1/4 tsp salt
1/4 tsp pepper
    1 tsp chopped fresh or dried rosemary

1 Preheat the broiler. Lay the squash face up on a broiler pan. Push a toothpick sideways through the onion slices to keep them together and lay on the pan. Add the tomato halves, face up.

2 Spray the vegetables lightly with olive oil pan spray and scatter salt, pepper, and rosemary over all.

3 Broil 4 inches from the broiler 3 minutes. Turn, spray the other side, and broil 3 minutes more. Broilers differ so watch carefully to see that the vegetables don't burn. This can also be done on a barbecue grill.

Per serving: 70 calories, 1 g fat, 0 g saturated fat, 0% calories from saturated fat, 15 g carbohydrates, 4 g fiber, 153 mg sodium
Exchanges: 3 Vegetable

And the Beet Goes On

SERVING SIZE: 1/4 recipes, SERVES: 4

1 bunch beets
    (4 large or 8 small beets) with greens

1/2 cup 100% orange juice
1/4 tsp salt

1 Wash the beets and their leaves well. Cut the greens off the beets leaving an inch of stem.

2 Cut the greens into 1/4-inch pieces. Set aside.

3 Cover the beets with water in a saucepan and cook whole until tender; 30 to 45 minutes depending on their size. Drain and run under cold water to cool. Peel and cut into quarters.

4 Place the greens in a large skillet with the 100% orange juice, cover and bring to a boil. Reduce the heat and cook 3 or 4 minutes until nearly tender. Toss in the quartered beets and continue cooking, uncovered, until they are heated through and the liquid is almost gone. Season with salt and serve.

Per serving: 72 calories, 0 g fat, 0 g saturated fat, 0% calories from saturated fat, 16 g carbohydrate, 4 g dietary fiber, 345 mg sodium
Exchanges: 3 Vegetable

Rosemary Braised Brussels Sprouts

SERVING SIZE: 1/4 of recipe, SERVES: 4

- 1 lb smallest possible Brussels sprouts
- 1 cup low-sodium chicken or vegetable broth
- 1 tsp dried or fresh rosemary
- 1/4 tsp salt
- 1 tsp arrowroot or cornstarch mixed with 1 Tbsp broth or water (slurry)

1 Strip the outer leaves off the Brussels sprouts. If they are very small, cook whole. Cut in half if they're larger than 3/4-inch in diameter.

2 Bring the broth to a boil. Add the rosemary, salt, and prepared sprouts. Bring back to a boil, reduce the heat, and simmer 7 to 10 minutes or until tender but still bright green.

3 Stir in the slurry and heat until the sauce is glossy and slightly thickened. Serve with a little sauce spooned over.

Per serving: 54 calories, 1 g fat, 0 g saturated fat, 0% calories from saturated fat, 12 g carbohydrate, 2 g dietary fiber, 187 mg sodium
Exchanges: 2 Vegetable

Colorful Mashed Potatoes

SERVING SIZE: 1/6 of recipe, SERVES: 6

2 medium Yukon Gold potatoes cut in chunks (2 cups)	1 cup chopped carrots
1 1/2 cup low-fat milk	1/4 tsp caraway seeds
2 tsp olive oil	1 cup chopped broccoli
1 cup chopped sweet onions	1/4 tsp salt
	1/4 tsp pepper

1 Boil potatoes 10 to 15 minutes, or until very soft. Mash and stir in the milk.

2 Heat oil in a skillet, and sauté onions 2 minutes. Add carrots and caraway, cover, and cook until almost tender, about 10 minutes. Add broccoli, and cook 5 minutes. Carrots and broccoli should both be tender and bright in color.

3 Stir in mashed potatoes, salt, and pepper. Heat through and serve

Per serving: 119 calories, 3 g fat, 0 g saturated fat, 0% calories from saturated fat, 22 g carbohydrate, 3 g dietary fiber, 168 mg sodium
Exchanges: 1 Starch, 1 Vegetable, 1/2 Fat

Zucchini with Herbs and Lemon

SERVING SIZE: 1/4 of recipe, SERVES: 4

2 medium zucchini (3/4 lb)	3/4 cup low-sodium chicken or vegetable stock (pages 463, 473)
1 tsp non-aromatic olive oil	pinch of saffron
1/2 cup finely sliced onion	1 Tbsp freshly squeezed lemon juice
1 clove garlic, peeled, bashed, and chopped	1/2 tsp arrowroot mixed with 1 tsp water (slurry)
1/4 tsp dried oregano	
1/4 tsp dried basil	
1/4 tsp dried thyme	

1 Trim the ends off the zucchini and cut in half lengthwise and then in half crosswise. Set aside.

2 Heat the oil in a high-sided skillet, add the onions, and cook for a minute before adding the garlic and herbs. Stir and cook for 3 minutes. Add the zucchini, salt, pepper, and chicken stock. Cover and cook on medium high for 7 minutes. Stir in the saffron, lemon juice, and slurry. Serve when the sauce is slightly thickened and glossy.

Per serving: 35 calories, 1 g fat, 0 g saturated fat, 0% calories from saturated fat, 5 g carbohydrate, 1 g dietary fiber, 98 mg sodium, 2 g protein
Exchanges: 1 Vegetable

Ratatouille

SERVING SIZE: 1/6 of recipe, SERVES: 6

2 small eggplants (2 lb), cut
  in 2-inch cubes
  olive oil pan spray
1 Tbsp extra virgin olive oil, divided
1 sweet onion, cut in 1-inch chunks
4 cloves garlic, bashed and chopped
1 red bell pepper, seeded and cut
  in 1/2-inch strips
1 green bell pepper, seeded and cut
  in 1/2-inch strips

3 medium zucchini, cut
  in 1-inch chunks
1 (28 oz) can tomatoes diced
  in juice or 3 cups fresh,
  peeled and diced
1 Tbsp dried oregano
1/4 tsp salt
1/4 tsp pepper
1/4 cup chopped fresh parsley
1/4 cup chopped fresh basil

1 Preheat oven to 400°F. Place the eggplant cubes in a baking dish, spray lightly with olive oil pan spray, and bake 20 minutes or until tender. Set aside.

2 Heat 1 tsp of the oil in a high-sided skillet on medium high. Sauté the onions 2 minutes, add the garlic and cook 1 minute more. Stir in the red and green peppers and zucchini and cook until wilted, about 10 minutes. Add the tomatoes, oregano, salt, and pepper and cook 10 minutes.

3 Stir in the eggplant and simmer 10 more minutes or until everything is tender. Add the remaining 2 tsp olive oil and basil and stir. Serve hot or at room temperature as a side dish, on toasted Italian bread or over polenta, pasta, or rice.

Per serving: 127 calories, 3 g fat, 0 g saturated fat, 0% calories from saturated fat, 24 g carbohydrate, 3 g dietary fiber, 332 mg sodium, 1 g protein
Exchanges: 5 Vegetable

Fabulous Fennel

SERVING SIZE: 1/4 of recipe, SERVES: 4

1 tsp non-aromatic olive oil
1 cup chopped onion
1 leek, white part only, sliced
4 small fennel bulbs or 2 large,
  trimmed of stems and fronds

1 cup low-sodium vegetable broth
  (see page 473)
1/4 tsp salt
1/4 tsp pepper
4 Tbsp chopped fronds

1 Heat the oil in a high-sided skillet on medium high. Sauté the onion
2 minutes or until it starts to wilt. Add the leek and fennel and stir to coat
with oil about 1 minute. Pour in the broth, salt, and pepper. Bring to a boil,
reduce the heat, and simmer 20 minutes.

2 Continue cooking until the fennel is tender. Stir in the reserved fronds and
serve. This is a wonderful side dish with fish.

Per serving: 48 calories, 0 g fat, 0 g saturated fat, 0% calories from saturated fat,
11 g carbohydrate, 2 g dietary fiber, 193 mg sodium
Exchanges: 2 Vegetable

Steamed Asparagus

SERVING SIZE: 1/6 of recipe, SERVES: 6

2 lb fresh asparagus, trimmed
1/8 tsp salt
1/4 tsp freshly ground black pepper

1 sprig of fresh tarragon
1 lemon, juiced (about 2 Tbsp)

1 Partially fill a saucepan or steamer pot with water and bring to a boil.
Double a piece of waxed paper and arrange it so that it covers half the openings in your steamer basket or platform. Place the heads of the asparagus
spears over the waxed paper and the stems over the open holes. (This allows
the thick stems to get more steam and cook more quickly than the tender
spears.)

2 Sprinkle the asparagus with the salt and pepper, then lay the sprig of
tarragon over the top.

3 Place the steamer over the boiling water, cover, and steam for 8 minutes, or
until crisp-tender. The thickness of the asparagus will determine the time
necessary to cook it.

4 Remove from the heat, sprinkle with the lemon juice, and serve immediately.

Per serving: 52 calories, 1 g fat, 0 g saturated fat, 0% calories from saturated fat, 9 g carbohydrate, 4 g dietary fiber, 2 g protein
Exchanges: 2 Vegetable

Braised Onions and Parsnips

SERVING SIZE: 1/4 of recipe, SERVES: 4

> 1 tsp non-aromatic olive oil
+> 1/2 cup chopped onions
> 1 clove garlic, bashed and chopped
<C 4 medium parsnips (1 1/2 lb), peeled and cut in 1/2-inch chunks
1/4 tsp salt
1/4 tsp pepper
1 sprig fresh rosemary (optional)
1/2 cup low-sodium chicken or vegetable broth

1 Heat the oil in a high-sided skillet on medium high. Sauté the onions until they start to wilt, about 2 minutes, and then add the garlic to cook 1 minute more. Stir in the parsnips, salt, and pepper.

2 Lay the rosemary over the parsnips and pour in the broth. Cover and cook until they are tender, about 5 minutes. Remove the rosemary and serve.

<C **To Cut Carb**
+> Chopped Onions: increase to 2 medium, cut into quarters.
<C Parsnips: reduce to 4 med/small (1 lb peeled weight), continue as per Step 2.

Per serving: 137 calories, 2 g fat, 0 g saturated fat, 0% calories from saturated fat, 30 g carbohydrate, 6 g dietary fiber, 224 mg sodium
Exchanges: 2 Starch

Low Carb
Per serving: 133 calories, 2 g fat, 0 g saturated fat, 0% calories from saturated fat, 29 g carbohydrate, 6 g dietary fiber, 222 mg sodium
Exchanges: 1 1/2 Starch, 1 Vegetable

Zucchini Fritters

SERVING SIZE: 2 3-inch pancakes, SERVES: 4

5 Tbsp pancake flour
1/4 tsp pepper
1/4 cup grated Parmesan cheese
1/2 cup egg substitute or 2 eggs,
    slightly beaten

2 Tbsp chopped zucchini
2 Tbsp chopped sweet onion
2 Tbsp diced green chilis

1 Combine the pancake flour, pepper, and Parmesan cheese in a bowl. Stir in the eggs. Add the zucchini, onion, and chilis and stir to blend.

2 Heat a nonstick skillet on medium high. Spray with olive oil. Drop batter onto the hot pan with a large kitchen spoon. Fry on one side about 3 minutes, turn, and cook until the vegetables are tender, about 3 more minutes.

Per serving (with egg substitute): 94 calories, 2 g fat, 1 g saturated fat, 10% calories from saturated fat, 11 g carbohydrate, 1 g dietary fiber, 314 mg sodium
Exchanges: 1/2 Starch, 1 Very Lean Meat, 1 Vegetable

Chilled Steamed Asparagus

SERVING SIZE: 1/4 of recipe, SERVES: 4

1 lb (or more) fresh asparagus
1 Tbsp Parmesan cheese
   or
2 tsp freshly squeezed lemon juice and a sprinkling of fresh dill or tarragon
   or
2 Tbsp Treena's Vinaigrette or low-fat salad dressing

1 Pop ends off the asparagus stems. They snap at the point the stalk gets tough, so you won't have any stringy ends. Place in a steamer over boiling water for 3 to 5 minutes or until crisp tender and still beautifully green.

2 Toss into a bowl of cold water to stop the cooking. Drain and chill.

3 Dust with Parmesan cheese and eat whole as finger food or

4 Cut on the diagonal into 2-inch pieces and toss with lemon juice and fresh herbs or

5 Cut on the diagonal into 2-inch pieces, toss with the vinaigrette and serve as a side salad on a leaf of butter lettuce garnished with a couple of cherry tomatoes.

Per serving step 3: 31 calories, 1 g fat, 0 g saturated fat, 0% calories from saturated fat, 4 g carbohydrate, 0 g dietary fiber, 35 mg sodium
Per serving step 4: 26 calories, 0 g fat, 0 g saturated fat, 0% calories from saturated fat, 5 g carbohydrate, 0 g dietary fiber, 12 mg sodium
Per serving step 5: 48 calories, 3 g fat, 0 g saturated fat, 0% calories from saturated fat, 5 g carbohydrate, 0 g dietary fiber, 60 mg sodium
Exchanges: 1 Vegetable, (step 5) 1/2 Fat

Carrot and Parsnip Puree

SERVING SIZE: 1/4 of recipe, SERVES: 4

<C 1 lb carrots, peeled and thinly sliced
<C 1 lb small parsnips, peeled and thinly sliced
1/4 tsp salt

1/4 tsp pepper
3 Tbsp sesame seeds

1 Preheat the oven to 350°F. Steam the carrots and parsnips 15 minutes or until very soft. Mash roughly and stir in the salt and pepper.

2 Place in a baking dish, and scatter sesame seeds over the top. Bake in the preheated oven 20 minutes or until good and hot, and the sesame seeds are nice and brown.

<C **To Cut Carb**
<C Carrots: reduce to 10 oz (1 1/4 cup).   +> Add rutabaga, 10 oz (1 cup).
<C Parsnips: reduce to 8 oz (1 cup).

Per serving: 160 calories, 4 g fat, 1 g saturated fat, 5% calories from saturated fat, 31 g carbohydrate, 8 g dietary fiber, 192 mg sodium
Exchanges: 1 1/2 Starch, 1 Vegetable, 1/2 Fat

Low Carb
Per serving: 126 calories, 4 g fat, 1 g saturated fat, 7% calories from saturated fat, 22 g carbohydrate, 6 g dietary fiber, 184 mg sodium
Exchanges: 1/2 Starch, 3 Vegetable, 1/2 Fat

Sautéed Red, Yellow, and Green Bell Peppers

SERVING SIZE: 1/4 of recipe, SERVES: 4

1 tsp olive oil
1 cup sliced sweet onion
2 cloves garlic, chopped
1 red bell pepper, cored and
  cut in strips
1 yellow bell pepper, cored and
  cut in strips

1 green bell pepper, cored and
  cut in strips
1/4 tsp salt
1/4 tsp pepper
2 Tbsp chopped parsley

1 Heat the oil in a skillet on medium high. Fry the onion 2 minutes or until it starts to wilt but not brown. Add the garlic and pepper strips and sauté until tender, about 10 minutes. Stir in the salt, pepper, and parsley.

2 Serve as a side dish to barbecued meats, in omelets or heaped on small garlic rubbed toast rounds (bruschetta).

Per serving: 60 calories, 1 g fat, 0 g saturated fat, 0% calories from saturated fat, 12 g carbohydrate, 3 g dietary fiber, 143 mg sodium
Exchanges: 2 Vegetable

Cauliflower with Carrot "Cheese" Sauce

SERVING SIZE: 1/4 of recipe, SERVES: 4

4 cups cauliflower florets
3 carrots, peeled and sliced in
  1/2-inch rounds (1 1/2 cups)
1/2 cup evaporated skim milk
1/4 cup water
1 tsp Dijon mustard

1/2 tsp Worcestershire Sauce
1 Tbsp lemon juice
1/4 tsp salt
  pinch cayenne
  pinch cumin
1/4 cup grated Parmesan cheese

1 Steam cauliflower 12 minutes or until tender but not mushy. Set aside.

2 Cook the carrots in the evaporated milk and water 10–15 minutes or until very soft. Whip them in a blender with the mustard, Worcestershire sauce, and lemon juice for 2 or 3 minutes or until smooth and glossy. Add salt, cayenne, and cumin and whip to mix.

3 Place the cauliflower in a baking dish. Spoon the sauce over the cauliflower, and scatter the grated cheese over the top. Brown under the broiler and serve.

Per serving: 103 calories, 3 g fat, 1 g saturated fat, 9% calories from saturated fat, 14 g carbohydrate, 5 g dietary fiber, 340 mg sodium
Exchanges: 3 Vegetable, 1/2 Fat

Sautéed Onions

SERVING SIZE: 1/4 of recipe, SERVES: 4

1 tsp olive oil	1/4 tsp salt
4 medium onions, peeled and sliced	1/4 tsp pepper
<C 1 Tbsp maple syrup	2 Tbsp chopped fresh basil
2 Tbsp balsamic vinegar	

1 Heat the oil in a large high-sided skillet on medium high. Sauté the onions 2 minutes. Add the syrup, vinegar, salt, and pepper and continue cooking, stirring often, until the onions are golden, tender, and cooked down, 20 to 25 minutes. Stir in the basil.

2 These onions can be served on their own as a side dish, mixed with other vegetables, over rice or pasta, or even on baked beans.

<C **To Cut Carb**
<C Maple Syrup: reduce to 1 tsp and add 2 tsp Splenda.

Per serving: 86 calories, 1 g fat, 0 g saturated fat, 0% calories from saturated fat, 18 g carbohydrate, 3 g dietary fiber, 151 mg sodium
Exchanges: 2 Vegetable, 1/2 Carbohydrate

Low Carb
Per serving: 78 calories, 1 g fat, 0 g saturated fat, 0% calories from saturated fat, 16 g carbohydrate, 3 g dietary fiber, 150 mg sodium
Exchanges: 3 Vegetable

Spring Vegetable Sauté

SERVING SIZE: 1/4 of recipe, SERVES: 4

1 tsp olive oil	3/4 cup sugar snap peas
1/2 cup sliced sweet onion	1/2 cup quartered radishes
1 clove garlic, finely chopped	1/4 tsp salt
3/4 cup quartered tiny new potatoes	1/4 tsp pepper
3/4 cup baby carrots, cut in half diagonally	1 Tbsp chopped fresh dill weed or
3/4 cup asparagus pieces	1/2 tsp dried

1 Heat the oil in a high-sided skillet. Cook the onion 2 minutes, add the garlic and cook another minute. Stir in the potatoes and carrots, cover, turn the heat to low, and cook until almost tender, about 4 minutes. If the vegetables start to brown, add a Tbsp or 2 of water.

2 Now add the asparagus, peas, radishes, salt, pepper, and dill. Cook, stirring often, until just tender, about 4 minutes more. Try this with a piece of barbecued fish for a complete spring meal.

Per serving: 65 calories, 1 g fat, 0 g saturated fat, 0% calories from saturated fat, 12 g carbohydrate, 3 g dietary fiber, 178 mg sodium, 2 g protein
Exchanges: 1/2 Starch, 1 Vegetable

Broccoli, Carrot,
Sweet Pepper Stir-Fry

SERVING SIZE: 1/4 of recipe, SERVES: 4

      1 tsp non-aromatic olive oil
      1 clove garlic, bashed and chopped
      1 tsp chopped ginger
      4 green onions, white and green parts separated, both parts cut in 1/4-inch slices
      1 cup carrots, peeled and cut in 1/4-inch diagonal slices
    1/2 red sweet pepper, cut in 2-inch strips
  1 1/2 cups broccoli stems, peeled and cut in 1/4-inch matchsticks
    1/4 tsp salt

1 Heat the oil in a skillet big enough to hold all the ingredients. Fry the garlic, ginger, and onion in the hot oil for 30 seconds.

2 Add the carrots, peppers, and broccoli stems, and reduce the heat to medium. Cook, stirring, 3 or 4 minutes or until the vegetables are tender but still crisp. Season with salt and serve.

Per serving: 35 calories, 1 g fat, 0 g saturated fat, 0% calories from saturated fat, 5 g carbohydrate, 2 g dietary fiber, 164 mg sodium
Exchanges: 1 Vegetable

Pineapple Fried Rice

SERVING SIZE: 1/6 of recipe, SERVES: 6

1 Tbsp non-aromatic olive oil
1 tsp finely grated lemon zest
1 jalapeno, seeded and chopped
3 cloves garlic, bashed and chopped
1/3 cup chopped red bell pepper
1/2 cup chopped celery
4 tsp grated ginger root
3 cups cooked (1 cup raw) long-grain brown rice, chilled

1 cup chopped fresh pineapple
12 mint leaves, rolled and cut into strips
1/4 cup loosely packed cilantro leaves, chopped
1 Tbsp Thai fish sauce or soy sauce
1 tsp rice vinegar
1 tsp toasted sesame oil

1 This is a stir-fry, so have all the ingredients ready at hand. Warm the oil in a large frying pan over medium-high heat. Sauté the lemon zest, jalapeno, and garlic for 30 seconds. Add the red pepper, celery, and ginger and stir-fry for another 30 seconds.

2 Add the chilled rice and cook until heated through, stirring occasionally to keep from sticking. Stir in the pineapple, mint, and cilantro. Sprinkle the fish sauce, vinegar, and sesame oil over the top. Stir to mix and serve immediately.

Per serving: 157 calories, 4 g fat, 1 g saturated fat, 6% calories from saturated fat, 28 g carbohydrate, 2 g dietary fiber, 38 mg sodium, 2 g protein
Exchanges: 2 Starch, 1/2 Fat

Steamed then Broiled Fennel

SERVING SIZE: 1/4 of recipe, SERVES: 4

4 small fennel bulbs or 2 large	1/4 tsp pepper
1/4 tsp salt	2 Tbsp lemon juice

1 Preheat the broiler. Trim off the stems, fronds, and any discolored outside layers of the bulb. Chop and save a few of the fronds to scatter over the top of the finished dish. Cut small bulbs in half lengthwise or large bulbs in 4 thick slices.

2 Place the fennel slices in a steamer and steam over boiling water for 8 to 10 minutes or until tender but still crisp.

3 Lay them in a single layer on a broiler pan. Season with salt and pepper and brush lemon juice on both sides. Spray lightly with olive oil pan spray and broil about 3 inches from the heat source until golden brown. Turn and brown the other side. Divide among 4 hot plates and scatter the reserved fronds over the top.

Per serving: 29 calories, 0 g fat, 0 g saturated fat, 0% calories from saturated fat, 7 g carbohydrate, 0 g dietary fiber, 191 mg sodium
Exchanges: 1 Vegetable

Broccoli & Green Beans with Ginger Green Sauce

SERVING SIZE: 1/4 of recipe, SERVES: 4

Green Sauce:

2 cups tightly packed, fresh spinach leaves	1/2 tsp grated fresh ginger (optional)
1/2 cup low-sodium vegetable broth	2 cups green beans, sliced into bite-sized pieces (use fresh or frozen)
1/4 tsp reduced-sodium soy sauce	2 cups broccoli florets, cut into bite-sized pieces (use fresh or frozen)
1/2 tsp sesame oil	
2 tsp rice wine vinegar or white vinegar	

Puree green sauce ingredients in the blender until the sauce is bright and very smooth. Meanwhile, use the stove or microwave to steam green beans and broccoli just until each is bright green and tender-crisp. To serve, drizzle some green sauce on each plate, and top with a 1/4 cup pile of hot green beans and a 1/4 cup pile of hot broccoli.

Per serving: 54 calories, 2 g fat, 0 g saturated fat, 0% calories from saturated fat, 8 g carbohydrate, 2 g dietary fiber, 133 mg sodium, 3 g protein, 0 mg cholesterol
Exchanges: 2 Vegetable

Saffron Rice

SERVING SIZE: 1/6 of recipe, SERVES: 6

1/2 tsp light olive oil
3/4 cup chopped onion
1 cup long-grain white rice
1 3/4 cups low-sodium fish or vegetable stock (pages 468, 473)

1/4 tsp salt
1 pinch of powdered saffron

This is close to reasonable/moderate at the upper end of the carbohydrate scale and therefore needs to be matched with another very low carbohydrate choice on the same plate.

1 Warm the oil in a saucepan over medium-high heat. Sauté the onion until translucent, 2 or 3 minutes. Add the rice and cook until it turns chalky white, another 2 or 3 minutes.

2 Pour in the stock and season with the salt and saffron. Cover, bring to a boil, then reduce the heat as low as possible. Cook for 20 minutes, remove from the heat, and set aside for 5 minutes before serving.

Per serving: 157 calories, 1 g fat, 0 g saturated fat, 0% of calories from saturated fat, 33 g carbohydrate, 1 g dietary fiber, 4 g protein
Exchanges: 2 Starch

Sesame Grilled Asparagus

SERVING SIZE: 8 stalks, SERVES: 4

32 stalks fresh asparagus
 1 Tbsp soy sauce
 1 Tbsp rice vinegar
 1 tsp sugar

1/2 tsp toasted sesame oil
    pinch dried crushed chilis (optional)
 1 tsp toasted sesame seeds

1 Preheat the barbecue to about 400°F. Wash the asparagus and snap off the tough ends. It will break at the place it starts to get tough and stringy.

2 Combine the soy sauce, vinegar, sugar, sesame oil, and chilis. Brush on the asparagus and marinate at least 15 minutes. Lay on the grill and cook, turning once until tender, up to 10 minutes.

3 Serve sprinkled with the sesame seeds.

Per serving: 39 calories, 1 g fat, 0 g saturated fat, 0% calories from saturated fat, 5 g carbohydrate, 3 g dietary fiber, 250 mg sodium
Exchanges: 1 Vegetable

Sautéed Asian Pears

SERVING SIZE: 1 pear, SERVES: 4

4 Asian or regular pears (1 1/2 lb)
   pinch ground ginger
1 Tbsp sugar
1 Tbsp chopped crystallized ginger

1 Tbsp lemon juice
1 tsp non-aromatic olive oil
2 tsp toasted sesame seeds

1 Peel and core the pears and cut into 1/4-inch slices. Toss with the ground ginger, sugar, crystallized ginger, and lemon juice.

2 Heat the oil in a skillet on medium-high heat. Sauté the pear slices, stirring until they are tender and the sugar has caramelized, about 5 minutes. Sprinkle with sesame seeds and serve.

Per serving: 92 calories, 2 g fat, 0 g saturated fat, 0% calories from saturated fat, 19 g carbohydrate, 5 g dietary fiber, 1 mg sodium
Exchanges: 1 Fruit, 1/2 Fat

Roasted Beets

SERVING SIZE: 1 beet, SERVES: 4

4 beets
2 Tbsp fresh lime juice   1 Tbsp honey
1/4 tsp cardamom   1 tsp non-aromatic olive oil

1 Preheat the oven to 400°F. Peel the beets and cut into 1-inch chunks.

2 Combine the lime juice, cardamom, honey, and oil. Place the beets in a baking dish and toss with the lime juice mixture.

3 Lay a sheet of aluminum foil over the top and bake 30 minutes. Remove the foil and bake 20 minutes longer or until the beets are glazed and tender.

Per serving: 82 calories, 1 g fat, 0 g saturated fat, 0% calories from saturated fat, 17 g carbohydrate, 4 g dietary fiber, 89 mg sodium
Exchanges: 3 Vegetable

Spinach-Stuffed Red Bell Peppers

SERVING SIZE: 1/2 pepper, SERVES: 4

2 large red bell peppers, seeded and cut in half lengthwise   1/4 tsp salt
2 lb fresh spinach or 2 packages chopped frozen spinach   1/4 tsp pepper
   1/4 tsp nutmeg

1 Place the pepper halves in a steamer and steam 3 minutes over boiling water. Set aside.

2 Wash the spinach and discard the stems. Chop and season with salt, pepper, and nutmeg. Steam until wilted, about 3 minutes. Press out excess water and fill the pepper halves.

3 Steam the stuffed peppers 3 minutes or until heated through. Cut each half into 2 wedges and serve.

Per serving:74 calories, 1 g fat, 0 g saturated fat, 0% calories from saturated fat, 15 g carbohydrate, 6 g dietary fiber, 242 mg sodium
Exchanges: 3 Vegetable

Steamed Green Beans

SERVING SIZE: 1/4 of recipe, SERVES: 4

1 lb green beans
1 clove garlic, bashed and chopped
1/4 cup low-sodium vegetable or
   chicken stock (pages 473, 463)
1/4 tsp arrowroot or cornstarch
1/4 tsp salt
1/4 tsp pepper
   pinch nutmeg

1 Remove the stem ends of the green beans and the tips if you want to. (I kind of like to leave them on.) Place them in a steamer, sprinkle with garlic, and steam over boiling water for 6 minutes or until tender.

2 While the beans are cooking, combine the stock, arrowroot, salt, pepper, and nutmeg in a small saucepan. Heat until glossy and slightly thickened. Pour over the cooked beans, toss, and serve.

Per serving: 42 calories, 0 g fat, 0 g saturated fat, 0% calories from saturated fat, 9 g carbohydrate, 4 g dietary fiber, 153 mg sodium, 2 g protein
Exchanges: 2 Vegetable

Szechuan Spinach

SERVING SIZE: 2 cups, SERVES: 4

8 cups well washed spinach leaves or
   one box of frozen spinach
1 Tbsp light soy sauce
1 Tbsp rice vinegar
1 tsp sugar
1 tsp toasted sesame oil
   pinch of dried, crushed chilis
1/2 tsp finely chopped fresh ginger
2 sliced green onions (scallions)

1 Place spinach leaves in a colander and pour lots of boiling water over the top to wilt the spinach. Drain well.

2 Combine the soy sauce, vinegar, sugar, sesame oil, chilis, and ginger. Toss with the spinach and green onions to coat well. Let sit 30 minutes.

Per serving: 20 calories, 1 g fat, 0 g saturated fat, 0 % calories from saturated fat, 2 g carbohydrate, 6 g dietary fiber, 322 mg sodium
Exchanges: 1 Vegetable

Sautéed Shredded Carrots with Dill

SERVING SIZE: 1/4 of recipe, SERVES: 4

1 tsp non-aromatic olive oil
4 cups shredded carrots
1 tsp dried dill weed

1/4 tsp salt
1 Tbsp fresh dill weed (optional)

1 Heat the oil in a high-sided skillet on medium high. Add the carrots and dried dill and sauté, stirring often until tender, about 6 minutes.

2 Stir in the salt and fresh dill weed, if you are using it, and serve.

Per serving: 58 calories, 1 g fat, 0 g saturated fat, 0% calories from saturated fat, 11 g carbohydrate, 3 g dietary fiber, 179 mg sodium
Exchanges: 2 Vegetable

Braised Fennel in Spicy Tomato Juice

SERVING SIZE: 1 fennel bulb, SERVES: 4

4 small fennel bulbs
1 tsp fennel seeds

1 cup spicy tomato-vegetable juice

1 Preheat the oven to 350°F. Trim the fennel bulbs, saving the stems to flavor soups or fish stews. Cut lengthwise into quarters.

2 Lay the bulbs in a glass or ceramic baking dish. Scatter fennel seeds over the top and pour in the tomato juice. Bake, covered, 45 minutes, basting with the pan juices 2 or 3 times.

3 Serve as a side dish for fish, chicken, pork, or lamb.

Per serving: 87 calories, 1 g fat, 0 g saturated fat, 0% calories from saturated fat, 20 g carbohydrates, 5 g dietary fiber, 210 mg sodium
Exchanges: 4 Vegetable

Braised Chestnuts

SERVING SIZE: 1/4 of recipe, SERVES: 4

  2 cups water packed canned chestnuts, drained (be sure they are not in a sugar syrup)
  1 cup low-sodium chicken broth or dry red wine
1/4 tsp dried thyme
1/4 tsp dried sage
  2 tsp arrowroot or cornstarch mixed with 2 Tbsp water (slurry)
  1 Tbsp chopped fresh parsley

1 Simmer the chestnuts in the broth or wine with the thyme and sage 20 minutes. Stir in the slurry and stir to thicken and clear.

2 Add the parsley and serve with a holiday bird or other roast.

Per serving: 117 calories, 1 g fat, 0 g saturated fat, 0% calories from saturated fat, 24 g carbohydrate, 48 mg sodium, 2 g dietary fiber
Exchanges: 1 1/2 Starch

Steamed Mature Bok Choy

SERVING SIZE: 1/4 of recipe, SERVES: 4

  1 large bok choy   1/4 tsp pepper
1/4 tsp salt   1 Tbsp freshly squeezed lemon juice

1 Cut the thick white stems from the green leaves. Cut off the bottom of the stalk to separate the stems. Wash and trim.

2 Steam the white parts 3 minutes, turn, season with salt and pepper, and steam 3 more minutes. Divide among 4 hot plates.

3 Lay the leaves in the steamer, season with the remaining salt and pepper and steam 2 minutes. Lay on the plates with the stems, sprinkle with lemon juice, and serve.

Per serving: 9 calories, 0 g fat, 0 g saturated fat, 0% calories from saturated fat, 1 g carbohydrate, 1 g dietary fiber, 106 mg sodium, 4 g protein
Exchanges: Free Food

Thai Spiced Parsnips

SERVING SIZE: 1/4 of recipe, SERVES: 4

2 tsp non-aromatic olive oil
1 red chili
2-inch peeled ginger root,
  cut in thin slices
1 lb medium parsnips, peeled and
  cut in 1/4-inch slices

1 cup low-sodium vegetable broth
1/4 tsp salt
1 tsp arrowroot or cornstarch mixed
  with 1 Tbsp of water (slurry)
2 Tbsp chopped spearmint
1 Tbsp toasted sesame seeds

1 Heat the oil in a high-sided skillet on medium high. Sauté the chili and ginger slices for 2 minutes to break out the flavors. Add the parsnips and cook until golden brown, about 5 minutes.

2 Pour the broth into the pan, cover, and cook until the parsnips are tender. Add the salt, remove the chilis and stir in the slurry. Heat to thicken and serve topped with the mint and sesame seeds.

Per serving: 134 calories, 4 g fat, 1 g saturated fat, 7% calories from saturated fat, 24 g carbohydrate, 6 g dietary fiber, 277 mg sodium
Exchanges: 1 1/2 Starch, 1/2 Fat

Diamond Cut Roasted Potato

SERVING SIZE: 1 potato, SERVES: 4

4 small russet potatoes
1/2 tsp olive oil
1 Tbsp lemon juice

1/4 tsp salt
1/4 tsp white pepper

1 Scrub potatoes, puncture with a fork, and microwave 10 minutes on high. Cut in half lengthwise. Make 3 shallow diagonal cuts on the face of the potatoes. Make 3 more going the other way to make a diamond pattern.

2 Preheat the broiler. Combine olive oil, lemon juice, salt, and pepper. Brush this mixture on potatoes and broil until the tops are crisp and brown.

Per serving: 114 calories, 1 g fat, 0 g saturated fat, 0% calories from saturated fat, 22 g carbohydrate, 4 g dietary fiber, 307 mg sodium
Exchanges: 1 1/2 Starch

Steamed Kale

SERVING SIZE: 1/4 lb, SERVES: 4

1 lb kale	1/4 tsp pepper
1/4 tsp salt	1 Tbsp lemon juice

1 Wash the kale in a sink full of cold water. Remove the heavy stems and place the leaves in a steamer. Sprinkle with salt, pepper, and lemon juice and steam over boiling water for 4 to 6 minutes, or until tender.

For a holiday dinner or just for added color on a dull winter day, add 1/2 cup chopped red bell pepper to the kale before steaming.

Per serving: 28 calories, 0 g fat, 0 g saturated fat, 0% calories from saturated fat, 5 g carbohydrate, 3 g dietary fiber, 165 mg sodium, 2 g protein
Exchanges: 1 Vegetable

Spinach Defrosted in Broth

SERVING SIZE: 1/3 of recipe, SERVES: 3

1 cup low-sodium chicken or vegetable broth (pages 463, 473)	1/8 tsp ground nutmeg
1 (10 oz) package frozen spinach (1 1/2 cups)	2 tsp cornstarch mixed with 2 Tbsp water (slurry)

1 Bring the broth to a boil in a small saucepan. Add the spinach, cover, reduce the heat to low, and cook for 10 minutes.

2 Add nutmeg. Pour in the slurry to thicken and heat for 30 seconds. Serve with a colorful vegetable like carrots or tomatoes.

Per serving: 34 calories, 0 g fat, 0 g saturated fat, 0% calories from saturated fat, 6 g carbohydrate, 2 g dietary fiber, 97 mg sodium
Exchanges: 1 Vegetable

Beets and Greens in Orange Juice

SERVING SIZE: 1/4 of recipe, SERVES: 4

1 bunch beets (4 large or 8 small beets)
  with greens

1/2 cup orange juice
1/4 tsp salt

1 Cut the greens off the beets leaving an inch of stem. Wash the greens in lots of water, drain, remove the stems, and cut across the leaves into 1/2-inch strips. Set aside.

2 Scrub the beets, cover with water in a saucepan, and cook whole until tender, 30 to 45 minutes depending on their size. Drain and run under cold water to cool. Peel and cut into quarters.

3 Place the greens in a large skillet with the orange juice, cover and bring to a boil. Reduce the heat and cook 3 or 4 minutes until nearly tender. Toss in the quartered beets and continue cooking, uncovered, until they are heated through and the liquid is almost gone. Season with salt and serve.

Per serving: 72 calories, 0 g fat, 0 g saturated fat, 0% calories from saturated fat, 16 g carbohydrate, 4 g dietary fiber, 345 mg sodium
Exchanges: 3 Vegetable

Baby Squash Sauté

SERVING SIZE: 1/4 of recipe, SERVES: 4

1 lb mixed baby squash
1/2 tsp extra virgin olive oil
1 tsp chopped garlic

2 Tbsp chopped parsley
1/4 tsp salt
1/4 tsp pepper

1 Wash and trim off the stem end of the squash and dry on paper towels. Cut the larger ones in half.

2 Heat the oil in a skillet over medium-high heat. Fry the squash until tender, 8 to 10 minutes. Stir in the garlic, parsley, salt, and pepper. Cook 1 minute longer then serve.

Per serving: 30 calories, 1 g fat, 0 g saturated fat, 0% calories from saturated fat, 4 g carbohydrate, 1 g dietary fiber, 144 mg sodium
Exchanges: 1 Vegetable

Tabbouleh

SERVING SIZE: 1/4 of recipe, SERVES: 4

1/2 cup dry bulgur
  4 cups cold water
  4 Roma tomatoes
  1 red bell pepper
1/2 cup chopped parsley

  1 Tbsp extra virgin olive oil
  3 Tbsp lemon juice
1/2 tsp salt
1/4 tsp pepper

1. Cover the bulgur with the boiling water and soak 30 minutes.

2. While it's soaking, chop the tomatoes and bell pepper in small pieces.

3. After 30 minutes, pour the bulgur into a sieve lined with a tea towel. Pick up the corners of the towel and squeeze the bulgur until it's quite dry. Tip into a bowl and add the chopped vegetables, parsley, oil, lemon juice, salt, and pepper. Mix thoroughly and let sit 30 minutes to mellow.

Per serving: 132 calories, 4 g fat, 1 g saturated fat, 7% calories from saturated fat, 23 g carbohydrate, 6 g dietary fiber, 298 mg sodium
Exchanges: 1 Starch, 1 Vegetable, 1/2 Fat

Savory Poached Pears

SERVING SIZE: 1/4 of recipe, SERVES: 4

  1 cup nonalcoholic red wine
1/2 cup cider vinegar
  6 whole cloves

  6 allspice berries
  1 (3-inch) cinnamon stick
  2 pears, peeled, halved, and cored

1. Heat the wine, vinegar, cloves, and allspice in a saucepan. Add the pear halves and simmer 30 minutes or until the pears are tender and red in color. Serve with beef, venison, turkey, or any flavorful meat.

Per serving: 49 calories, 0 g fat, 0 g saturated fat, 0% calories from saturated fat, 13 g carbohydrate, 2 g dietary fiber, 0 mg sodium
Exchanges: 1 Fruit

Carrots and Snow Peas with Mint

SERVING SIZE: 1/4 of recipe, SERVES: 4

  4 medium carrots
1/2 cup low-sodium chicken or vegetable broth
  1 cup fresh or frozen snow peas with the strings removed from each side
  2 Tbsp chopped fresh mint
1/4 tsp salt
1/4 tsp pepper
1/2 tsp cornstarch or arrowroot mixed with 1/4 cup broth or water (slurry)

1 Peel the carrots and cut diagonally in 1/4-inch widths. Heat the broth in a skillet, add the carrots, cover and cook 5 minutes or until tender but still a bit crisp. Stir in the peas and cook uncovered until crisp-tender, 2 minutes.

2 Toss in the mint, salt, and pepper, and thicken with the slurry if you like.

Per serving: 35 calories, 0 g fat, 0 g saturated fat, 0% calories from saturated fat, 8 g carbohydrate, 2 g dietary fiber, 169 mg sodium
Exchanges: 1 Vegetable

Mashed Sweet Potatoes

SERVING SIZE: 1/6 of recipe, SERVES: 6

  4 small to medium orange-colored sweet potatoes, to make 2 cups
  2 tsp fresh thyme leaves or 3/4 tsp dried thyme
1/4 tsp salt
1/4 tsp pepper

1 Peel and cut the sweet potatoes into 1/2-inch slices. Cook in a steamer over boiling water until tender, about 20 minutes. When they are very soft, tip into a bowl and mash with a fork or potato masher. Stir in thyme, salt, and pepper and serve.

Per serving: 99 calories, 0 g fat, 0 g saturated fat, 0% calories from saturated fat, 23 g carbohydrate, 2 g fiber, 59 mg sodium, 2 g protein
Exchanges: 1 1/2 Starch

Stir-Fried Bok Choy

SERVING SIZE: 2 cups, SERVES: 4

1 head bok choy (8 cups)
1 tsp non-aromatic olive oil
1 clove garlic, peeled and sliced

1 tsp chopped ginger root
1 green onion, chopped
1 Tbsp Chinese hoisin or light soy sauce

1 Cut 2 inches off the bottom of the head of bok choy. Separate the leaves and wash carefully. Drain and dry on paper towels. Separate the stems from the leaves. Cut the stems across into 1/4-inch slices and the leaves into a separate heap of 1/4-inch strips. You should have 8 cups.

2 Heat the oil in a large skillet on medium high. Drop in the garlic, ginger, and onion and cook 30 seconds. Add the bok choy stems and stir-fry 3–5 minutes. Toss in the leaves and cook 1 minute longer. Add the hoisin or soy sauce and stir to coat the bok choy. Serve immediately.

Per serving: 33 calories, 1 g fat, 0 g saturated fat, 0% calories from saturated fat, 4 g carbohydrate, 2 g dietary fiber, 235 mg sodium
Exchanges: 1 Vegetable

Steamed Broccoli

SERVING SIZE: 1/4 of recipe, SERVES: 4

1 bunch (1 1/2 lb) broccoli
1/4 tsp salt

1/2 tsp dried basil
1 tsp lemon juice

1 Remove the tough bottom of each stalk and discard. Cut off the stalks where they meet the florets. Peel the stems, cut in 1/4-inch diagonal slices and lay in a steamer (or save for a soup later).

2 Cut apart the florets and lay on top of the stems. Season with salt and scatter the basil and lemon juice over the top. Steam 5 to 7 minutes and serve immediately. Five minutes will probably be enough time to cook the florets without the stems.

Per serving: 42 calories, 1 g fat, 0 g saturated fat, 0% calories from saturated fat, 8 g carbohydrate, 0 g dietary fiber, 182 mg Sodium, 2 g protein
Exchanges: 2 Vegetable

Rutabaga Puree

SERVING SIZE: 1/4 of recipe, SERVES: 4

4 small rutabagas (1 1/2 lbs)
1 small russet potato (optional)
  up to 1/2 cup low-fat milk or broth

1/4 tsp salt
1/4 tsp white pepper

1 Peel the rutabagas and potato and cut in quarters. Steam over boiling water for 25 minutes or until very soft. Adding potato will make a thicker puree.

2 Place in a processor to puree, adding just enough milk to get the texture you want. Season with salt and pepper and reheat before serving.

Per serving: 63 calories, 1 g fat, 0 g saturated fat, 0% calories from saturated fat, 12 g carbohydrate, 2 g dietary fiber, 173 mg sodium, 2 g protein
Exchanges: 2 Vegetable

Celery Root and Potato Purée

SERVING SIZE: 1/6 of recipe, SERVES: 6

1 small celery root (about 1 lb unpeeled)
2 large russet potatoes
3 Tbsp finely sliced fresh celery leaves

1/4 tsp salt
1/4 cup yogurt cheese (page 475)
1/4 tsp white pepper

1 Scrub the celery root with a vegetable brush. Cut off the top and bottom and discard. Peel the celery root with a knife, making sure to cut out all the brown spots and any woody parts near the center. Slice thickly, and then cut into 1-inch pieces.

2 Peel the potatoes, and cut into 1-inch slices. Put the celery root, potatoes, salt, and 2 cups of water into a medium saucepan. Cover and bring to a boil, then simmer for 25 minutes, or until very soft.

3 Strain the vegetables, and mash well. Stir in the yogurt cheese, white pepper, and sliced celery leaves. Cover until ready to serve.

Per serving: 155 calories, 0 g fat, 0 g saturated fat, 1% of calories from fat, 35 g carbohydrate, 3 g dietary fiber
Exchanges: 1 1/2 Starch, 2 Vegetable

Collards with a Spicy Twist

SERVING SIZE: 1/4 of recipe, SERVES: 4

1 lb bunch collard greens	1/2 tsp dried thyme
1/2 tsp non-aromatic olive oil	pinch cayenne pepper
2 oz Canadian bacon, chopped	1 tsp lemon juice

1 Wash greens and remove heavy stems. Stack one third of the leaves on top of each other and roll into a "cigar." Cut into 1/4-inch ribbons. Repeat with the rest of the greens.

2 Heat oil in a large skillet on medium high. Fry bacon until it starts to color. Add collards, thyme, and cayenne, and stir to mix well. Cover and cook, stirring occasionally, 7 minutes or until the greens are tender but still bright green.

3 Sprinkle on lemon juice and serve.

Per serving: 49 calories, 1 g fat, 0 g saturated fat, 0% calories from saturated fat, 6 g carbohydrate, 4 g dietary fiber, 207 mg sodium
Exchanges: 1 Very Lean Meat, 1 Vegetable

Beet and Potato Puree

SERVING SIZE: 1/4 of recipe, SERVES: 4

2 medium russet potatoes	1/4 tsp salt
1 can beets or 3 medium cooked peeled beets	1/4 tsp pepper

1 Peel the potatoes and cut in eighths. Cook for 15 minutes in boiling water. Add the beets and cook until the potatoes are tender, about 5 minutes more. Drain.

2 Mash the potatoes and beets together and stir in the salt and pepper. I like a rather lumpy mash for its interesting texture, but if you want it completely smooth, you can whiz it in a processor.

Per serving: 75 calories, 0 g fat, 0 g saturated fat, 0% calories from saturated fat, 17 g carbohydrate, 2 g fiber, 178 mg sodium
Exchanges: 1 Starch

Broccoflower

SERVING SIZE: 1/4 of recipe, SERVES: 4

  1 head (4 cups) broccoflower, broccoli, or cauliflower
1/4 tsp salt
  1 Tbsp lemon juice (optional)

1 Wash and cut the broccoflower into small florets. Place in a pot of water on top of a steaming basket. Season with salt, place the lid on the pot, and steam for about 6 minutes, until tender.

2 Serve on a dish with a splash of lemon juice.

Per serving: 21 calories, 0 g fat, 0 g saturated fat, 0% calories from saturated fat, 4 g carbohydrate, 2 g dietary fiber, 154 mg sodium
Exchanges:1 Vegetable

Herb Broiled Artichokes

SERVING SIZE: 1 artichoke bottom, SERVES: 4

  4 canned artichoke bottoms
1/4 tsp dried tarragon or 1 tsp chopped fresh
1/4 tsp dried basil or 1 tsp chopped fresh
  1 Tbsp chopped fresh parsley
  1 Tbsp chopped fresh chives
     extra virgin olive oil
     pan spray
1/4 cup Mango Chutney (optional) (page 472)

1 Turn the broiler on to preheat. Lay the artichoke bottoms on a broiler pan. Combine the tarragon, basil, parsley, and chives in a bowl. Coat the artichokes lightly with the pan spray. Scatter the herbs over the top and spray again.

2 Cook under the hot broiler until heated through and slightly browned. Garnish with a Tbsp of chutney and set on top of a scoop of rice or couscous.

Per serving: 54 calories, 1 g fat, 0 g saturated fat, 0% calories from saturated fat, 11 g carbohydrate, 0 g dietary fiber, 34 mg sodium
Exchanges: 2 Vegetable

Okra Simmered with Bacon and Tomatoes

SERVING SIZE: 1/4 of recipe, SERVES: 4

1/2 tsp olive oil
 1 cup chopped onion
 2 (2 oz) slices chopped
   Canadian bacon

 1 lb fresh or frozen okra
 1 cup canned tomatoes or
   peeled and seeded fresh ones
1/4 tsp pepper

1 Heat the oil in a high-sided skillet on medium high. Sauté the onion with the Canadian bacon until soft, about 10 minutes, lowering the heat to keep from scorching.

2 Trim the caps off the okra and cut into 1/2-inch slices. Add to the onions and bacon with the tomatoes and cook 10 minutes more or until the okra is tender. Season with pepper and serve.

Per serving: 89 calories, 2 g fat, 0 g saturated fat, 0% calories from saturated fat, 11 g carbohydrate, 5 g dietary fiber, 316 mg sodium, 7 g protein
Exchanges: 1 Lean Meat, 2 Vegetable

Broiled Tomatoes

SERVING SIZE: 1/6 of recipe, SERVES: 6

9 medium round tomatoes
  (not plum tomatoes)

1/8 tsp salt
1/8 tsp freshly ground black pepper

1 Preheat the broiler. Spray a broiling pan with cooking spray.

2 Cut the tomatoes in half across the girth and dry the cut surfaces gently with a paper towel. Sprinkle with salt and pepper and set on the oiled pan.

3 Broil for 5 minutes or until soft and lightly browned.

Per serving: 39 calories 1 g fat, 0 g saturated fat, 0% calories from saturated fat 9 g carbohydrate, 2 g dietary fiber
Exchanges: 2 Vegetable

Pan Roasted Parsnips

SERVING SIZE: 1/2 parsnip, SERVES: 4

1 tsp non-aromatic olive oil
1/2 cup roughly chopped onions
1 clove garlic, peeled, bashed, and chopped
2 (1/4 lb) parsnips, peeled
1/4 tsp salt
1/4 tsp white pepper
6-inch sprig fresh rosemary
1/2 cup low-sodium chicken or vegetable stock (pages 463, 473)

1 Cut the parsnips lengthwise into quarters and slice crosswise into 1/4-inch-thick wedges. Pour the oil into a high-sided skillet on medium high. Add the onions, garlic, parsnips, salt, and pepper and stir to mix thoroughly. Sauté 2 to 3 minutes or until the vegetables just start to brown.

2 Bury the rosemary sprig in the cooking vegetables, pour in the chicken stock, cover, and cook for 5 minutes or until they are as tender as you like them. Remove the rosemary and serve.

Per serving: 164 cal, 2 g fat, 0 saturated fat, 0% calories from saturated fat, 37 g carbohydrate,167 mg sodium, 3 g protein
Exchanges: 2 Starch

Cabbage Sauté with Caraway

SERVING SIZE: 1, SERVES: 1

1 tsp non-aromatic olive oil
1 large onion, sliced
1 lb (small) cabbage, shredded
1/4 tsp salt
1/4 tsp pepper
1 tsp caraway seed

1 Heat the oil in a high-sided skillet on medium high. Add the onion and cook, stirring occasionally until golden, 8 minutes.

2 Stir in the cabbage, salt, pepper, and caraway seed. Cook, stirring, for about 12 minutes or until tender. Serve with a slice of ham and a few boiled red potatoes.

Per serving: 71 calories, 2 g fat, 0 g saturated fat, 0% calories from saturated fat, 13 g carbohydrate, 4 g dietary fiber, 168 mg sodium
Exchanges: 3 Vegetable

Harvest Succotash

SERVING SIZE: 1/4 of recipe, SERVES: 4

Succotash

2 tsp non-aromatic olive oil
<C 1 medium onion, chopped
(1 1/2 cups)
3 cloves garlic, bashed and
chopped
1 Tbsp mild chili powder
1/4 tsp salt

<C 2 cups frozen corn kernels
<C 2 cups frozen baby lima beans
1 cup low-sodium chicken or
vegetable broth
2 tsp arrowroot or cornstarch
mixed with 2 Tbsp water (slurry)

Garnish

2 Tbsp chopped cilantro (optional)
2 Tbsp toasted sunflower seeds

1 Heat the oil in a high-sided skillet on medium high. Sauté the onion 3 minutes then add the garlic and cook 1 minute more or until the onions are soft but not browned. Season with the chili powder and salt.

2 Add the corn, lima beans, and stock. Bring to a boil, reduce the heat, and simmer 10 minutes. Stir in the slurry and heat to thicken, about 30 seconds.

3 Serve topped with the cilantro and sunflower seeds.

<C **To Cut Carb**

<C Onions: reduce to 1/2 cup.
<C Corn: reduce to 1 cup.
<C Lima beans: reduce to 1 cup.
+> Add 2 cups of your favorite vegetable.

Per serving: 228 calories, 5 g fat, 1 g saturated fat, 3% calories from saturated fat, 40 g carbohydrate, 8 g dietary fiber, 221 mg sodium, 10 g protein
Exchanges: 2 Starch, 2 Vegetable, 1/2 Fat

Low Carb

Per serving: 154 calories, 5 g fat, 1 g saturated fat, 3% calories from saturated fat, 24 g carbohydrate, 5 g dietary fiber, 207 mg sodium, 6 g protein
Exchanges: 1 Starch, 1 Vegetable, 1 Fat

Steamed, Microwaved, or Grilled Corn on the Cob in the Husk

SERVING SIZE: 1/4 of recipe, SERVES: 4

4 ears corn with husks   1 1/2 tsp arrowroot or cornstarch
1/2 cup chicken stock

> Warmth speeds the conversion of sugars to starch which results in a less sweet ear of corn. Corn should be stored in the refrigerator and not more than one day. It's best eaten the day it's picked.

1. Gently pull back the husks around the corn without pulling them clear off. Remove and discard the silk. Pull the husks back up around the corn and tie at the top with kitchen string or a piece of wire if you're going to grill it.

2. Steam in a single layer over boiling water in a large flat steamer 15 minutes.

3. Microwave in a single layer on high 9–12 minutes (fewer ears will take less time).

4. To grill over hot coals, soak first in cold water for 15 minutes then grill, turning once, 15 minutes for small ears, up to 30 minutes for very large ones.

5. Allow to cool a little before removing the husks. If you are doing it in the kitchen before serving, run each ear under cold water to cool the husks enough to handle.

6. Combine the broth and arrowroot and cornstarch. Heat until it clears and thickens. Brush on the corn in place of butter.

Per serving: 145 calories, 2 g fat, 1 g saturated fat, 6% calories from saturated fat, 35 g carbohydrate, 2 g fiber, 68 mg sodium
Exchanges: 2 Starch

Baked Sweet Onions

SERVING SIZE: 1 onion, SERVES: 4

4 medium sweet onions
1/4 cup balsamic vinegar
1/4 cup water

1 tsp arrowroot or corn starch mixed
with 2 tsp water (slurry)

1 Preheat the oven to 350°F. Cut off both ends of the onions and peel. Place in a small casserole dish. Combine the vinegar and water and pour over onions. Bake, uncovered, 1 hour or until tender.

2 Place an onion on each of 4 hot plates and pour the juice into a small saucepan. Stir in the slurry and heat until the liquid is clear and glossy. Serve as a sauce over the onions.

Per serving: 73 calories, 0 g fat, 0 g saturated fat, 0% calories from saturated fat, 17 g carbohydrate, 3 g dietary fiber, 5 mg sodium
Exchanges: 3 Vegetable

Baked Winter Squash

SERVING SIZE: 1/4 of recipe, SERVES: 4

4 serving size pieces winter squash
(2 acorns, 1 butternut, 2 delicatas, or
2 lb larger squash, such as hubbard)
olive oil spray

1/4 tsp salt
1/4 tsp pepper
1 tsp dried tarragon or thyme

1 Preheat the oven to 350°F. Cut the acorns, delicatas or butternut in half and scoop out the seeds and pulp. Leave the acorns or delicatas in halves. Cut the butternut in quarters and cut the larger squash in serving size pieces.

2 Lay the squash pieces on a baking sheet. Spray lightly with the olive oil spray. Season with salt and pepper and scatter the tarragon or thyme over the top. Bake about an hour, depending on the thickness of the squash, or until soft when pierced with a fork.

Per serving: 88 calories, 1 g fat, 0 g saturated fat, 0% calories from saturated fat, 20 g carbohydrate, 4 g dietary fiber, 149 mg sodium
Exchanges: 1 Starch

Thai Style Vegetables

SERVING SIZE: 1/4 of recipe, SERVES: 4

1 tsp Thai curry paste
1/3 cup low-sodium chicken or
    vegetable broth or water
1 tsp non-aromatic olive oil
1 cup small cauliflower florets

1 cup thinly sliced carrots
2 cups small broccoli florets
1 Tbsp Thai fish sauce or light soy sauce
1 tsp lime zest
2 Tbsp freshly squeezed lime juice

1 Dissolve the curry paste in the broth and set aside. Heat the oil in a skillet large enough for the whole recipe. Stir fry the cauliflower and carrots 3 minutes. Add the broccoli and stir to coat with oil. Pour in the reserved curry mixture and fish sauce. Cover and cook on medium heat 6 minutes or until tender.

2 Stir in the zest and lime juice. Serve with rice and a nice piece of grilled fish or chicken.

Per serving: 57 calories, 1 g fat, 0 g saturated fat, 0% calories from saturated fat, 9 g carbohydrate, 4 g dietary fiber, 478 mg sodium
Exchanges: 2 Vegetable

Microwaved Celery Hearts

SERVING SIZE: 1/2 celery heart, SERVES: 4

2 celery hearts
2 cups low sodium broth of your choice

1 Trim the celery heart and cut in half lengthwise. Place in a microwave-safe pan. Add the broth, cover with waxed paper, and cook on high in the microwave for 10 minutes. Turn the celery over and cook for another 5 minutes.

2 Drain and serve. Save the broth for another dish.

Per serving: 15 calories, 0 g fat, 0 g saturated fat, 0% calories from saturated fat, 1 g carbohydrate, 1 g fiber, 45 mg sodium, 2 g protein
Exchanges: Free Food

Roasted Green Beans

SERVING SIZE: 1/4 of recipe, SERVES: 4

1 lb green beans (or asparagus, sliced
  sweet onions, sliced eggplant, etc.)
  olive oil pan spray

1/4 tsp salt
1/4 tsp pepper
  1 Tbsp balsamic vinegar (optional)

1 Preheat the oven to 425°F. Lay the vegetables in a single layer on a lightly greased baking sheet. Spray the vegetables lightly with the pan spray and dust with salt and pepper.

2 Roast 10 minutes or until the vegetables are tender. Sprinkle with balsamic vinegar (if you are using it) and serve.

Per serving: 38 calories, 0 g fat, 0 g saturated fat, 0% calories from saturated fat, 9 g carbohydrate, 4 g dietary fiber, 146 mg sodium
Exchanges: 2 Vegetable

Broiled Mixed Vegetables

SERVING SIZE: 1/4 of recipe, SERVES: 4

1 (2 lb) package frozen mixed vegetables
  of your choice
2 tsp olive oil

1/4 tsp salt
1/4 tsp pepper
1/4 tsp rosemary

1 Preheat the broiler. Place a rack with very small open squares on a broiler pan or baking sheet.

2 Place the frozen vegetables, oil, salt, pepper, and rosemary in a plastic bag. Shake to coat the vegetables with the oil and seasonings. Spread on the broiler rack.

3 Broil 6 minutes 4 inches from the heat source.

Per serving: 148 calories, 2 g fat, 0 g saturated fat, 0% calories from saturated fat, 23 g carbohydrate, 5 g dietary fiber, 255 mg sodium
Exchanges: 1 1/2 Starch, 1/2 Fat

Simmered Radishes

SERVING SIZE: 1/4 of recipe, SERVES: 4

3 bunches red round radishes
1 cup low-sodium chicken or
   vegetable broth

2 tsp cornstarch mixed with 2 Tbsp water
1/4 tsp freshly ground black pepper

1 Trim the radishes leaving a little of the green stems and cutting off the root end. Place in a saucepan with the broth, bring to a boil, cover, reduce the heat, and simmer until tender, about 10 minutes.

2 Stir in the cornstarch slurry and heat to thicken and clear. Dust with pepper and serve as a side dish with meat.

Per serving: 8 calories, 0 g fat, 0 g saturated fat, 0% calories from saturated fat, 1 g carbohydrate, 0 g fiber, 22 mg sodium
Exchanges: Free Food

Butternut Squash Baked with Tamari

SERVING SIZE: 1/6 of recipe, SERVES: 6

1 butternut squash (3 lb) or acorn squash
1 Tbsp low sodium tamari or soy sauce

1/4 tsp pepper

1 Preheat the oven to 350°F. Cut the squash in half lengthwise. Scoop out and discard the seeds and pulp. Cut each half, again lengthwise, into 3 wedges. If you are using acorn squash, cut each half into 2 wedges.

2 Set the squash wedges into a baking dish. Brush with the tamari and season with pepper. Coat lightly with olive oil cooking spray. Bake 45 minutes or until the squash is soft.

Per serving: 81 calories, 0 g fat, 0 g saturated fat, 0% calories from saturated fat, 20 g carbohydrate, 3 g dietary fiber, 509 mg sodium
Exchanges: 1 Starch

Braised Leeks

SERVING SIZE: 1 large or 2 small leeks, SERVES: 4

8 small leeks or 4 large
1 tsp extra virgin olive oil

1 cup low-sodium vegetable broth
(see page 473)

1 Cut off the curly root ends and the green leaves of the leeks. Discard the roots and save the greens for stocks. Remove the 2 outer sheaths that trap the dirt as the leek grows. Wash carefully, dislodging any dirt hiding in the next few sheaths. If you have to use large leeks, cut them in half lengthwise and clean carefully.

2 Heat the oil in a skillet on medium high. Fry the leeks to brown slightly. Pour in the stock, bring to a boil, reduce the heat, and simmer, covered, 15 minutes or until tender.

Per serving: 51 calories, 1 g fat, 0 g saturated fat, 0% calories from saturated fat, 9 g carbohydrate, 4 g dietary fiber, 27 mg sodium
Exchanges: 2 Vegetable

Spicy Roasted Sweet Potato Wedges

SERVING SIZE: 1/4 lb, SERVES: 4

1 lb orange sweet potatoes
1/2 tsp olive oil or olive oil pan spray
1/4 tsp cumin

1/4 tsp mild chili powder
pinch cayenne pepper (optional)

1 Preheat the oven to 350°F. Peel the sweet potatoes and cut in thin wedges or sticks. Lay on a greased baking sheet and brush or spray with oil.

2 Combine the seasonings in a small bowl and dust over the top. Roast 30 minutes in the preheated oven.

Per serving: 128 calories, 28 g fat, 0 g saturated fat, 0% calories from saturated fat, 28 g carbohydrate, 4 g dietary fiber, 13 mg sodium
Exchanges: 1 Starch

Grilled Portabello Mushrooms with Tomato Jalapeño Sauce

SERVING SIZE: 1 mushroom, SERVES: 6

Mushrooms

2 cloves garlic, bashed, and finely chopped
1/4 tsp cayenne pepper
1/8 tsp ground allspice
1/4 tsp salt

1 tsp olive oil
1 Tbsp lemon juice
6 medium portabello mushrooms, cleaned with stems removed

Sauce

1/2 tsp light olive oil
2 cups roughly chopped sweet onion
3 jalapeño peppers, cored, seeded, and roughly chopped
3 small (or 2 large) Italian plum tomatoes, such as Roma, quartered
1 (14 1/2 oz) can crushed tomatoes in purée
1/8 tsp salt
1/8 tsp ground allspice
1 bay leaf
1 Tbsp arrowroot mixed with 1/2 cup nonalcoholic red wine or water (slurry)

1 Combine the garlic, cayenne, allspice, salt, olive oil, and lemon juice in a bowl. Season the mushrooms with the marinade in a shallow dish. Set aside while you make the sauce. Heat the barbecue grill or broiler.

2 Warm the oil in a medium frying pan over medium heat. Sauté the onions until slightly browned, 3–5 minutes. Stir in the jalapeños, tomatoes (both fresh and canned), salt, allspice, and bay leaf. Cook for 10 minutes over low heat. Press the tomato sauce through a sieve into a saucepan, discarding the pulp. Add the slurry to the sauce and stir over medium heat until thickened. Remove from the heat and keep warm until ready to serve.

3 Place the mushrooms on the hot grill or broiler pan and cook about 3 minutes per side. Cut the mushrooms into slices and fan out on 6 plates. Pour any juices from the broiler pan and cutting board into the tomato sauce. Spoon the sauce over the mushrooms.

Per serving: 90 calories, 0 g fat, 0 g saturated fat, 0% calories from saturated fat, 17 g carbohydrate, 5 g dietary fiber, 261 mg sodium, 5 g protein
Exchanges: 3 Vegetable

Grapefruit, Orange, Kiwi Salad in Grapefruit Shells

SERVING SIZE: 1 shell, SERVES: 4

2 whole red grapefruit
1 cup fresh or canned orange segments

1 cup peeled kiwi wedges
1/4 cup chopped chives

1 Cut the grapefruit in half. Remove the fruit in one piece by separating the fruit from the shell with a spoon. Cut each in half. You should have 2 cups.

2 Combine the grapefruit with the orange segments, kiwi wedges, and chives. Spoon into the shells and top with a crossed sprig of chives or a chive flower.

3 Serve with pork or chicken.

Per serving: 112 calories, 1 g fat, 0 g saturated fat, 0% calories from saturated fat, 26 g carbohydrate, 5 g dietary fiber, 2 mg sodium
Exchanges: 2 Fruit

Green Bean Rice Pilau

SERVING SIZE: 1/6 of recipe, SERVES: 6

<C 3 cups low-sodium chicken or
      vegetable stock (pages 463, 473)
    3 cardamom pods
    1 cinnamon stick, 1 1/2 inches long
1/8 tsp black peppercorns
1/4 tsp ground turmeric
    2 whole cloves
    1 tsp light olive oil
<C 1 cup finely diced onion

    2 cloves garlic, peeled, bashed,
      and chopped
<C 1 cup long-grain white rice
    1 bay leaf
1/4 tsp salt
1 1/2 cups green beans,
      cut into 1/4-inch slices
1/4 tsp ground cardamom
<C 1/4 cup raisins

1 Preheat the oven to 400°F.

2 Warm the stock in a small saucepan over medium-high heat. Pulverize the cardamom pods, cinnamon stick, peppercorns, turmeric, and cloves in a coffee mill or crush them with a mortar and pestle. Add the spice mixture to the stock and bring to a boil. Reduce the heat and simmer for about 30 minutes.

3 Heat 1/2 tsp of the oil in a medium ovenproof saucepan. Sauté the onion and garlic for 1 minute over medium heat. Add the rice and continue to cook for an additional 3 minutes.

4 Pour the seasoned stock through a strainer into the pan with the rice. Add the bay leaf and 1/8 tsp of the salt. Stir well and place, uncovered, in the preheated oven. Bake for 20 minutes, or until the rice is tender and the liquid is absorbed.

5 Heat the remaining 1/2 tsp of oil in a large sauté pan. Add the green beans, remaining 1/8 tsp of salt, and ground cardamom. Cook for 6–8 minutes, or until tender. You may need to add just a little water so the beans won't brown, but don't let them lose their bright green color.

6 After the rice has finished baking, stir in the green beans and raisins and serve immediately.

<C To Cut Carb

<C Stock: reduce to 2 cups.
<C Onions: reduce to 1/2 cup.
<C Raisins: reduce to 1 Tbsp.

<C Rice: reduce to 2/3 cup, replace with brown rice at step 4, bake for 40 minutes.

Per serving: 166 calories, 1 g fat, 0 g saturated fat, 0% calories from saturated fat, 35 g carbohydrate, 2 g dietary fiber, 111 mg sodium, 4 g protein
Exchanges: 1 1/2 Starch, 1 Vegetable, 1/2 Fruit

Low Carb
Per serving: 109 calories, 2 g fat, 0 g saturated fat, 0% calories from saturated fat, 21 g carbohydrate, 2 g dietary fiber, 107 mg sodium, 3 g protein
Exchanges: 1 Starch, 1 Vegetable

Steamed Pattypan

SERVING SIZE: 1/4 of recipe, SERVES: 4

4 2 1/2-inch to 3-inch pattypan squash, cut in half top to bottom
1 Tbsp chopped fresh basil or 1 tsp dried

1/4 tsp salt
1/4 tsp pepper

(*Continued*)

Lay the squash halves in a steamer and season with salt, pepper, and basil. Steam over boiling water 6 minutes or until tender but still firm.

Per serving: 28 calories, 0 g fat, 0 g saturated fat, 0% calories from saturated fat, 6 g carbohydrates, 2 g fiber, 141 mg sodium, 1 g protein
Exchanges: 1 Vegetable

Caramelized Onions

SERVING SIZE:1/4 of recipe, SERVES: 4

1 tsp olive oil
1 lb onions, peeled and sliced

Heat the oil in a heavy skillet on medium heat. Cook, stirring occasionally, until soft and browned, about 20 minutes. Serve as a side dish or as an addition to salad, spaghetti sauce, or vegetables and rice.

Per serving: 53 calories, 1 g fat, 0 g saturated fat, 0% calories from saturated fat, 10 g carbohydrate, 2 g dietary fiber, 3 mg sodium
Exchanges: 2 Vegetable

Steamed Broccoflower

SERVING SIZE: 1 cup, SERVES: 4

1 head (4 cups broccoflower)   1 Tbsp lemon juice (optional)
1/4 tsp salt

Cut the broccoflower into small florets, season with salt, and steam over boiling water for 6 minutes or until tender. Serve with a little lemon juice if you like.

Per serving: 21 calories, 0 g fat, 0 g saturated fat, 0% calories from saturated fat, 4 g carbohydrate, 2 g dietary fiber, 154 mg sodium
Exchanges: 1 Vegetable

Steamed Baby Bok Choy

SERVING SIZE: 1/4 of recipe, SERVES: 4

1/4 tsp salt
1/4 tsp pepper

4 baby bok choy (up to 5 inches long)

Cut the bok choys in half lengthwise. Lay them in a large steamer and season with salt and pepper. Steam, covered, 3 minutes. Serve immediately.

Per serving: 9 calories, 0 g fat, 0 g saturated fat, 0% calories from saturated fat, 1 g carbohydrate, 1 g dietary fiber, 106 mg sodium
Exchanges: Free Food

Citrus Vegetables

SERVING SIZE: 1/4 of recipe, SERVES: 4

2 Tbsp fresh lime juice
1/2 Tbsp olive oil
1/2 tsp chopped fresh oregano

4 cups sliced steamed vegetables such as zucchini, corn, and tomatoes

Mix lime juice with oil. Add oregano, and pour over vegetables.

Per serving: 73 calories, 0 g fat, 0 g saturated fat, 0% calories from saturated fat, 14 g carbohydrate, 2 g dietary fiber, 9 mg sodium
Exchanges: 1/2 Starch, 1 Vegetable

Steamed Collards

SERVING SIZE: 1/4 of recipe, SERVES: 4

1 lb bunch collards
1/4 tsp dried basil
1/4 tsp cayenne pepper (optional)
1 Tbsp lemon juice

1/4 tsp salt
1/4 tsp pepper
   (omit if using cayenne pepper)

(*Continued*)

1. Wash and remove heavy stems of the greens. Pile a few of the leaves on top of each other, roll into a cylinder, and cut across into strips. Repeat with the rest.

2. Place in a steamer, add the basil, optional cayenne, lemon juice, salt, and pepper. Steam 4 to 6 minutes or until tender but still nice and green.

Per serving: 28 calories, 0 g fat, 0 g saturated fat, 0% calories from saturated fat, 6 g carbohydrate, 4 g dietary fiber, 161 mg sodium
Exchanges: 1 Vegetable

Sautéed Mushrooms with Lemon and Dill

SERVING SIZE: 1/4 of recipe, SERVES: 4

1 lb 1-inch diameter white or
   brown mushrooms
2 Tbsp freshly squeezed lemon juice

1/2 tsp dried dill weed
1/8 tsp cayenne pepper

1. Remove the stems from the mushrooms and save for stocks. Clean the mushrooms with a dry cloth or soft brush.

2. Place, round side down, in a hot nonstick skillet big enough to hold them in a single layer. Sprinkle with lemon juice, dill, and cayenne and cook on medium for 3 minutes. Turn, stirring, 1 more minute or until they lose their chalky, raw look.

Per serving: 21 calories, 0 g fat, 0 g saturated fat, 0% calories from saturated fat, 4 g carbohydrate, 1 g dietary fiber, 5 mg sodium
Exchanges: 1 Vegetable

Main Dishes

Waimea Fried Rice

SERVING SIZE: 1/6 of recipe, SERVES: 6

Rice

1 cup long-grain brown rice
1 stalk lemon grass
1 Tbsp light olive oil with a dash
    of toasted sesame oil
1 Tbsp finely diced jalapeño chilis,
    seeds and membranes removed
3 cloves of garlic, peeled, bashed,
    and finely chopped
    heaping 1/3 cup red pepper, cut in
    1/4-inch dice

1/2 cup celery, cut in 1/4-inch dice
  4 tsp grated fresh ginger root
  1 cup chopped fresh pineapple,
    cut in 1/4-inch dice
 12 mint leaves, finely chopped
1/4 cup loosely packed cilantro leaves,
    finely chopped
  1 tsp toasted sesame oil
  1 Tbsp Thai fish sauce or tamari
  1 tsp rice wine vinegar

Garnish

6 sprigs fresh mint

6 sprigs cilantro

1   Boil the brown rice in 4 cups of water for 25 minutes or until just tender.
    Drain through a sieve and rinse with cold water to wash the starch off and
    start the chilling process. Spread in a flat metal pan and set in the refrigera-
    tor to chill at least 30 minutes.

2   Remove the tough outside layer of the lemon grass, cut off the immediate
    root end and the dry top part. Start slicing from the root end to get the most
    tender part of the stalk. Slice thinly and chop fine so the flavor will be
    spread throughout. You should have about 1/4 cup.

3   Remember that this is a very quick dish so it's important to have all the
    elements of the recipe ready at hand. Heat the oil in a large frying pan on
    medium-high heat. Stir in the lemon grass, garlic, and chilis and cook for
    30 seconds to release the aromatic oils. Add the red peppers, celery, and
    ginger and stir fry for another 30 seconds. Add the chilled rice, and cook
    until heated through. Stir the pineapple, mint, and cilantro into the hot rice.
    Sprinkle the oil, fish sauce, and vinegar over the top, stir to mix, and serve
    immediately.

4   Garnish with sprigs of mint and cilantro and serve alongside Roasted
    Chicken with Pineapple Curry Sauce (page 268).

Per serving: 157 calories, 4 g fat, 1 g saturated fat, 6% of calories from fat, 28 g
carbohydrate, 2 g dietary fiber, 38 mg sodium, 3 g protein
Exchanges: 1 1/2 Starch, 1 Vegetable, 1/2 Fat

Turkey Picadillo and Cuban Black Beans with Baked Plantain

SERVING SIZE: 1/6 of recipe, SERVES: 6

Sofrito

<C 4 cups roughly chopped sweet onions

1 large green bell pepper, roughly chopped

7 cloves garlic

1 Tbsp distilled vinegar

Picadillo

1 tsp non-aromatic olive oil

1 1/2 lb extra lean ground turkey

1/4 tsp salt

1 tsp ground cumin

1 Tbsp tomato paste

1 Tbsp capers

10 large black olives

<C 2 Tbsp raisins

2 Tbsp fine sliced cilantro

<C 3 cups boiled white or brown rice (optional)

Cuban Black Beans

1 tsp non-aromatic olive oil

1/4 cup sofrito

1 tsp cumin

1 tsp brown sugar

1 Tbsp vinegar

<C 2 cups home cooked or canned black beans, drained and rinsed

1 1/2 cups nonalcoholic dry white wine

4 bay leaves

1/4 tsp salt

Baked Plantain

<C 2 plantains

To Prepare the Sofrito and Picadillo

To make the sofrito place the onions, peppers, garlic, and vinegar in a blender. Start the blender at the chop level then increase speed to puree. Whiz until smooth. This will keep in the refrigerator for a week and can be used to add flavor to soups, stews, and casseroles.

2 Heat 1/2 tsp of the oil in a skillet or chef's pan on medium high. Sauté 3 Tbsp of the sofrito, 1 Tbsp of the tomato paste, and the cumin together until the mix is thick and dark. Reserve on a plate and rinse the pan.

3 Heat the remaining oil and brown the turkey, mashing it as you go to keep it loose. Stir in the remaining sofrito and tomato paste along with the capers, olives, and raisins. Serve with Cuban Black Beans and baked plantain for a comforting Cuban meal. It will look fresh and interesting if you scatter everything with fine sliced cilantro.

To Prepare the Cuban Black Beans

4 Heat the oil in a chef's pan or large saucepan on medium high. Fry the sofrito and cumin, stirring, 2 minutes. Add the sugar, vinegar, beans, wine, bay, and salt. Simmer until thick, about 25 minutes.

5 Serve with the picadillo.

To Prepare the Baked Plantains

6 Preheat the oven to 375°F. Slit the skin of 2 ripe plantains from end to end. Lay in a baking dish slit side up and bake 1 hour or until tender. Peel, slice on the diagonal, and serve with the picadillo and beans.

<C **To Cut Carb**

<C Onions: reduce to 3 cups.	<C Black beans: reduce to 1 1/2 cups.
<C Raisins: reduce to 1 Tbsp.	<C Plantain: reduce to only one
<C Brown rice: reduce to 1 cup.	(now a small garnish).

Per serving (without rice): 370 calories, 4 g fat, 0 g saturated fat, 0% calories from saturated fat, 52 g carbohydrate, 10 g dietary fiber, 364 mg sodium, 35 g protein
Exchanges: 2 1/2 Starch, 3 Very Lean Meat, 3 Vegetable

Low Carb
Per serving: 302 calories, 4 g fat, 0 g saturated fat, 0% calories from fat, 35 g carbohydrate, 7 g dietary fiber, 361 mg sodium, 33 g protein
Exchanges: 1 1/2 Starch, 3 Very Lean Meat, 3 Vegetable
Per serving: 157 calories, 4 g fat, 1g saturated fat, 6% of calories from fat, 28 g carbohydrate, 2 g dietary fiber, 38 mg sodium, 3 g protein
Exchanges: 1 1/2 Starch, 1 Vegetable, 1/2 Fat

Thai Chicken Stir-Fry with Coconut Sauce

SERVING SIZE: 1/4 of recipe, SERVES: 4

Stir-fry

1 tsp non-aromatic olive oil
1 Tbsp finely chopped ginger
1 tsp chopped garlic
1 Tbsp finely chopped lemon grass
12 oz boneless, skinless chicken
    breast, cut in 2-inch × 1-inch
1/4 plus 1/8 tsp salt

1/2 tsp freshly ground black pepper
1/2 Napa cabbage, washed,
    trimmed, and cut into
    1/4-inch strips
1/2 cup enoki mushrooms or
    quartered white mushrooms
1/2 red bell pepper, cut in thin strips

Sauce

1 cup coconut cream (page 465)
1 Tbsp Thai fish sauce or light
    soy sauce
1 tsp grated lime zest (optional)

1/2 cup low-sodium chicken stock
    (page 463)
1 tsp cornstarch
1/8 tsp cayenne pepper

Vegetarian Option

12 oz firm light tofu, cut into 2-inch x 1-inch strips
1/2 cup low-sodium vegetable stock (page 473)

Replace the chicken with the tofu and treat the same way as you would
the chicken. Use vegetable stock instead of chicken stock and soy sauce
in place of fish sauce and you have a lovely vegetarian stir-fry.

---

1 Heat 1/2 tsp of the oil in large high-sided skillet on medium high. Add the
ginger, garlic and lemongrass, stirring to release flavors. Toss in the
chicken, sprinkle with 1/4 tsp of the salt and pepper and cook until white on
the outside, about 2 minutes. Tip into a warm bowl, cover, and set aside.

2 Heat the remaining 1/2 tsp oil and stir-fry the cabbage, mushrooms, and red
bell peppers until wilted but still crisp, about 2 minutes. Sprinkle with the
remaining salt and pepper and add the chicken.

3 Combine the sauce ingredients and pour over the stir-fry, stir to mix, and heat to thicken. Serve with rice.

Per serving: 229 calories, 6 g fat, 3 g saturated fat, 11% calories from saturated fat, 20 g carbohydrate, 5 g dietary fiber, 697 mg sodium, 24 g protein
Exchanges: 3 Very Lean Meat, 2 Vegetable, 1 Fat, 1/2 Carbohydrate

Vegetarian
Per serving: 167 calories, 6 g fat, 3 g saturated fat, 16% calories from saturated fat, 21 g carbohydrate, 5 g dietary fiber, 623 mg sodium, 8 g protein
Exchanges: 1 Very Lean Meat, 2 Vegetable, 1 Fat, 1/2 Carbohydrate

Vegetable Stir-Fry with Passion Fruit Vinaigrette

SERVING SIZE: 1/6 of recipe, SERVES: 6

1 tsp non-aromatic olive oil
6 green onions, white parts sliced, green parts cut on the diagonal
4 carrots, peeled and cut on the diagonal in 1/4-inch slices (1 cup)
1 yellow bell pepper, cut in 2-inch strips
1 red bell pepper, cut in 2-inch strips

3 cups broccoli flowerettes, cut small
1 cup bean sprouts
1 recipe Passion Fruit Vinaigrette (page 460)
6 large butter lettuce leaves

1 Warm a high-sided skillet over medium-high heat and add the oil. Sauté the white parts of the onions for 1 minute to release their flavor. Add the carrots and red and yellow peppers and continue cooking for 1 minute. Stir in the broccoli and reduce the heat to low. Cover the pan and cook for 2 or 3 more minutes.

2 Add the sprouts and green parts of the onions and cook until just heated through. Pour the vinaigrette over the hot vegetables and stir until it bubbles, thickens, and develops a glossy sheen.

3 Lay a lettuce leaf on each of 6 plates and divide the stir-fry among them.

Per serving: 74 calories, 1 g fat, 0 g saturated fat, 0% calories from saturated fat, 15 g carbohydrate, 5 g dietary fiber, 41 mg sodium
Exchanges: 2 Vegetable, 1/2 Fruit

Roasted Chicken with Pineapple Curry Sauce

SERVING SIZE: 1/6 of recipe, SERVES: 6

Chicken

2 (9 inch) stalks fresh
lemongrass

1 (4 inch) piece ginger root,
finely sliced

6 cloves garlic, peeled, bashed, and
chopped

2 (3 1/2 lb) whole chickens, rinsed
and dried

Pineapple Curry Sauce

1 tsp light olive oil

3/4 cup finely diced sweet onion

1 Tbsp India Ethmix (page 477) or good Madras curry

1 Tbsp peeled and grated ginger root

2 large cloves garlic, peeled, bashed, and finely chopped

1 Tbsp finely sliced lemongrass

3/4 cup low-sodium chicken or vegetable stock (pages 463, 473)

1/3 cup frozen pineapple juice concentrate

1/4 cup yogurt cheese (page 475)

1/2 tsp coconut extract

1 Tbsp fish sauce

To Prepare the Chickens

1 Preheat the oven to 350°F.

2 Remove the tough outside layer of the lemongrass stalk and cut off the root end and the dry top. Starting from the root end, cut the most tender, bulb-like part of the stalk into thin diagonal slices.

3 Combine the lemongrass, ginger, and garlic and divide between the cavities of the two chickens. Turn the chickens breast down on a plate so that the seasonings fall against the inside of the breasts. Insert a vertical poultry roaster into each chicken and stand upright. Tie the legs together with cotton string and tuck the wings behind the breast. Set the chickens in a 9-inch × 13-inch baking dish. (If you don't have a vertical roaster, lay the chickens on a rack in a roasting pan. Tie the legs together with cotton string and tuck the wings behind the breast.)

4 Whichever roasting method you are using, pour 1 1/2 cups of warm water into the bottom of the baking dish. Bake in the preheated oven for 45 minutes to 1 hour, or until the chickens reach 140°F in the thickest part of the thigh. (The chickens in the roasting pan may take an extra 10 minutes.) Remove from the oven and set aside for 10 minutes. The final internal temperature should be 160°F.

To Prepare the Sauce

5 Warm the oil in a medium saucepan over medium heat. Sauté the onion and India Ethmix until the onion is soft and translucent, about 5 minutes. Stir in the ginger, garlic, and lemongrass and cook for 3 more minutes.

6 Add the chicken stock and pineapple juice concentrate, stirring to incorporate. Cook for an additional 3 minutes. Strain the sauce through a sieve into a small saucepan using a purée press or the back of a spoon.

7 Whisk together the yogurt cheese, coconut extract, and Thai fish sauce in a 2-cup glass measuring cup. Pour a little of the hot pineapple sauce into the yogurt mixture and stir to warm the yogurt cheese. Add the tempered yogurt cheese to the sauce and whisk until smooth. Cover and set aside to keep warm.

To Assemble the Dish

8 Remove the chickens from the roasting pan and pour the cooking juices into a fat strainer. Remove the vertical roasters if you were using them. Remove and discard the skin. Cut the legs and breast meat away from the carcasses. Put aside 1 leg and 1 breast for another meal. Slice the meat from the remaining breasts and legs and arrange on a warmed plate. Cover and keep warm.

9 Pour the de-fatted pan juices into a small saucepan and boil vigorously until the liquid is reduced to about 1/4 cup. Allow to cool for a minute, then stir into the curry sauce.

10 Arrange slices of chicken on a warmed plate and spoon curry sauce over the meat. Serve Vegetable Stir-Fry with Passion Fruit Vinaigrette (page 267) alongside.

Per serving: 297 calories, 8 g fat, 2 g saturated fat, 6% calories from saturated fat, 12 g carbohydrate, 1 g dietary fiber, 44 g protein
Exchanges: 4 Lean Meat, 1 Carbohydrate

Sicilian Baked White Fish

SERVING SIZE: 1 fillet, SERVES: 4

1 tsp non-aromatic olive oil
2 cups chopped onion, 1/4-inch pieces
1 (4-inch) sprig fresh rosemary or 1 tsp dried
3 cloves garlic, bashed and chopped
2 ribs celery, chopped
2 (14 1/2 oz) cans diced tomatoes in puree
1/2 cup nonalcoholic dry white wine
1/4 cup roughly chopped green olives

2 Tbsp capers
1/8 tsp crushed chilis
1/8 tsp freshly ground black pepper
4 (6 oz) cod or other firm white fish fillets
1/2 tsp extra virgin olive oil
1 Tbsp arrowroot mixed with
2 Tbsp nonalcoholic white wine (slurry)
1 Tbsp chopped fresh parsley

Vegetarian Option

1 lb reduced-fat tofu

Replace the fish with the tofu. Cut the tofu into 4 oz servings and treat them exactly as you would the fish.

---

1 Preheat the oven to 375°F. Heat the oil in a high-sided skillet on medium high. Cook the onions with the sprig of rosemary for 1 minute. Add the garlic and celery and cook 2 minutes. Pour in the tomatoes and wine and simmer 4 minutes.

2 Stir in the olives, capers, chilis, and pepper. Bury the fish fillets in the sauce, cover, and bake for 8 minutes or until the fish flakes.

3 Divide the fish fillets among 4 hot plates. Stir the olive oil and slurry into the sauce and heat to thicken slightly. Spoon over the fish fillets, sprinkle with chopped parsley, and serve with a crusty Italian bread like the Italian Bread with Roasted Vegetables (see page 198).

Per serving: 289 calories, 4 g fat, 1 g saturated fat, 3% calories from saturated fat, 18 g carbohydrate, 3 g dietary fiber, 937 mg sodium, 45 g protein
Exchanges: 5 Very Lean Meat, 4 Vegetable, 1/2 Fat

Vegetarian

Per serving: 140 calories, 4 g fat, 1 g saturated fat, 6% calories from saturated fat, 20 g carbohydrate, 3 g dietary fiber, 947 mg sodium, 6 g protein
Exchanges: 4 Vegetable, 1 Fat

Three Sisters Stew

SERVING SIZE: 1/4 of recipe, SERVES: 4

Stew

1 tsp non-aromatic olive oil
1 medium sweet onion, thinly sliced
2 cups fresh green beans, tipped, tailed, cut in 1-inch pieces
2 cups low-sodium vegetable broth (page 473)
1 zucchini, cut in 1-inch chunks
1 (15 oz) can garbanzo beans, rinsed and drained

1 cup fresh, frozen or canned corn kernels
1 poblano chili, roasted, peeled, and cut in 1-inch pieces
1/2 cup prepared green salsa
1/2 cup prepared red salsa
1/2 cup chopped cilantro
2 Roma tomatoes, peeled and halved

Dumplings

Scant 1/2 cup dry masa harina
1/3 cup water
1 tsp non-aromatic olive oil
2 Tbsp chopped cilantro

1/4 cup parmesan cheese
3/4 cup low-fat cottage cheese
1/4 cup egg substitute or 1 whole egg

1 Heat the oil in a chef's pan or large saucepan on medium high. Sauté the onion until it begins to wilt, about 2 minutes. Add the green beans and stock and simmer 5 minutes. Stir in the zucchini, garbanzo beans, corn, and green and red salsas.

2 Drop tsp-size dumpling into the simmering soup and simmer 10 minutes more or until the dumplings are cooked and the green beans are tender. Stir in the chili pieces and tomato halves and heat through. Divide among 4 hot bowls and garnish with the chopped cilantro.

Per serving: 315 calories, 8 g fat, 2 g saturated fat, 6% calories from saturated fat, 47 g carbohydrate, 11 g dietary fiber, 797 mg sodium, 14 g protein
Exchanges: 2 1/2 Starch, 2 Vegetable, 1 1/2 Fat

Shrimp Gumbo

SERVING SIZE: 1/4 of recipe, SERVES: 4

<C   1 lb medium shrimp
         1 cup uncooked long grain
           white rice
         3 tsp non-aromatic olive oil,
           divided
     1/4 lb Canadian bacon, cut in
           1/2-inch dice (scant 3/4 cup)
<C 1 1/2 cups chopped onion
         2 cloves garlic, bashed and
           chopped
>   1 cup celery, cut in 1/2-inch
           slices

      1 large red bell pepper, cut in
   1/4-inch dice (generous cup)
      3 Tbsp tomato paste
   1/4 cup all-purpose flour
      2 cups frozen or fresh sliced okra
         (1/2-inch slices)
      2 cups shrimp shell stock
   1/4 tsp cayenne pepper
   1/2 tsp dried thyme
      2 bay leaves
      1 tsp gumbo filé

1 Shell and devein the shrimp, reserving the shells. Pour 4 cups water over the shells in a large saucepan and bring to a boil. Reduce the heat and simmer 2 minutes. Strain, and use 2 cups of the liquid to cook the rice, boil, then cover and reduce to a simmer for about 15 minutes until all moisture is absorbed. Save the rest for the gumbo.

2 Heat 1 tsp of the oil in a skillet or chef's pan on medium high. Sauté the Canadian bacon 2 minutes. Add the onions and cook until they start to wilt, 2 minutes. Add the garlic, celery, and red pepper and continue to sauté 3–4 minutes. Pull the vegetables to the side of the pan and add the tomato paste. Cook, stirring, until it darkens and coats the vegetables. Remove to a plate.

3 Heat the remaining oil in the same pan. Shake the okra in the flour in a bag. Pour into a strainer to remove extra flour. Brown the floured okra in the hot oil. Return the vegetables to the pan and add the remaining shrimp liquid. Season with the cayenne, thyme and bay and simmer until the okra is tender, about 10 minutes. Stir in the shrimp and cook until pink. Add the filé and simmer 5 minutes until thickened. *Do not* boil after adding filé. The gumbo will be pretty thick so this shouldn't be a problem.

4 Divide the rice among 4 hot soup plates and pour the gumbo over the top. Garnish with chopped fresh parsley if you like.

Sea Bass with Mango Chutney,
page 322

Mesclun Salad with Fruit, page 181

Turkey Pot Pie, page 316

Manhattan Clam Chowder, page 144,
Creamy Clam Chowder, page 164

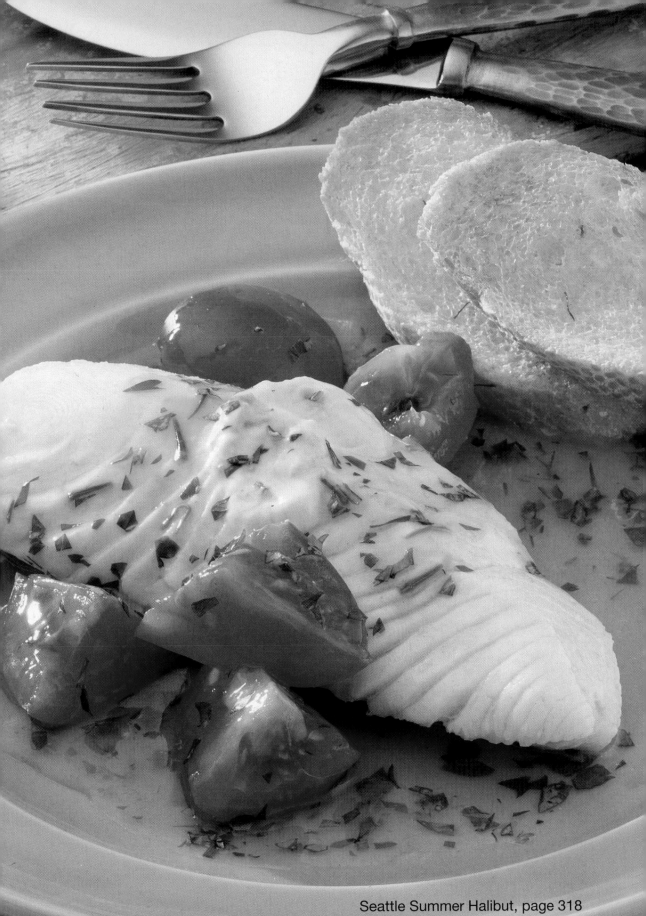

Seattle Summer Halibut, page 318

Nora's Shrimp and Mushroom
Risotto, page 294

Jerk Marinated Lamb, page 314, served over sweet potatoes and kale

Pineapple Nieve, page 431

Per serving: 419 calories, 7 g fat, 2 g saturated fat, 4% calories from saturated fat, 60 g carbohydrate, 6 g fiber, 570 mg sodium
Exchanges: 3 Starch, 2 Lean Meat, 3 Vegetable

Low Carb
Per serving: 330 calories, 7 g fat, 1 g saturated fat, 4% calories from saturated fat, 40 g carbohydrate, 5 g dietary fiber, 582 mg sodium
Exchanges: 1 1/2 Starch, 2 Lean Meat, 3 Vegetable

BLT with a Difference

SERVING SIZE: 1 sandwich, SERVES: 1

1/2 oz thinly sliced Canadian bacon
2 slices whole-wheat bread
1 tsp mayonnaise dressing

2 leaves romaine
<C 1 whole tomato, sliced thinly
(3/4 cup)

1 Heat a dry skillet on medium high. Lay the Canadian bacon in the pan and fry until a little brown on both sides. Toast the bread and spread with the dressing.

2 Lay a lettuce leaf on one side of the prepared toast. Now layer half the tomato slices, the Canadian bacon, the rest of the tomato slices, and the other lettuce leaf on top. Cover with the remaining bread slice, cut into 4 pieces and serve.

<C **To Cut Carb**
<C Bread: as with all our sandwiches, you can go open-faced with one slice or you could cut off the crusts and use them as salad croutons.

Per serving: 223 calories, 7 g fat, 1 g saturated fat, 5% calories from saturated fat, 33 g carbohydrate, 5 g dietary fiber, 506 mg sodium
Exchanges: 2 Starch, 1 Vegetable, 1 Fat

Low Carb
Per serving: 154 calories, 6 g fat, 1 g saturated fat, 6% calories from saturated fat, 20 g carbohydrate, 4 g dietary fiber, 359 mg sodium
Exchanges: 1 Starch, 1 Vegetable, 1 Fat

Steamed Prawns and Oysters

SERVING SIZE: 1/6 of recipe, SERVES: 6

Ginger Drizzle Sauce

1/2 tsp light olive oil
  1 tsp fresh ginger root, peeled and cut into fine matchsticks

1/2 cup dry white wine
  (I prefer nonalcoholic chardonnay)

Main Ingredients

  1 head savoy cabbage, cut into 1/2-inch strips
1/4 tsp salt
1/4 tsp freshly ground black pepper
  1 tsp fresh ginger root, peeled and cut into fine matchsticks

18 medium prawns, peeled and deveined
18 extra-small oysters, on the half shell

Vegetarian Option: Steamed Heart of Palm and Mushrooms

 6 heart of palm
36 button mushrooms

2 Tbsp fresh lemon juice

Cut the heart of palm in half lengthwise and place in a steamer with the mushrooms. Cover and steam for 7 minutes. Season with the lemon juice and a light dusting of salt and pepper.

To Prepare the Sauce

1 Warm the oil in a small saucepan over medium-high heat. Sauté the ginger for 1 minute. Stir in the wine and set aside until ready to serve.

To Prepare the Shellfish and Cabbage

2 Scatter the cabbage on the bottom platform of a two-tiered steamer or place in a steamer insert. Sprinkle with the salt, pepper, and ginger. Cover and steam for 2 minutes.

3 Reduce the heat to low and lay the prawns over the top of the partially cooked cabbage. Place the oysters in the second platform and stack it on top. Cover and steam both levels for 2 minutes. If you do not have a two-tiered steamer, steam the prawns over the cabbage for 2 minutes, then transfer to covered bowls to keep warm while you steam the oysters.

To Serve

4 Spread a bed of cabbage on each salad plate, then arrange the oysters and prawns around a small bowl of "drizzle sauce" on each plate. Serve immediately.

Per serving: 175 calories, 4 g fat, 1 g saturated fat, 5% calories from saturated fat, 12 g carbohydrate, 2 g dietary fiber, 23 g protein
Exchanges: 3 Very Lean Meat, 2 Vegetable, 1/2 Fat

Vegetarian
Per serving: 70 calories, 1 g fat, 0 g saturated fat, 0% calories from saturated fat, 16 g carbohydrate, 3 g dietary fiber
Exchanges: 3 Vegetable

Crustless Spinach Ricotta Quiche

SERVING SIZE: 1/6 of recipe, SERVES: 6

12 cups well-washed fresh spinach or
2 packages frozen spinach, thawed
2 tsp olive oil
1/2 cup finely chopped onions
1 cup low-fat ricotta cheese
1/2 cup egg substitute or
   2 whole eggs, beaten

1/2 tsp dried dill weed
1/4 tsp pepper
1/4 tsp salt
   pinch nutmeg (optional)
3 plum tomatoes, seeds and juice
   removed, chopped (1 cup)
1 Tbsp grated Parmesan cheese

1 Preheat oven to 350°F. Grease a 9-inch pie plate. Steam fresh spinach until just wilted. (Frozen spinach just needs to be thawed.) Press water out of cooked or thawed spinach, and set aside.

2 Heat oil in a small skillet, and cook onions until soft but not brown. Combine ricotta cheese, egg substitute, dill, pepper, and nutmeg in a large bowl. Add prepared spinach, tomatoes, and onions. Mix thoroughly, and tip into pie pan.

3 Sprinkle Parmesan cheese over the top, and bake until set, about 30 minutes. Let the quiche cool for 5 or 10 minutes before serving.

Per serving: 115 calories, 3 g fat, 1 g saturated fat, 8% calories from saturated fat, 9 g carbohydrate, 6 g dietary fiber, 327 mg sodium
Exchanges: 1 Lean Meat, 2 Vegetable

Steamed Chicken with a Peanut Dipping Sauce

SERVING SIZE: 1/4 of recipe, SERVES: 4

Chicken

4-lb roasting chicken
2 green onions, cut in half lengthwise
1 Tbsp chopped ginger
1/4 tsp salt

1/4 tsp freshly ground pepper
8 baby bok choy, carefully washed and trimmed

Dipping Sauce

1/2 tsp light olive oil
4 cloves garlic, bashed and chopped
2 tsp grated ginger
1 cup nonalcoholic, fruity white wine
1 Tbsp low sodium tamari or soy sauce
1 Tbsp light brown sugar
1/2 tsp Shanghai Ethmix (page 477)

3 Tbsp creamy natural peanut butter, oil poured off before use
1 Tbsp arrowroot mixed with
2 Tbsp water, slurry
<C 1/2 French baguette (8 oz), cut into 8 slices
12 cilantro leaves, chopped

1 Wash and dry the chicken with paper towels. Cut off the legs, thighs and breast meat and set aside. Save the carcass and wings to make stock. Lay the onion pieces around the bottom of a bundt pan or kugelhopf pan. Season the breast and thigh pieces with the chopped ginger, salt, and pepper. Lay them on the onions. Set the bundt pan in a Dutch oven with enough hot water to come about a third of the way up the side. Cover and boil for 15 minutes. Open and add the breast pieces and simmer, covered, 30 minutes more.

2 While the chicken is steaming, make the dipping sauce. Heat the oil in a small saucepan on medium and fry the garlic and ginger for a minute or two to release the flavorful oils. Add 3/4 cup of the wine, tamari, brown sugar, and Shanghai Ethmix. Remove from the heat and add the peanut butter, stirring until smooth. Set aside and keep warm.

3 When the chicken is done, remove it to a plate and keep warm. Strain the accumulated juices into a fat separator and pour the defatted liquid into a small saucepan. Lay the bok choy evenly around the bundt pan and return it to the Dutch oven. Cover and steam 5 minutes. Pour the slurry into the liquid in the saucepan and heat until it thickens and clears. Thin the dipping sauce with the remaining wine.

4 Remove the skin from the chicken, discard, and divide the chicken among 4 hot plates. Place 2 baby bok choy and 2 slices of bread on each plate. Divide the sauces among 8 small dishes so each person gets a dish of each. Scatter the cilantro over the chicken and serve.

<C **To Cut Carb**

<C French Bread: reduce to one slice per serving.

Per serving: 486 calories, 14 g fat, 3 g saturated fat, 5% calories from saturated fat, 41 g carbohydrate, 3 g dietary fiber, 790 mg sodium, 48 g protein
Exchanges: 2 Starch, 5 Lean Meat, 1/2 Carbohydrate

Low Carb
Per serving: 418 calories, 14 g fat, 3 g saturated fat, 5% calories from saturated fat, 27 g carbohydrate, 2 g dietary fiber, 620 mg sodium, 45 g protein
Exchanges: 1 Starch, 5 Lean Meat, 1/2 Carbohydrate

Vegetable Wraps with Chicken and Hummus

SERVING SIZE: 1/4 of recipe, SERVES: 4

1 cup diced cooked chicken
1/2 cup chopped cucumber
1/2 cup chopped red bell pepper
1/2 cup chopped raw sugar snap peas
1/2 cup chopped arugula

1/2 cup hummus
4 (8 inch) wraps or flour tortillas
4 lettuce leaves (leaf or butter lettuce works best)

1 Combine the chicken, cucumber, bell pepper, peas, arugula, and hummus in a bowl. (You can add different vegetables according to the season and your family's preferences.)

2 Lay the wraps on the counter and cover each with a lettuce leaf. Divide the vegetable mixture among them and spread, leaving at least a half-inch border around the edge. Roll up tightly, tucking in the edges as you roll. Cut in half and wrap in plastic food film.

Per serving: 190 calories, 3 g fat, 1 g saturated fat, 5% calories from saturated fat, 25 g carbohydrate, 10 g dietary fiber, 355 m sodium, 16 g protein
Exchanges: 1 1/2 Starch, 1 Lean Meat, 1 Vegetable

Beef and Beer Stew with Ginger and Lemon

SERVING SIZE: 1/4 of recipe, SERVES: 4

   1 lb stew meat from a blade roast, cut in 1-inch cubes
1 1/2 tsp non-aromatic olive oil
   1 inch peeled ginger root, cut in thin slices
   4 shallots, chopped
   2 cloves garlic, peeled, bashed, and chopped
   1 Tbsp finely grated lemon zest
   4 tsp tomato paste
   1 (12 oz) can nonalcoholic beer, amber if possible
1/8 tsp ground cinnamon
1/4 tsp freshly ground black pepper
   2 Turkish bay leaves
   3 medium carrots, peeled and roll cut
   2 medium turnips, peeled and cut in 1-inch chunks
   3 small chayote squash, cut in 1/2-inch chunks
   1 Tbsp Thai fish sauce (nam pla)
   1 tsp arrowroot mixed with 1 Tbsp water (slurry)
   1 tsp each chopped fresh parsley, cilantro and spearmint, and red pepper
     flakes (optional), mixed

Vegetarian Option

To make a similar dish without meat, eliminate the beef. Stir fry the
ginger, shallots, garlic, and lemon zest for a minute. Add the tomato
paste, cook to darken, and then add the beer, cinnamon, pepper, and bay
leaves. Double the vegetables, adding 6 carrots, 4 turnips, and 6 chayote
squash. Season with 1 Tbsp of soy sauce, bring to a boil, cover, and set
in the preheated oven for 45 minutes or until the vegetables are tender.
Thicken and serve as in step 4.

---

1 Preheat the oven to 350°F. Heat 1 Tbsp of the oil in a high-sided skillet on
medium high. Just as it starts to smoke, drop in the chunks of stew meat and
allow to brown on one side only without stirring. The meat is ready when it
is nice and brown on one side and has started to lighten in color around the
edges, around 3 minutes. Remove the meat to a plate and set aside.

2 Add the remaining 1/2 tsp oil to the pan without cleaning it out and reduce the heat to medium. Stir-fry the ginger, shallots, garlic, and lemon zest together for about a minute. Add the tomato paste, stirring until it darkens. Return the meat and any accumulated juices to the pan and pour in the beer. Stir in the cinnamon, pepper, and bay leaves. Cover and bake for 1 hour and 45 minutes or until the meat is almost tender.

3 Add the vegetables and fish sauce, cover and continue baking for 45 minutes to an hour or until the vegetables are soft.

4 Stir in the slurry, allow to thicken and serve over rice. Dust each serving liberally with the minced fresh herbs. For those who can't resist spicy heat, a sprinkle of crushed red peppers will do nicely.

Per serving: 244 calories, 7 g fat, 2 g saturated fat, 7% calories from saturated fat, 13 g carbohydrate, 3 g dietary fiber, 485 mg Sodium
Exchanges: 3 Lean Meat, 3 Vegetable

Vegetarian
Per serving: 109 calories, 2 g fat, 0 g saturated fat, 0% calories from saturated fat, 22 g carbohydrate, 5 g dietary fiber, 289 mg sodium
Exchanges: 4 Vegetable, 1/2 Fat

Pinto Bean Taco

SERVING SIZE: 1 taco, SERVES: 4

4 corn tortillas
1 tsp non-aromatic olive oil
1 cup chopped onion
1 (15-oz) can pinto beans, drained and rinsed

1/2 cup salsa
1/2 cup grated reduced-fat Monterey Jack cheese
2 Roma tomatoes, cored and sliced
1 cup shredded romaine lettuce

1 Place the tortillas in a brown paper bag and heat in the microwave or 10 minutes at 350°F in a conventional oven.

2 Heat the oil in a skillet and add the onion. Cook until soft, then stir in the beans and salsa. Heat through.

3 Lay the tortillas on 4 plates. Divide the bean mixture among the tortillas and sprinkle on the cheese to melt on the hot beans. Lay on the tomato slices, top with lettuce, and fold the tortilla around the filling if you can! If you can't, eat with a knife and fork.

Per serving: 200 calories, 4 g fat, 1 g saturated fat, 5% calories from saturated fat, 32 g carbohydrate, 6 g dietary fiber, 633 mg sodium
Exchanges: 1 1/2 Starch, 2 Vegetable, 1/2 Fat

Green Risotto

SERVING SIZE: 1/4 of recipe, SERVES: 4

1 tsp olive oil	1/2 cup nonalcoholic wine (optional)
1/2 cup chopped onions	or 1/2 cup water
1/2 cup chopped fennel bulb	
<C 3/4 cup Arborio rice	<C 1 cup peas
<C 3 1/2 cups low-sodium vegetable broth, divided (page 473)	+> 1 Tbsp chopped parsley
	2 Tbsp Parmesan cheese

1 Heat the oil in a large saucepan on medium high. Fry the onion and fennel 3 minutes. Add the rice and cook, stirring, 2 more minutes. Add 1/2 cup stock and the nonalcoholic wine or water and cook, stirring occasionally, until the liquid is gone.

2 Keep adding the liquid (saving 1/2 cup for the peas) about a half cup at a time and cook until it disappears. The end result should be quite creamy and the rice should be tender.

3 In a separate pan heat the peas, parsley, and the remaining 1/2 cup stock. Pour into a blender and whiz until smooth. Stir into the risotto and add the Parmesan cheese.

<C To Cut Carb

<C Arborio rice: reduce to 1/2 cup.   <C Peas: reduce to 1/2 cup.
<C Vegetable broth: decrease to 2 1/2 cups.   +> Parsley: increase to 3 Tbsp.

Per serving: 191 calories, 2 g fat, 1 g saturated fat, 3% calories from saturated fat, 36 g carbohydrate, 4 g dietary fiber, 379 mg sodium
Exchanges: 2 Starch, 1 Vegetable

Low Carb
Per serving: 166 calories, 2 g fat, 1 g saturated fat, 4% calories from saturated fat, 30 g carbohydrate, 5 g dietary fiber, 308 mg sodium
Exchanges: 1 1/2 Starch, 1 Vegetable, 1/2 Fat

Spaghetti with Mustard Greens and Italian Sausage

SERVING SIZE: 1/4 of recipe, SERVES: 4

<C 1/2 lb dry spaghetti
    1 tsp olive oil
<C 1 cup chopped onion
    2 cloves garlic, bashed and chopped
    2 low fat chicken Italian sausages cut in small pieces (about 4 oz)

+> 1/4 tsp fennel seeds
    8 cups chopped mustard green leaves (2 bunches) or 2 packages frozen
    1/4 tsp salt
    1/4 tsp salt
    1 Tbsp balsamic vinegar
    1/2 tsp crushed red pepper
    2 Tbsp grated Parmesan cheese

1. Cook the spaghetti according to package directions. Drain and keep warm in a colander over a bowl of hot water.

2. Heat the oil in a high-sided skillet on medium high. Sauté the onion 2 minutes or until it begins to turn translucent. Add the garlic and cook 1 more minute. Toss in the sausage and fennel seeds and cook 2 minutes or until lightly browned on the outside.

3. Stir in the mustard greens, cover, and cook on low until they wilt but are still bright green, about 5 minutes. Toss with the spaghetti and season with salt, pepper, balsamic vinegar, and red pepper. Serve when heated through with Parmesan cheese sprinkled over the top.

<C To Cut Carb

<C Spaghetti: reduce to 1/4 lb of whole wheat pasta.
<C Onion: reduce to 1/2 cup (4 oz).
+> Fennel: increase by 1 cup (chopped) and add it at step 2.

Per serving: 349 calories, 5 g fat, 1 g saturated fat, 3% calories from saturated fat, 53 g carbohydrate, 6 g dietary fiber, 202 mg sodium
Exchanges: 3 Starch, 1 Lean Meat, 2 Vegetable

Low Carb
Per serving: 241 calories, 5 g fat, 1 g saturated fat, 4% calories from saturated fat, 31 g carbohydrate, 6 g dietary fiber, 211 mg sodium
Exchanges: 1 1/2 Starch, 1 Lean Meat, 2 Vegetable, 1/2 Fat

Swordfish Sydney

SERVING SIZE: 1/6 of recipe, SERVES: 6

Rice Pilaf

	1/2 tsp light olive oil		1/4 tsp white pepper
<C	1 cup finely diced onion	<C	3 cups low-sodium chicken or
<C	1 1/2 cups long-grain white rice		vegetable stock
	1/2 tsp salt		(pages 463, 473)

Fish

1 tsp light olive oil

1 Tbsp fresh lemon juice

1/2 tsp powdered lemon myrtle or dried lemon thyme

1/4 tsp salt

1/2 tsp white pepper

1/2 tsp mountain pepper, optional

2 1/4 lb swordfish, cut into 6 slices

1 tsp paprika

6 fresh bay leaves

1 Preheat the oven to 450°F.

To Prepare the Rice Pilaf

2 Warm the oil in a medium saucepan over medium-high heat. Sauté the onion for 3 minutes, or until soft but not browned.

3 Stir in the rice, salt, and pepper. Cook for an additional 2 minutes, stirring often. Add the stock.

To Prepare the Fish

4 You will need 6 pieces of baking parchment measuring 12 inches × 16 inches. Stack the pieces in a neat pile and fold them in half, short end to short end, so that you have an 8-inch × 12-inch rectangle. Using the folded edge as the center, draw a half-heart shape on the parchment, making the dimensions as large as possible. (After the paper is cut and unfolded, a whole heart will emerge.) Cut along the outline through all the layers.

5 Combine the oil and lemon juice and brush on a cookie sheet. Sprinkle the lemon myrtle, salt, white pepper, and optional mountain pepper evenly over the oiled pan.

6 Lay the fish fillets on top of the seasonings, then turn them over, so that the rub adheres to both sides of the fish.

7 Unfold one of the parchment hearts and lay flat. Spoon 1/3 cup of the cooked rice onto the right-hand side of the heart. Lay the seasoned fish on top of the rice. Sprinkle the fillet with paprika and top with a bay leaf. Fold the left half of the heart over the fish and align the edges of the parchment. Starting with a small section at the top of the heart, fold the edges together, crease, and fold again, as if making a narrow hem. Work your way around the curve of the heart a small section at a time. Each new section will overlap the end of the previous section, like a series of pleats. When you have finished the folds, give the rim a good pinch to seal the package thoroughly. Repeat with the remaining packages.

8 Place on a baking sheet lightly coated with cooking spray. Store in the refrigerator until ready to cook. Spray the tops of the packages lightly before baking.

9 Bake in the preheated oven for 8–12 minutes, depending on whether the packages have been chilled. Open one of the packets to check for doneness–the fish should be just barely cooked through, since it will continue cooking as you prepare the plates for serving.

To Serve

10 Place a package in the center of a warmed dinner plate. Cut a large X across the top of the paper with scissors and roll back the parchment to reveal the ingredients. Serve Cauliflower with Carrots (page 208) on the side or your own favorite vegetable.

<C **To Cut Carb**
<C Onion: reduce to 1/2 cup.
<C Rice: reduce to 3/4 cup and substitute with brown rice. At step 3 increase cooking time to 30 minutes until tender.
<C Stock: reduce to 2 cups.

Per serving: 413 calories, 9 g fat, 0 g saturated fat, 0% calories from saturated fat, 41 g carbohydrate, 1 g dietary fiber, 501 mg sodium
Exchanges: 2 1/2 Starch, 5 Very Lean Meat, 1 Fat

Low Carb
Per serving: 318 calories, 9 g fat, 0 g saturated fat, 0% calories from saturated fat, 20 g carbohydrate, 1 g dietary fiber, 481 mg sodium
Exchanges: 1 1/2 Starch, 5 Very Lean Meat, 1 Fat

Warmly Aromatic Sri Lankan Chicken Curry

SERVING SIZE: 1/4 of recipe, SERVES: 4

Marinade

- 1 tsp non-aromatic olive oil
- 2 cloves garlic, peeled, bashed, and chopped
- 2 tsp Sri Lankan curry powder (see below)

- 1 Tbsp rice vinegar
- 1 Tbsp nonalcoholic red wine
- 1 Tbsp Worcestershire sauce

Curry

- 2 boneless, skinless chicken breasts
- 2 boneless, skinless chicken legs and thighs
- 1 tsp non-aromatic olive oil
- 1 large onion roughly chopped
- 2 cloves garlic, bashed, and chopped
- 1 tsp Sri Lanka curry (see below)
- 1 tsp brown sugar
- 1/2 tsp salt
- 1 serrano chili, finely sliced with seeds

- 2 Roma tomatoes, chopped in 1/4-inch pieces
- 1 cup low-sodium chicken stock (page 463)
- 1 cup nonalcoholic red wine
- 1 Tbsp cornstarch mixed with 2 Tbsp nonalcoholic red wine (slurry)
- 1/4 cup yogurt cheese (page 475)
- 2 Tbsp chopped fresh spearmint
- 2 Tbsp chopped fresh cilantro
- 2 Tbsp chopped fresh parsley

Vegetarian Option

1 1/2 lb Yukon Gold or red potatoes, peeled and quartered
1 cup low-sodium vegetable stock

Replace the chicken in the recipe with the potatoes. Make the marinade as in step 1, strain, and set aside. Fry the onion, add garlic, curry, brown sugar, salt, and chili. Simmer until onions are soft and stir in tomatoes and potatoes. Pour in vegetable stock and wine. Simmer 45 minutes and proceed with step 3 and 4.

---

1 Heat the oil in a high-sided skillet on medium and sauté the garlic 1 minute. Add the curry and stir to mix and warm. Pour in the vinegar, wine, and Worcestershire sauce, stir and cook 1 minute. Strain through a fine sieve. If you have a flavor injector (an inexpensive syringe with side-perforated nylon needles), fill it with the marinade and inject into the chicken. If you don't have one, cut a few shallow slits in the flesh and rub the marinade in. Set the chicken aside while you prepare the rest of the dish.

2 Rinse the pan, add the oil, and heat on medium high. Fry the onion until it starts to wilt, about 2 minutes, then add the garlic, curry, brown sugar, salt and the chili. Reduce the heat and cook until the onions are soft, 12–15 minutes. Stir in the tomatoes. Lay the chicken pieces on top, pour in the stock and wine, cover, and simmer 45 minutes.

3 Push the chicken pieces aside and stir the slurry into the liquid. Let it boil for 30 seconds to cook the starch. Stir some of the hot liquid into the yogurt cheese to temper it, then pour it into the pan. Combine the fresh herbs and add half to the curry.

4 Serve on a bed of rice. Scatter the remaining spearmint, cilantro, and parsley over the whole plate.

Sri Lankan Curry Powder

1 tsp ground nutmeg	1/2 tsp ground red pepper
1/2 tsp ground cinnamon	1/8 tsp ground cloves
1/2 tsp freshly ground black pepper	1/2 tsp ground mustard
1/2 tsp ground cardamom	

Combine the spices in a small bowl for use in the dish.

Per serving: 357 calories, 10 g fat, 2 g saturated fat, 5% calories from saturated fat, 21 g carbohydrate, 3 g dietary fiber, 782 mg sodium
Exchanges: 4 Lean Meat, 3 Vegetable, 1/2 Carbohydrate

Vegetarian
Per serving: 263 calories, 3 g fat, 1 g saturated fat, 3% calories from saturated fat, 53 g carbohydrates, 3 g fiber, 809 mg sodium
Exchanges: 2 Starch, 1/2 Carbohydrate, 3 Vegetable

Venison Canterbury

SERVING SIZE: 1/6 of recipe, SERVES: 6

Blackberry Sauce

1 Tbsp honey
3/4 cup finely sliced shallots
   (about 3 medium cloves)
1 Tbsp freshly grated ginger root
1/2 cup plus 2 Tbsp orange juice
2 1/2 cups blackberries, fresh or frozen
1 Tbsp balsamic vinegar

2 fresh sage leaves
1 sprig fresh thyme, about
   3-inches long
1 Tbsp arrowroot
1/2 cup low-sodium beef or
   vegetable stock
   (pages 466, 473)

Venison

1/4 tsp salt
1 tsp freshly ground black pepper
1/2 tsp rubbed sage
1/2 tsp dried thyme

1 1/2 lb boneless leg of venison,
   cut into 12 medallions
1 tsp light olive oil

Vegetarian Option: Browned Eggplant Canterbury

2 Tbsp light olive oil   18 thick slices eggplant

Warm the oil in a medium skillet over medium-high heat. Cook the eggplant slices for 2 or 3 minutes per side, or until browned and tender. Spoon the reserved blackberry sauce over the top.

---

1 Preheat the oven to 350°F.

To Prepare the Sauce

2 Bring the honey to a boil in a small saucepan over medium-high heat. When it is thick and bubbling, add the shallots and ginger. Cook for a few minutes, stirring frequently, until the shallots are soft and lightly browned.

3 As the sauce thickens, add 1/2 cup of the orange juice, a little at a time. When you have about a quarter of a cup of orange juice left, pour it in all at

once. Stir in the blackberries, balsamic vinegar, sage leaves, and thyme sprig. Simmer gently for 3 or 4 minutes, or until the berries are heated through and give up their juice.

4 Pour the sauce through a fine strainer set over a small saucepan. Press with a purée press or the back of a spoon, discarding the seeds and pulp. You should have about 1 cup of juice.

5 Mix the arrowroot with the remaining 2 Tbsp of orange juice to make a slurry. Add the slurry and the stock to the blackberry juice and set aside without heating while you cook the meat. (Vegetarian Option: Use vegetable stock here and set aside 1/4 cup of sauce per vegetarian serving before proceeding to the next step.)

To Prepare the Venison

6 Measure the salt, pepper, sage, and thyme into a large paper or plastic bag. Add the venison medallions and shake to coat.

7 Heat the oil in a large ovenproof frying pan. When the pan is very hot, brown the venison medallions for 1 minute. Turn and brown the other side for 1 minute. Bake in the preheated oven for 4 minutes while you finish the sauce.

8 Warm the sauce over medium heat, stirring frequently, until thickened and clear. Pour over the venison, stirring to capture the flavorful bits on the bottom of the frying pan.

To Serve

9 Place two medallions of venison on each warmed dinner plate and spoon any extra sauce over the meat. Arrange portions of Mashed Sweet Potatoes (page 241) and Spinach Defrosted in Broth (page 238) on the side.

Per serving: 202 calories, 6 g fat, 3 g saturated fat, 9% of calories from fat, 13 g carbohydrate, 0 g dietary fiber, 24 g protein
Exchanges: 3 Very Lean Meat, 1 Fruit, 1 Fat

Vegetarian
Per serving: 116 calories, 4 g fat, 1 g saturated fat, 7% of calories from fat, 20 g carbohydrate, 5 g dietary fiber, 0 g protein
Exchanges: 1 Vegetable, 1 Fruit, 1 Fat

Spiced Spinach and Shrimp

SERVING SIZE: 1/6 of recipe, SERVES: 6

    1 stalk fresh lemongrass (about 3 inches)
    1 tsp finely chopped fresh thyme
1/4 tsp salt
1/4 tsp freshly ground black pepper
    2 cloves garlic, peeled, bashed, and chopped
1 1/2 tsp light olive oil
  12 medium shrimp (8 oz), peeled and rinsed
    3 serrano chilis, cored, seeded, and finely diced
    3 (2 oz) thin slices Canadian bacon, very finely diced
1/4 tsp ground nutmeg
    1 bunch green onions, sliced in 1/4-inch rounds, white parts separated from green parts (1/2 cup whites and 1 cup greens)
    3 bunches spinach, carefully washed, stems removed (12 cups)
    1 Tbsp roughly chopped fresh parsley
    1 tsp arrowroot
    2 tsp balsamic vinegar

Spicy Garnish

1 serrano chili, cored, seeded, and finely chopped   Balsamic vinegar
1 Tbsp roughly chopped fresh parsley

Vegetarian Option

6 red bell peppers, roasted

Leave out the shrimp in step 3 and the Canadian bacon in step 4.
Lay 2 shrimp-sized strips of roasted red bell pepper over the top of the spinach.

To Prepare the Shrimp

1   Remover the tough outside layer of the lemongrass and cut off the root end and the dry top. Slice from the root end and use only the tender bulb. Slice thinly so that the flavor can spread through the dish.

2 In a small bowl, combine the lemongrass, thyme, salt, pepper, and half of the chopped garlic.

3 Warm 1 tsp of the oil in a high-sided skillet over high heat. Add the shrimp and one-third of the garlic herb mixture. Toss just until the shrimp begin to turn pink, about 1 minute. Add 1 tsp of the diced chilis and cook 30 seconds more. Transfer the contents of the skillet to a warmed plate, cover with a lid, and set aside. The shrimp will finish cooking from the retained heat under the lid.

To Prepare the Spinach

4 Return the skillet to the stove without washing it and add the remaining 1/2 tsp of oil. Cook the Canadian bacon, 1/8 tsp of the nutmeg, and the remaining garlic-herb mixture for 1 minute, stirring constantly. Stir in the rest of the diced chilis and sliced onion whites.

5 Add 1/3 (about 4 cups) of the spinach to the skillet and toss the ingredients with two spoons to coat the spinach with oil and seasonings. Cover and cook for 60 seconds. Add half the remaining spinach, again tossing to cover with oil, then cover tightly and cook for 60 seconds. Repeat with the last batch of spinach. The skillet will be full in the beginning but will cook down after each addition. When all the spinach has finished cooking, the leaves will no longer be crisp but will remain bright green.

6 Scatter the green parts of the onions over the top of the spinach and sprinkle with the remaining nutmeg. Cover and warm through. Stir in the parsley and remove from heat.

7 Transfer the spinach to a strainer set over a bowl. Press as much liquid as possible out of the spinach and return the liquid to the skillet. Keep spinach warm.

8 Combine the arrowroot and balsamic vinegar to make a slurry. Add the slurry to the spinach liquid in the skillet and stir over medium heat until the mixture is slightly thickened. Add the shrimp and cook until heated through.

To Serve

9 Arrange two small mounds of spinach on individual salad plates. Set two shrimp in the center of each spinach mound and spoon a little of the thickened sauce over the shrimp.

(Continued)

10 To garnish, sprinkle the chopped chili and parsley over the spinach and around the rim of the plate. Pass a cruet of balsamic vinegar for the greens.

Per serving: 78 calories, 2 g fat, 0 g saturated fat, 0% calories from saturated fat, 6 g carbohydrate, 4 g dietary fiber
Exchanges: 1 Very Lean Meat, 1 Vegetable, 1/2 Fat

Vegetarian
Per serving: 52 calories, 2 g fat, 0 g saturated fat, 0% calories from saturated fat, 7 g carbohydrate, 4 g dietary fiber
Exchanges: 1 Vegetable, 1/2 Fat

Kiwi, Tuna Kebabs

SERVING SIZE: 1/4 of recipe, SERVES: 4

8 kiwifruit, peeled and halved
1 lb tuna or firm white fish, in 1-inch cubes
1/2 tsp non-aromatic olive oil
1 tsp chopped garlic
1/4 cup plus 2 Tbsp unsweetened pineapple juice

2 Tbsp low-sodium tamari or light soy sauce
1 tsp brown sugar
1 tsp Chinese 5 spice
2 Tbsp natural creamy peanut butter
1 tsp grated ginger root

Garnish

2 Tbsp chopped cilantro or parsley

1 Preheat barbecue or broiler. String kiwi halves and fish cubes on skewers. (For wood skewers, soak in warm water for 10–15 minutes before using.)

2 Heat oil in skillet and sauté garlic and ginger for a few seconds. Add 1/4 cup pineapple juice, tamari, brown sugar, Chinese 5 spice, and peanut butter. Heat, stirring until smooth.

3 Brush sauce on kebabs, and broil 3 minutes. Turn and grill 3 minutes more. Lay on a bed of rice. Thin remaining sauce with the rest of the juice and drizzle over each serving. Scatter cilantro or parsley on top.

Per serving: 295 calories, 6 g fat, 18% calories from fat, 1 g saturated fat, 3% calories from saturated fat, 29 g carbohydrate, 6 g dietary fiber, 381 mg sodium
Exchanges: 4 Lean Meat, 1 Fruit

Steak and Oyster Pie

SERVING SIZE: 1 wedge, SERVES: 8

1/2 recipe Basic Pie Crust (page 479)
  1 (10 oz) jar medium oysters, cut in 1-inch pieces
  1 tsp non-aromatic olive oil, divided
  1 medium onion, cut in 1-inch chunks
  4 carrots, peeled, cut in half lengthwise, and sliced in 1/2-inch slices
1/2 lb turnips, peeled and cut in 1/2-inch chunks
3/4 lb medium mushrooms, halved (3 cups)
3/4 lb lean chuck steak, trimmed of all fat and cut in 1/2-inch chunks
  2 heaping tsp tomato paste
  2 cups low-sodium canned or homemade beef stock (page 466)
1/4 tsp salt
1/8 tsp pepper
   Bouquet garni (page 467)
  2 Tbsp arrowroot mixed with 1/4 cup beef broth or water (slurry)

1 Preheat the oven to 400°F. Make the whole pie crust recipe and freeze half for another use. Roll the crust into a 9-inch circle. Wrap it around your rolling pin and transfer to a baking sheet. Make a scalloped edge by pinching it all around with your fingers. Cut into 8 equal wedges and bake 10 minutes or until light gold and crisp. Set aside. Drain and chop the oysters, reserving the juice.

2 Heat 1/2 tsp of the oil in a high-sided skillet on medium high. Sauté the onions briskly to color for 2 to 3 minutes. Add the carrots, turnips and mushrooms and sauté 1 more minute. Turn out onto a plate.

3 Heat the remaining oil in the same skillet on high. Toss in the meat and brown on 1 side, 3 minutes. When it's nice and brown, stir in the tomato paste and cook until the paste darkens, 2 minutes. Add the vegetables to the meat, pour in the stock, oyster liquid, and salt and pepper. Add the bouquet garni, cover and simmer 1 1/2 hours or until the meat is tender.

4 Remove the bouquet garni. Stir in the slurry to thicken the sauce. Add the chopped oysters. Lay the cooked crust wedges on top and bake 5 minutes more before serving.

Per serving: 276 calories, 12 g fat, 3 g saturated fat, 8% calories from saturated fat, 21 g carbohydrate, 2 g dietary fiber, 257 mg sodium, 21 g protein
Exchanges: 1/2 Starch, 2 Lean Meat, 3 Vegetable, 1 Fat

Taiwanese White Fish Stew with Ginger and Tofu

SERVING SIZE: 1/4 of recipe, SERVES: 4

    1 3/4cup low-sodium chicken stock (page 463)
    1 Tbsp light brown sugar
    2 Tbsp light soy sauce
    2 Tbsp balsamic vinegar
  1/8 tsp ground cayenne pepper
  3/4 lb low-fat extra firm tofu, cut in 1-inch squares
  3/4 lb halibut (or other firm white fish) steaks cut 1-inch thick
    2 tsp non-aromatic olive oil
    6 whole scallions, white parts cut in 2-inch lengths, greens cut in rings
    1 Tbsp finely chopped ginger
    3 cloves garlic, bashed and chopped
    2 medium carrots, peeled and cut on the diagonal in 1/8-inch slices
  3/4 lb small white mushrooms, cleaned and stems trimmed
  1/8 tsp salt
  1/8 tsp freshly ground black pepper
1 1/2 Tbsp arrowroot mixed with 3 Tbsp water (slurry)

Vegetarian Option

1 3/4 low-sodium vegetable stock
  3/4 lb low-fat extra firm tofu, cut in 1-inch squares

Replace the chicken stock with vegetable stock. Double the amount of tofu and leave out the fish.

If the fish you choose has bones, combine the stock, brown sugar, soy sauce, balsamic vinegar, and cayenne in a high-sided skillet and bring to a boil. Cut the halibut into pieces 1 1/2 inches long and 2 inches wide, skin attached, and set aside. Place the bones in the pot with the stock mixture, cover, and simmer while you prepare the rest of the ingredients, not longer than 20 minutes. If there are no bones, just combine the ingredients in a bowl, cut the fish, and set both aside.

2 Cut the tofu into 1-inch cubes, pour boiling water over them, and soak 15 minutes. This adds considerably to its firm texture.

3 Pour the stock through a strainer into a measuring cup, discard the fish bones, and rinse the pan. Heat 1 tsp of the oil in the same pan on medium high. Sauté the onion whites, garlic, ginger, carrots, and mushrooms for 2 minutes, taking care not to brown the garlic. Remove to a plate.

4 Without washing the pan, add another tsp of oil, heat, and drop the fish pieces in one by one. Season with the salt and pepper and fry 1 minute on either side. Scatter the vegetables over the fish, drain the tofu, and add to the pan. Pour in the stock. Cover and simmer 5 minutes. Add the green onion tops, pour in the slurry, and stir while it thickens.

5 Divide among four covered warm bowls. At the table, lift the lids in unison and just watch the eyes twinkle at the wonderful aromas.

Per serving: 249 calories, 8 g fat, 1 g saturated fat, 4% calories from saturated fat, 18 g carbohydrate, 2 g dietary fiber, 524 mg sodium, 26 g protein
Exchanges: 1/2 Starch, 3 Lean Meat, 2 Vegetable

Vegetarian
Per serving: 207 calories, 8 g fat, 0 g saturated fat, 0% calories from saturated fat, 20 g carbohydrate, 2 g dietary fiber, 532 mg sodium
Exchanges: 1/2 Starch, 1 Lean Meat, 2 Vegetable, 1 Fat

Mardi's Tomato Sandwich

SERVING SIZE: 1 sandwich, SERVES: 4

4 Tbsp low-fat butter flavored margarine
8 slices whole-wheat bread
8 Bibb lettuce leaves

3 medium vine-ripened tomatoes, cored and sliced
1/4 tsp salt
1/4 tsp pepper

1 Spread margarine on the bread. Lay a lettuce leaf on each piece to protect the bread from the inevitable sog of the tomatoes. Cover one side of each sandwich with the tomato slices, dust with salt and pepper, close, and cut into quarters.

Per serving: 175 calories, 6 g fat, 1 g saturated fat, 5% calories from saturated fat, 27 g carbohydrate, 4 g dietary fiber, 499 mg sodium, 3 g protein
Exchanges: 2 Starch, 1/2 Fat

Nora's Shrimp and Mushroom Risotto

SERVING SIZE: 1/6 of recipe, SERVES: 6

Rice

1 tsp non-aromatic olive oil	2 cups nonalcoholic dry white wine, divided
1/4 cup minced shallots	
5 large cloves garlic, bashed and chopped	<C 3 cups low-sodium chicken stock, divided (page 463)
<C 1 1/2 cups arborio rice	1/4 tsp saffron threads

Main Ingredients

4 tsp non-aromatic olive oil, divided	1/2 bunch spinach, stemmed and cut in thin strips
3 cloves garlic, bashed and chopped	
1/2 lb cremini mushrooms, wiped and sliced in 3 pieces	<C 1 cup frozen petit peas
	1 cup low-sodium chicken stock (page 463)
1 tsp wild mushroom powder	
2 Tbsp freshly squeezed lemon juice, divided	1 cup nonalcoholic dry white wine
1/2 tsp salt	2 Tbsp chopped chives or parsley for garnish
1/4 tsp freshly ground pepper	
1 lb medium shrimp, shelled and deveined	6 Tbsp fresh grated Parmesan cheese (optional, adds 2 grams of fat per serving)

1. Heat the oil in a skillet or chef's pan on medium high. Sauté the shallots until tender and transparent, about 3 minutes. Add the garlic and cook 1 minute more. Stir in the rice and cook until it starts to look translucent, about 2 minutes. Combine the wine and stock and heat. Add 1 cup of the liquid, bring to a boil, reduce the heat, add the saffron and simmer until the liquid is absorbed. Keep adding liquid 1 cup at a time, stirring frequently, until the rice is al dente, about 20 minutes. You may not need all the liquid to achieve al dente rice. If you have some left, use it at the end to reheat the risotto. Spread the rice on a baking sheet and cool.

2. Heat 3 tsp of the oil in the pan on medium high. Add the garlic to break out the flavors, 30 seconds, and toss in the mushrooms. Sprinkle with the mushroom powder and sauté until tender, 2 minutes. Season with the lemon juice, salt, and pepper. Tip out onto a plate.

3 Heat the remaining oil. Sauté the shrimp 2 minutes or until pink. Pour in the stock and wine. Return the mushrooms, and risotto to the pan to heat through. Stir in the peas and spinach and cook 2 minutes or until bright green. Sprinkle with the remaining lemon juice. Divide among 6 hot soup plates. Garnish with chives or parsley.

<C **To Cut Carb**
<C Arborio rice: reduce to 1 cup.   <C White wine: reduce to 1 1/2 cups.
<C Chicken stock: reduce to 2 cups.   <C Peas: reduce to 2/3 cup.

Per serving: 321 calories, 5 g fat, 1 g saturated fat, 3% calories from saturated fat, 48 g carbohydrate, 4 g dietary fiber, 411 mg sodium
Exchanges: 2 1/2 Starch, 1 Very Lean Meat, 1 Vegetable, 1/2 Fat, 1/2 Carbohydrate

Low Carb
Per serving: 257 calories, 5 g fat, 1 g saturated fat, 4% calories from saturated fat, 35 g carbohydrate, 3 g dietary fiber, 404 mg sodium
Exchanges: 1 1/2 Starch, 1 Very Lean Meat, 1 Vegetable, 1/2 Fat, 1/2 Carbohydrate

Arugula and Halibut

SERVING SIZE: 1/4 of recipe, SERVES: 4

4 cups arugula, radicchio, endive, escarole, romaine lettuce or a mixture of these
4 tsp low-fat vinaigrette dressing
4 (4 oz) halibut fillets

1/4 tsp salt
1/4 tsp pepper
2 Tbsp lemon juice

1 Wash the greens and spin dry. Tear into bite size pieces and toss with the vinaigrette. Divide among 4 dinner plates.

2 Season the fish with salt and pepper. Grill, skin side up, 3 to 5 minutes. Turn and cook 3 to 5 minutes more. You can gauge the time by measuring the thickness of the fish and cooking 10 minutes per inch.

3 Remove the skin as you take the halibut off the pan. Set the fillets on the greens and sprinkle with lemon juice. Tiny, new red potatoes go wonderfully with this dish.

Per serving: 139 calories, 3 g fat, 0 g saturated fat, 0% calories from saturated fat, 3 g carbohydrate, 0 g dietary fiber, 249 mg sodium
Exchanges: 3 Very Lean Meat, 1 Vegetable, 1/2 Fat

Jambalaya

SERVING SIZE: 1/6 of recipe, SERVES: 6

2 cups low-sodium chicken broth (page 463)	1 Tbsp tomato paste
1/2 lb medium shrimp, peeled and deveined	1 large red bell pepper, cut in 1 1/2-inch strips
<C 1 cup long-grain white rice	3 oz Canadian bacon, cut in 1 1/2-inch strips
1/8 tsp salt +>	1 large rib celery, cut in 1 1/2-inch strips
3 bay leaves	1/4 tsp cayenne pepper
1 1/2 tsp non-aromatic olive oil, divided	1/4 tsp thyme
3 spicy low-fat chicken sausages (12 oz)	pinch cloves
<C 1 large sweet onion, cut in half and sliced stem to root	8 Roma tomatoes, peeled, seeded, and chopped or 1 (28 oz) can diced tomatoes in juice
4 cloves garlic, bashed and chopped	1/4 cup chopped parsley

1 Bring the stock to a boil in a medium saucepan. Drop the shrimp in and cook 3 minutes. Remove shrimp and set aside. Measure the stock and add water to make 2 cups. Add the rice, salt, and bay leaves and cook 15 minutes or until tender and the liquid is gone. Set aside. Heat 1 tsp of the oil in a 10 1/2-inch chef's pan and fry the sausages, turning often, 11 minutes on medium high or until nearly done. Cut in rounds and set aside.

2 Pour the remaining 1/2 tsp oil into the pan and sauté the onion until it turns translucent, 3–4 minutes. Add the garlic and tomato paste and continue cooking until the paste darkens. Now toss in the celery, red pepper, and Canadian bacon and cook until the vegetables are crisp but tender. Season with cayenne, thyme, and cloves. Stir in the tomatoes, parsley, and reserved shrimp and cook until just heated through. Add the rice and mix well.

<C **To Cut Carb**

<C Long-grain rice: convert to long-grain brown rice, reduce to 3/4 cup. Cook at step 1 for 30 minutes. You may need to increase the stock by 1/2 cup.

<C Onion: reduce to only 1 cup (about 1/2 a large onion).

+> Celery: increase to 3 large ribs.

Per serving: 314 calories, 8 g fat, 2 g saturated fat, 5% calories from saturated fat, 38 g carbohydrate, 3 g fiber, 666 mg sodium, 23 g protein
Exchanges: 2 Starch, 2 Lean Meat, 2 Vegetable

Low Carb

Per serving: 287 calories, 8 g fat, 2 g saturated fat, 6% calories from saturated fat, 31 g carbohydrate, 4 g dietary fiber, 686 mg sodium. 23 g protein
Exchanges: 1 1/2 Starch, 2 Lean Meat, 2 Vegetable

Penne, Snap Peas, Roasted Peppers

SERVING SIZE: 1/4 of recipe, SERVES: 4

2 red peppers or 6 oz jarred roasted peppers, sliced into 2-inch strips

+> 2 cups sugar snap peas, lightly steamed

<C 1/2 pound penne pasta, cooked *al dente*

2 cups reduced-sodium vegetable stock

1 Tbsp virgin olive oil

2 tsp arrowroot or cornstarch

2 Tbsp Parmesan cheese

1 If using fresh peppers, preheat oven to 400°F. Spray a baking sheet and peppers with cooking spray. Place whole peppers on sheet and bake for 40–45 minutes, turning occasionally, until browned and soft. Remove peppers from oven with tongs and place in brown paper bag. Close bag and let peppers steam for 5 minutes. Remove peppers from bag and discard stem, seeds and skin. Slice into 2-inch strips.

2 Make the sauce by boiling the vegetable stock in a small saucepan. Continue to boil until reduced to one cup. Add olive oil and arrowroot or cornstarch; whisk until smooth and thickened.

3 In a heated bowl, toss together the pasta with the sugar snap peas, roasted red peppers, and sauce. Sprinkle with the Parmesan cheese and serve.

<C To Cut Carb

<C Penne Pasta: reduce to 4 oz.   +> Peas: increase to 3 cups.

Per serving: 306 calories, 6 g fat, 1 g saturated fat, 3% calories from saturated fat, 54 g carbohydrate, 5 g dietary fiber, 213 mg sodium, 10 g protein
Exchanges: 3 Starch, 2 Vegetable, 1/2 Fat

Low Carb

Per serving: 211 calories, 5 g fat, 1 g saturated fat, 4% calories from saturated fat, 34 g carbohydrate, 4 g dietary fiber, 214 mg sodium, 7 g protein
Exchanges: 1 1/2 Starch, 2 Vegetable, 1 Fat

Posole

SERVING SIZE: 1/6 of recipe, SERVES: 6

Stew

1 1/2 lb pork spareribs
   1/8 Tbsp plus 1/4 tsp salt
   1/4 tsp freshly ground black pepper
      1 chicken (about 31/2 lb)
   1/2 tsp light olive oil
      1 medium onion, roughly chopped (about 1 cup)
      2 cloves of garlic, peeled, bashed, and chopped

      3 bay leaves
<C 1 (29 oz) can yellow hominy, rinsed and drained
      1 bunch fresh kale, heavy stalks removed, thoroughly washed, and torn into 1-inch pieces (8 cups)

Garnish

1/2 cup fresh oregano leaves
   3 limes, halved
1/4 cup dried crushed red pepper flakes

1/2 cup finely diced onion
<C   6 corn tortillas

Vegetarian Option

6 cups low-fat vegetable stock
3 cups hominy
6 cups kale, torn into 1-inch pieces

1 lb cooked kidney beans
6 Tbsp grated Parmesan cheese

About 10 minutes before serving, bring the vegetable stock to a boil in a medium saucepan. Add the reserved hominy, kale, and the kidney beans and simmer for 5 minutes. Add the grated Parmesan cheese and serve in a warmed bowl. Garnish as you would the posole.

---

1 Preheat the oven to 350°F.

2 Season the ribs with 1/8 tsp of the salt and the pepper and place on a rack in a roasting pan. Add 1 cup of water to the pan, and roast in the preheated oven for 1 1/4 hours or until tender.

3 Rinse the chicken well and pat dry. Warm the oil in a Dutch oven or large iron casserole over medium-high heat. Sauté the onions and garlic until the onion starts to soften, about 2 minutes. Lay the chicken on top of the onions and pour 1/2 cup water over the chicken. Cover, and continue cooking for an additional 3 minutes. The chicken will be firm and white on the outside.

4 Turn the chicken over and cover with 10 cups of hot water. Add the bay leaves and the remaining 1/4 tsp of salt. Bring the liquid to a boil, reduce the heat, and cover the pot. Simmer for 1 hour. Turn off the heat, leave covered, and let sit for 20 minutes.

5 After the pork ribs have roasted, transfer them to a cutting board to cool. Add a little water to the roasting pan and deglaze with a flat-ended spurtle or wooden spoon, then pour the liquid into the pot with the chicken. Cut the meat off of the ribs and roughly dice to 1/4-inch pieces or smaller.

6 Transfer the chicken to a large plate. Remove the skin and return it to the pot. Separate the legs and wings from the bird and return the wings to the pot. Roughly chop the drumstick and thigh meat into pieces that can easily be eaten with a soup spoon. Remove the breast meat and cut into neat 1/2-inch cubes.

7 Return the carcass and any juices from the carving plate to the pot, along with the pork bones. Bring the stock to a vigorous boil for a few minutes to reduce the liquid by 50% and concentrate the flavors. Pour into a fat strainer a few cups at a time and allow the fat to rise to the surface. Pour the de-fatted stock (you should have 5 cups) into a large pot. Add the hominy, kale, pork, and chicken meat. (Vegetarian Option: Set aside 1/2 cup hominy and 1 cup kale per vegetarian serving.) Simmer for 5 minutes.

8 To serve, divide the posole among 6 warmed soup bowls. Pass small dishes of the fresh oregano leaves, lime halves, red pepper flakes, and diced onion for your guests to add according to their own tastes. Pass a basket of hot corn tortillas.

<c **To Cut Carb**

<c Yellow hominy: reduce to 3/4 can (22 oz).

<c Corn tortillas: reduce to only 3. This means just half a tortilla each, which does seem a trifle stingy, but at least it illustrates what we need to do to stay in control.

Per serving: 444 calories, 13 g fat, 4 g saturated fat, 7% calories from saturated fat; 38 g carbohydrate, 7 g dietary fiber, 540 mg sodium
Exchanges: 2 Starch, 4 Lean Meat, 2 Vegetable

(Continued)

Low Carb

Per serving: 397 calories, 12 g fat, 4 g saturated fat, 7% calories from saturated fat, 29 g carbohydrate, 5 g dietary fiber, 484 mg sodium
Exchanges: 1 Starch, 5 Lean Meat, 2 Vegetable

Vegetarian

Per serving: 265 calories, 4 g fat, 1 g saturated fat, 3% of calories from saturated fat, 49 g carbohydrate, 9 g dietary fiber
Exchanges: 2 1/2 Starch, 1 Vegetable, 1 Fat

Spinach Sauté

SERVING SIZE: 1/4 of recipe, SERVES: 4

2 bunches spinach, stemmed and washed 3 times
1/4 cup sun-dried tomatoes
1 tsp extra virgin olive oil
1 cup chopped onion
1 clove garlic, bashed and chopped

2 cups sliced mushrooms
1/4 tsp salt
1/4 tsp pepper
2 Tbsp toasted pine nuts
<C 2 cups cooked long grain white rice

1 Cut the spinach leaves in 1/2-inch strips and set aside for later. Cover the sun-dried tomatoes with hot water and soak 15 minutes. Drain and chop.

2 Heat the oil in a high-sided skillet on medium high. Shallow fry the onions 2 minutes. Add the garlic and reconstituted tomatoes and cook 1 minute more. Stir in the mushrooms and cook until they begin to wilt, 3 to 5 minutes.

3 Add the spinach, stirring to mix well. Cover and cook 3 minutes or until spinach wilts but is still bright green. Season with salt and pepper, spoon over rice, and scatter the pine nuts on top.

<C To Cut Carb

<C Rice: reduce to 1 1/2 cups cooked.

Per serving: 220 calories, 6 g fat, 1 g saturated fat, 4% calories from saturated fat, 36 g carbohydrate, 5 g dietary fiber, 309 mg sodium
Exchanges: 1 1/2 Starch, 3 Vegetable, 1/2 Fat

Low Carb

Per serving: 187 calories, 5 g fat, 1 g saturated fat, 3% calories from saturated fat, 30 g carbohydrate, 5 g dietary fiber, 286 mg sodium
Exchanges: 1 Starch, 3 Vegetable, 1/2 Fat

Vegetable Posole

SERVING SIZE: 1/6 of recipe, SERVES: 6

1 tsp non-aromatic olive oil
1 cup chopped onion
2 cloves garlic, bashed and chopped
  1 cup basic vegetable stock (page 473)
<C 1 (20 oz) can yellow hominy, rinsed
  and drained

6 cups trimmed and torn kale
<C 1 (15 oz) can low-sodium
  red kidney beans, rinsed
  and drained
1/3 cup grated Parmesan
  cheese

Garnish

1/2 cup fresh oregano leaves
  2 limes, cut in quarters
  dried crushed chili pepper flakes

1/2 cup chopped onions
<C 6 corn tortillas

1 Heat the oil in a Dutch oven on medium high. Fry the onion 2 minutes, add the garlic and cook 1 more minute. Pour in the stock and bring to a boil. Add the hominy, kale and kidney beans. Bring back to a boil, reduce the heat and simmer 5 minutes.

2 Stir in the Parmesan cheese and serve in bowls.

3 Pass the oregano leaves, limes, pepper flakes, and raw onions in individual bowls. Heat the tortillas and serve in a basket.

<C **To Cut Carb**

<C Hominy: reduce to 10 oz drained (1 1/4 cup).
<C Red kidney bean: reduce to 10 oz drained (1 1/4 cup).
<C Corn tortillas: reduce to 3 (one half per portion).

Per serving: 245 calories, 4 g fat, 1 g saturated fat, 3% calories from saturated fat, 43 g carbohydrate, 9 g dietary fiber, 210 mg sodium
Exchanges: 2 Starch, 2 Vegetable, 1/2 Fat

Low Carb
Per serving: 173 calories, 4 g fat, 1 g saturated fat, 5% calories from saturated fat, 29 g carbohydrate, 6 g dietary fiber, 141 mg sodium
Exchanges: 1 Starch, 2 Vegetables, 1/2 Fat

New England Boiled Dinner

SERVING SIZE: 1/6 of recipe, SERVES: 6

Meat

2 1/2 lb lean corned beef brisket   1/2 tsp mustard seeds
4 bay leaves   4 whole cloves
1/2 tsp black peppercorns   4 allspice berries

Vegetables

<C   1 lb carrots, peeled, cut in half lengthwise and crosswise
<C 12 oz parsnips, peeled, thick part cut in half, thin part left whole
     12 oz rutabagas, peeled, cut in 1/2-inch x 3-inch sticks
<C 12 tiny red potatoes, cut in half
     18 small onions, peeled (1 inch diameter)
>   1 small head cabbage, cut in sixths

1   Cover the corned beef with water in a large Dutch oven. Add the bay, peppercorns, mustard seeds, cloves, and allspice berries and bring to a boil. (For extra flavor, add a good handful of the peelings from the vegetables to the water.) Reduce the heat and simmer 2 hours or until the meat is tender but not falling apart.

2   Remove the meat, strain and defat the liquid and return both to the pan. Add all the vegetables except the cabbage and bring to a boil. Cook 20 minutes or until tender. The cabbage wedges can be steamed on top of the other vegetables if you have a steamer to fit your pan, or steamed separately 15 minutes or until tender.

3   Slice the meat across the grain in 1/2-inch slices and divide among 6 hot soup plates. Arrange the vegetables around the meat and pour a little of the liquid over the top. Sprinkle with chopped parsley and serve with mustard.

<C To Cut Carb

<C Carrots: reduce to 12 oz.   <C Potatoes: reduce to 6 only.
<C Parsnips: reduce to 8 oz.   <C Potatoes: reduce to 6 only.

Per serving: 379 calories, 13 g fat, 5 g saturated fat, 12% calories from saturated fat, 41 g carbohydrate, 10 g dietary fiber, 867 mg sodium
Exchanges: 1 1/2 Starch, 2 Medium Fat Meat, 4 Vegetable, 1/2 Fat

Low Carb
Per serving: 343 calories, 13 g fat, 5 g saturated fat, 12% calories from saturated fat, 32 g carbohydrate, 9 g dietary fiber, 864 mg sodium
Exchanges: 1 Starch, 2 Medium Fat Meat, 4 Vegetable, 1/2 Fat

Red & Green Holiday Risotto

SERVING SIZE: 1/4 of recipe, SERVES: 4

1 tsp olive oil	1/2 cup nonalcoholic wine
1/2 cup chopped onions	(optional) or 1/2 cup water
1/2 cup chopped fennel bulb	1 cup peas
1 cup chopped red pepper	1 cup zucchini
<C 3/4 cup arborio rice	1 Tbsp chopped parsley
1 cup water	2 Tbsp Parmesan cheese
2 1/2 cups low-sodium vegetable broth, divided	

1 Heat the oil in a large saucepan on medium high. Fry the onion, red pepper, and fennel 3 minutes. Add the rice and cook, stirring, 2 more minutes. Combine the water and broth and add 1/2 cup to the rice. Add the nonalcoholic wine or water and cook, stirring occasionally, until the liquid is gone.

2 Keep adding the liquid (saving 1/2 cup for the peas) about a 1/2 cup at a time and cook until it disappears. The end result should be quite creamy and the rice should be tender.

3 In a separate pan heat the peas, parsley, and the remaining 1/2 cup stock. Pour into a blender and mix until smooth. Stir into the risotto and add the Parmesan cheese.

<C **To Cut Carb**

<C Rice: reduce to 1/2 cup.

Per serving: 201 calories, 2 g fat, 1 g saturated fat, 3% calories from saturated fat, 38 g carbohydrate, 5 g dietary fiber, 291 mg sodium, 6 g protein
Exchanges: 2 Starch, 1 Vegetable, 1/2 Fat

Low Carb
Per serving: 163 calories, 2 g fat, 1 g saturated fat, 2% calories from saturated fat, 30 g carbohydrate, 5 g dietary fiber, 291 mg sodium, 6 g protein
Exchanges: 1 1/2 Starch, 1 Vegetable, 1/2 Fat

Spicy Pork and Potato Casserole with Coconut and Lemon Grass

SERVING SIZE: 1/4 of recipe, SERVES: 4

	1 1/2	tsp olive oil
	1	Tbsp Southeast Asian chili paste
<C	3	cups onion in 1-inch squares
	12	oz well trimmed pork tenderloin, cut in1-inch × 2-inch chunks
<C	1	lb red potatoes, skin on, cut in 1-inch chunks
	2	tsp grated lime zest
		6-inch piece lemon grass
	1/2	tsp coconut essence
	1/4	tsp salt
	2	cups low-sodium chicken stock
<C	1 1/2	cups young soy beans (edamame) or frozen baby lima beans
	2	cups broccoli flowerettes
	2	Tbsp lightly salted peanuts, chopped
	1/2	cup coconut cream (page 465)

1 Preheat the oven to 350°F.

2 Heat 1/2 tsp of the oil in a high-sided skillet on medium. Add the spice paste and cook for 1 minute. Stir in the onions and sauté until they soften and are covered with the spice paste, about 10 minutes. Bruise the lemon grass with the back of a knife to release the flavor and add to the onions with the lime zest and coconut essence. Remove to a bowl, scraping out all the onion, but leaving any residue in the pan. Add the remaining 1 tsp oil, increase the heat to medium high and brown the pork pieces on one side, 3 minutes.

3 Pour the stock into the pan with the pork and scrape up any brown bits on the bottom. Stir in the onions, potatoes, and 1/4 tsp of the salt. Cover and bake for 30 minutes. Uncover and continue to cook for an hour or until the meat and potatoes are very tender. Stir in the broccoli and cook 6 minutes. Add the beans and heat through on top of the stove. If baby lima beans are used, add them with the broccoli. Stir in the coconut cream, serve, and pass the spice paste for those, like Treena, who like it really hot!

<C Onions: reduce to 2 cups.
<C Potatoes: reduce to 8 oz (or 4 small red potatoes).
<C Soy (or lima) beans: reduce to 1/2 cup.

Per serving: 405 calories, 12 g fat, 3 g saturated fat, 5% calories from saturated fat, 45 g carbohydrate, 8 g dietary fiber, 489 mg sodium, 31 g protein
Exchanges: 2 Starch, 3 Lean Meat, 3 Vegetable

Low Carb

Per serving: 298 calories, 10 g fat, 3 g saturated fat, 9% calories from saturated fat, 27 g carbohydrate, 5 g dietary fiber, 482 mg sodium, 25 g protein
Exchanges: 1 Starch, 3 Lean Meat, 2 Vegetable

Southwest Swiss Chard and Bean Soup

SERVING SIZE: 1/4 of recipe, SERVES: 4

1 bunch Swiss chard (mixed color is fun, red is great, and white is fine)
1 tsp olive oil
1 1/2 cups chopped onion
2 cloves garlic, bashed and chopped
1 Tbsp mild chili powder
1 tsp ground cumin
3 cups low-sodium vegetable stock (page 473)
1 (15 oz) can pinto beans, drained and rinsed
1 (15 oz) can diced tomatoes
1/4 tsp salt

1 Wash the chard and remove the stems. Trim any discolored ends and cut the stems into 1/2-inch pieces. Stack the leaves and cut across into 1/2-inch strips.

2 Heat the oil in a high-sided skillet or large saucepan on medium high. Fry the onion until it starts to soften, 4 or 5 minutes. Add the garlic, chard stems, chili powder, and cumin and cook 1 minute more. Stir in the greens to coat with the spices.

3 Pour in the stock, beans, and tomatoes and bring to a boil. Reduce the heat and simmer 5 minutes or until the chard and stems are tender. Season with salt. Serve with a nice piece of corn bread and dream of the Grand Canyon.

Per serving: 160 calories, 3 g fat, 0 g saturated fat, 0% calories from saturated fat, 26 g carbohydrate, 8 g dietary fiber, 472 mg sodium, 7 g protein
Exchanges: 1 Starch, 2 Vegetable, 1/2 Fat

Taro and Chili Cakes

SERVING SIZE: 2 cakes, SERVES: 6

<C 1 3/4 lbs taro root or red potatoes
    1 tsp light olive oil
<C   1 large sweet onion, finely diced
    2 jalapeño peppers, cored,
      seeded, and finely diced

1/2 cup egg substitute
1/2 tsp salt
<C 1 large carrot, grated
  3 Tbsp chopped fresh parsley
1/2 cup all-purpose flour

1 Place the taro roots in a large steamer, cover, and steam for 30–40 minutes, or until very tender. Cover with cold water, then peel when cool enough to handle. Cut each taro root into several pieces and beat with an electric mixer until it has the consistency of smooth paste.

2 Preheat the oven to 450°F.

3 Warm the oil in a large frying pan over medium heat. Sauté the onion and jalapeños until very soft but not browned, about 10 minutes.

4 Add the egg substitute, salt, carrot, and parsley to the taro paste. Add the onion mixture and combine well.

5 Cover a large plate with the flour. Scoop about twelve 1/8-cup balls of the taro mixture onto the plate and dust with flour. Using the palm of your hand, flatten each ball into a patty about 1/2-inch thick. Lay the patties on a greased cookie sheet.

6 Lightly coat the tops of the cakes with cooking spray and bake in the pre-heated oven for 10 minutes. Turn the patties and bake for 10 minutes more, or until golden brown.

7 Serve two cakes per person.

<C **To Cut Carb**
<C Taro root: reduce to 1 lb.
<C Sweet Onions: reduce to 1/2 onion (1/3 cup chopped).
<C Carrots: reduce to 1/2 large (1/2 cup chopped).
<C Flour: reduce to 1/4 cup.

Per serving: 232 calories, 1 g fat, 0 g saturated fat, 0% calories from saturated fat, 51 g carbohydrate, 7 g dietary fiber, 259 mg sodium
Exchanges: 3 Starch, 1 Vegetable

Low Carb

Per serving: 143 calories, 1 g fat, 0 g saturated fat, 0% calories from saturated fat, 30 g carbohydrate, 4 g dietary fiber, 248 mg sodium
Exchanges: 2 Starch

Roasted Portabello Vegetable Hero

SERVING SIZE: 2 slices, SERVES: 4

2 Portabello mushrooms, stems removed and cut in half	1/2 tsp dried thyme
	1/4 tsp salt
1 medium zucchini, cut lengthwise in 1/2-inch slices	1/4 tsp pepper
	<C 1 (1 lb) loaf French bread
2 thick slices sweet onion	2 Tbsp roasted garlic
1 red bell pepper, cut in 1/2-inch rings	(see page 471)
2 jalapeños chilis, seeded and cut in strips	1 Tbsp Balsamic vinegar

1 Preheat the oven to 425°F. Lay the vegetables in one layer on a baking sheet. Sprinkle with thyme, salt, and pepper. Spray with olive oil pan spray and roast 20 minutes or until tender and golden.

2 Heat the bread in the oven during the last 10 minutes of vegetable cooking. Cut in half lengthwise and remove some of the center to make a hollow for the vegetables. Spread with roasted garlic, lay the vegetables in the hollow, and sprinkle with the Balsamic vinegar. Top with the other half of the bread and cut into 8 thick slices.

<C **To Cut Carb** ═══════════════════════════════

<C French bread loaf (or sub): use only half. This is an excellent example of the effect that large amounts of bread can have to make a fat *percentage* seem *very* reasonable. But just look at the carbs!!

Per serving: 290 calories, 1 g fat, 0 g saturated fat, 0% calories from saturated fat, 61 g carbohydrate, 5 g dietary fiber, 755 mg sodium
Exchanges: 3 Starch, 2 Vegetable

Low Carb

Per serving: 171 calories, 1 g fat, 0 g saturated fat, 0% calories from saturated fat, 36 g carbohydrate, 4 g dietary fiber, 458 mg sodium
Exchanges: 1 1/2 Starch, 2 Vegetable

Pork and Shrimp with Rice Noodles Philippine Style

SERVING SIZE: 1/6 of recipe, SERVES: 6

2 cups water
3/4 lb cooked shrimp
1 tsp peeled and chopped ginger root
1 red bell pepper
4 green onions
1/2 lb pork tenderloin, trimmed of all fat
1 tsp non-aromatic olive oil
4 cloves garlic, sliced
1/4 tsp turmeric

2 tsp fish sauce
2 Tbsp arrowroot mixed with
1/4 cup water (slurry)
3/4 lb firm light tofu, cubed
1/4 tsp pepper
1 Tbsp chopped cilantro
<C 3/4 lb thin rice noodles or angel hair pasta

Vegetarian Option

1/2 lb fresh shiitake mushrooms
1/2 lb green soy beans

2 tsp light soy sauce

Substitute the mushrooms for the shrimp. Remove the stems and add to the broth along with the ginger, pepper, and onion trim. Cut the caps into thin strips. Use the green soy beans (found in Asian markets) instead of the pork. Sauté the shiitakes and beans with the garlic and ginger and proceed as in step 3. Season with soy sauce instead of fish sauce. Finish the sauce, cook the noodles, and serve.

1 Heat the water in a saucepan. Finely chop 1/3 of the shrimp and add to the simmering water. Peel the ginger and cut into thin strips, adding the ginger trim to the broth. Core, trim, and chop the red pepper, tossing any trim into the simmering broth. Set aside the chopped pepper. Wash the onions and cut off and discard the root ends. Cut 3 inches off the green ends and add to the broth. Slice the rest and set aside. Simmer the broth for 15 minutes.

2 Cut the pork tenderloin in half lengthwise, then into 1/4-inch strips also lengthwise. Now cut across the strips making 1/4-inch cubes. Heat a large pot of water for the pasta while you make the sauce.

3 Heat the oil in a high-sided skillet on high. Add the pork, garlic, and ginger and cook for 3 minutes, or until the pork is lightly browned. Add the red

pepper, turmeric, and fish sauce and cook 1 minute longer. Strain the broth into the pan, add the slurry, and thicken. Stir in the tofu, remaining shrimp, cilantro, green onions, and pepper.

4 Cook the noodles 3 minutes, drain, and divide among 6 bowls. Spoon the sauce over the noodles and serve with red pepper flakes on the side for those who like a little heat.

<c **To Cut Carb**

<C Rice Noodles: reduce to 1/3 lb.

Per serving: 346 calories, 4 g fat, 1 g saturated fat, 2% calories from saturated fat, 55 g carbohydrate, 2 g dietary fiber, 439 mg sodium
Exchanges: 3 1/2 Starch, 2 Very Lean Meat

Low Carb
Per serving: 225 calories, 3 g fat, 1 g saturated fat, 4% calories from saturated fat, 27 g carbohydrate, 1 g dietary fiber, 379 mg sodium
Exchanges: 2 Starch, 2 Very Lean Meat

Vegetarian
Per serving: 324 calories, 4 g fat, 1 g saturated fat, 2% calories from saturated fat, 60 g carbohydrate, 4 g dietary fiber, 266 mg sodium
Exchanges: 3 1/2 Starch, 1 Vegetable, 1/2 Fat

Pasta Vegetable Toss

SERVING SIZE: 1/4 of recipe, SERVES: 4

<C 8 oz dry spaghetti
   1 tsp olive oil
<C 1 cup chopped onion
   2 cloves garlic, chopped
   1 cup red bell pepper
   1 cup zucchini, cut in strips

   1 cup crookneck squash, cut in strips
   1 cup no-added-salt tomato sauce
   1 tsp dried basil
   1 tsp dried oregano
1/4 cup grated Parmesan cheese

1 Cook the spaghetti according to package directions. Drain and keep warm in a colander over hot water.

2 Heat the oil in a high-sided skillet on medium-high. Fry the onion 2 minutes then add the garlic and cook 1 minute more. Stir in the red pepper, zucchini, crookneck squash, and kidney beans.

(Continued)

3 Pour in the tomato sauce, basil, and oregano and heat.

4 Serve topped with Parmesan cheese.

<C **To Cut Carb**

<C Pasta: reduce to 4 oz.   <C Onion: reduce to 4 oz (1/2 cup).

Per serving: 299 calories, 4 g fat, 2 g saturated fat, 6% calories from saturated fat, 55 g carbohydrate, 4 g dietary fiber, 70 mg sodium
Exchanges: 3 Starch, 2 Vegetable, 1/2 Fat

Low Carb
Per serving: 185 calories, 4 g fat, 1 g saturated fat, 5% calories from saturated fat, 32 g carbohydrate, 3 g dietary fiber, 67 mg sodium
Exchanges: 1 1/2 Starch, 2 Vegetable, 1/2 Fat

Grandma Yan's Porridge

Copyright by Yan Can Cook, Inc. 1999

SERVING SIZE: 1/8 of recipe, Serving: 8

1 1/2 cups uncooked long-grain rice
   1 Tbsp shredded ginger
  12 cups low-sodium chicken broth (page 463)

1/2 lb boneless chicken, cut into small pieces

Marinade

2 tsp cornstarch   1/8 tsp white pepper
1/4 tsp salt   1 tsp sesame oil

Garnishes

Chopped cilantro   Roasted peanuts
Thinly sliced green onion

1 In a large pot combine rice, ginger, and broth and bring to a boil. Reduce heat, cover, and simmer, stirring occasionally, until rice becomes very soft and creamy, about 1 1/2 hours.

2 While rice is cooking, combine marinade ingredients in a bowl; add chicken and stir to coat.

3 Add chicken and simmer, stirring occasionally, for 10 minutes. Stir in sesame oil.

4 To serve, ladle porridge into individual soup bowls and top with garnishes.

Per serving: 207 calories, 4 g fat, 1 g saturated fat, 4% calories from saturated fat, 34 g carbohydrate, 1 g dietary fiber, 178 mg sodium, 8 g protein
Exchanges: 2 1/2 Starch, 1/2 Fat

Double-the-Serving Stew

SERVING SIZE: 1/6 of recipe, SERVES: 6

2 Tbsp all-purpose flour	2 medium onions
3/4 tsp salt	2 stalks celery
1/2 tsp ground black pepper	2 medium potatoes
1 lb lean beef stew meat, cut into 1-inch cubes	2 medium turnips
1 Tbsp vegetable oil	4 carrots
3 cups low-fat, low-sodium beef broth, plus more as needed	2 cloves garlic, chopped
	1/2 tsp dried thyme
	1/4 cup fresh parsley, chopped

1 In a plastic bag, combine flour, salt, and pepper. Add meat and shake to coat. Heat oil in large saucepan or Dutch oven. Add meat and brown.

2 Prepare vegetables by cutting one onion, two celery stalks, one potato, one turnip and two carrots into large chunks. Add vegetables to meat along with garlic and thyme. Stir in broth, and bring to boil. Reduce heat and cover. Simmer for about 40 minutes or until meat is tender.

3 While meat is cooking, prepare remaining vegetables by cutting the onion, celery, potato, turnip and carrot into 1-inch cubes.

4 Remove simmered vegetables and blend until smooth. Return puree to pot. Thin with beef broth or water, if necessary. Add remaining uncooked onions, celery, potato, turnips, and carrots to pot. Bring to simmer and cover. Cook for 30 minutes or until vegetables are tender. Add parsley just before serving.

Per serving: 275 calories, 9 g fat, 3 g saturated fat, 10% calories from saturated fat, 28 g carbohydrate, 5 g dietary fiber, 484 mg sodium
Exchanges: 1 Starch, 2 Lean Meat, 3 Vegetable, 1/2 Fat

Texas Chili

SERVING SIZE: 1/6 of recipe, SERVES: 6

1 1/2 tsp non-aromatic olive oil, divided
   8 oz bottom round, cut in fine dice
   8 oz turkey thigh, cut in fine dice
   1 onion, cut into 1/4-inch dice
   1 (10 1/2 oz) can tomato puree
   2 jalapeño peppers, seeded
    and chopped
    (leave the seeds if you like it hot)
   1 (4 oz) can diced green chilis
   1 tsp ground cumin
   1 tsp dried oregano
 1/4 tsp cayenne pepper
   1 Tbsp cocoa

 1/4 tsp salt
1 1/2 cups nonalcoholic red wine
    (this can be replaced with
    beef stock)
1 1/2 cups low-sodium beef
    stock (page 466) or water
   3 cloves garlic, bashed and
    chopped
   1 Tbsp cornmeal
<C 1 1/2 cups cooked brown rice
<C   3 cups canned pinto beans,
    rinsed and drained

Garnish

1/2 cup finely chopped raw onions
1/2 cup chopped cilantro

6 Tbsp parmesan cheese

1 Mix 1 tsp of the oil with the diced beef. Drop into a hot pan to brown. When it's pretty well browned, about 2 minutes, add the turkey and continue cooking 2 more minutes. Tip out onto a plate.

2 Heat the remaining oil in the unwashed pan and sauté the onion until it starts to wilt, about 2 to 3 minutes. Add the jalapenos, diced chilis, cumin, oregano, cayenne, cocoa, and salt. Cook 1 minute longer. Pour in the wine and stock, bring to a boil, reduce the heat, and simmer 30 minutes.

3 Stir in the garlic and cornmeal. Cook 3 or 4 minutes until the chili thickens. Divide the rice and beans among 6 hot bowls. Ladle the chili over the top and pass the garnishes at the table.

<C **To Cut Carb**

<C Brown rice: reduce to 2/3 cup.   <C Pinto beans: reduce to 2 cups.

Per serving: 377 calories, 8 g fat, 3 g saturated fat, 5% calories from saturated fat, 48 g carbohydrate, 11 g dietary fiber, 877 mg sodium
Exchanges: 2 1/2 Starch, 2 Lean Meat, 2 Vegetable

Low Carb

Per serving: 302 calories, 8 g fat, 3 g saturated fat, 6% calories from saturated fat, 34 g carbohydrate, 8 g dietary fiber, 549 mg sodium
Exchanges: 1 1/2 Starch, 2 Lean Meat, 2 Vegetable

Vegetable Curry

SERVING SIZE: 1/4 of recipe, SERVES: 4

1 tsp non-aromatic olive oil	<C 1 cup petit peas, thawed
1/2 cup chopped onions	1/4 tsp salt
1 Tbsp curry powder	2 Tbsp 100% orange juice mixed
2 cups cauliflower florets	with 1 tsp arrowroot or
1 cup thinly sliced carrots	cornstarch (slurry)
<C 1/4 cup raisins	1/4 cup cashew nuts
<C 1/2 cup 100% orange juice	<C 2 cups cooked rice

1 Heat the oil in a high-sided skillet on medium high. Sauté the onions for 1 minute then add the curry powder and cook 2 minutes more. Stir in the potatoes, carrots, and raisins and toss to coat with curry. Pour in the juice, cover, and cook on medium for 20 minutes or until the vegetables are tender.

2 Stir in the peas and salt and heat through. Add the slurry and stir until thickened and clear. Serve over rice and scatter the cashews over the top.

<C **To Cut Carb**

<C Raisins: reduce to 1 Tbsp.

<C Orange juice: reduce to 1/4 cup.

<C Peas: reduce to 1/2 cup.

<C Rice: reduce to 1 cup and change to brown rice.

+> Add 1 cup of your favorite vegetable.

Per serving: 278 calories, 6 g fat, 1 g saturated fat, 3% calories from saturated fat, 50 g carbohydrates, 7 g fiber, 264 mg sodium
Exchanges: 2 Starch, 1 Vegetable, 1 Fruit, 1 Fat

Low Carb

Per serving: 194 calories, 6 g fat, 1 g saturated fat, 4% calories from saturated fat, 31 g carbohydrate, 6 g dietary fiber, 250 mg sodium
Exchanges: 1 Starch, 2 Vegetable, 1/2 Fruit, 1 Fat

Jerk Marinated Lamb

SERVING SIZE: 1/6 of recipe, SERVES: 6

1 tsp non-aromatic olive oil
2 scallions, chopped
2 large cloves garlic, bashed and chopped
1 1/2 Tbsp allspice berries, crushed or 1/2 tsp ground allspice
1/2 tsp crushed chilis (increase for heat)
1 tsp thyme
2-inch ginger root cut in slices
2 cups + 2 Tbsp nonalcoholic red wine
1/2 tsp + 1/8 tsp salt

1 1/2 lb lean lamb leg cut in 1-inch chunks
18 pearl onions, peeled or 1 can pearl onions
1 lb baby carrots
1 bunch collard greens, washed and stemmed
1/8 tsp ground red pepper (increase for heat)
1 Tbsp arrowroot
2 Tbsp nonalcoholic red wine or water

1 Heat 1/2 tsp of the oil in a chef's pan or high-sided skillet on medium high. Add the scallions, garlic, allspice, chilis, thyme, and ginger. Cook, stirring, 2 minutes. Pour in 1 cup of the wine and 1/2 tsp of the salt and continue cooking until the wine is almost gone, about 5 minutes. Strain into a bowl and rinse the pan with the other cup of wine and add to the bowl. Pour over the meat and marinate 8 hours or overnight. Drain, reserving the marinade, and pat dry.

2 Preheat the oven to 350°F. Heat the remaining oil in a chef's pan or high-sided skillet on high. Drop in the meat in one layer and do not disturb until browned on one side, 2–3 minutes. (You can peek as you start to see the bottom browning around the edges.) Tip the meat onto a plate and add the onions and carrots to the hot pan. Cook, stirring, 3 or 4 minutes or until they start to brown just a little. Pour the reserved marinade over the top and let it boil. Return the meat with any accumulated juices to the pan. Pour the reserved marinade over the top, cover, and bake in the preheated oven 1 hour.

3 Remove the pan from the oven. Drop the collard greens into the pan, sprinkle with the ground red pepper and remaining salt, and cover. Cook 5 minutes over medium heat. Remove to the plate with the meat and other vegetables, starting with a good layer of the collard greens. Thicken the remaining liquid with a slurry made from the arrowroot and remaining wine. Pour the sauce over the meat and vegetables and serve.

Per serving: 317 calories, 12 g fat, 4 g saturated fat, 11% calories from saturated fat, 15 g carbohydrate, 3 g dietary fiber, 380 mg sodium, protein 37 g protein
Exchanges: 4 Lean Meat, 3 Vegetable

Crab Cakes

SERVING SIZE: 1/4 of recipe, SERVES: 4

Crab Cakes

1/4 cup finely chopped sweet onion
1/4 cup finely chopped celery
1/4 cup finely chopped red bell pepper
1/4 cup chopped parsley
1/2 tsp dried thyme
16 unsalted saltines, crushed (3/4 cup)
1/2 cup nonfat yogurt cheese
1 tsp horseradish

pinch saffron
1 Tbsp freshly squeezed lemon juice
2 Tbsp egg substitute
1 lb lump crabmeat
1 Tbsp paprika
1 bunch watercress, stemmed
2 cups mixed salad greens
1/4 cup peanut vinaigrette

Peanut Vinaigrette

1 clove garlic, bashed and chopped
2 Tbsp non-aromatic olive oil
1/2 cup rice wine vinegar
1/2 tsp dry mustard

1 tsp brown sugar
2 Tbsp peanut butter
1/8 tsp cayenne

1 Combine onion, celery, pepper, parsley, thyme, cracker crumbs, yogurt, horseradish, saffron, lemon juice, and egg substitute. Stir the crab in gently.

2 Spray a baking sheet with olive oil spray. Sprinkle paprika over the pan. Pack the crab mixture tightly into a 1/3-cup measure, and then tap it out onto the pan. Flatten each cake to make 8 3/4-inch thick patties. Turn and sprinkle the other sides with more paprika.

3 Heat a large skillet. Spray with olive oil, and lay the patties in the hot pan. Sprinkle paprika lightly on the tops. Fry 3 minutes on each side. Combine watercress and salad greens, and divide among 4 plates. Drizzle with peanut dressing, and top with 2 crab cakes.

Per serving: 264 calories, 5 g fat, 1 g saturated fat, 3% calories from saturated fat, 20 g carbohydrate, 3 g dietary fiber, 55 mg sodium
Exchanges: 1/2 Starch, 4 Very Lean Meat, 2 Vegetable, 1/2 Fat

Turkey Pot Pie

SERVING SIZE: 1/4 of recipe, SERVES: 4

Pie Filling

1 tsp non-aromatic olive oil	1 1/2 cups homemade turkey or low-sodium chicken stock (page 463)
1/2 sweet onion, cut in 1/4-inch dice (1 cup)	
<C 2 carrots, cut in 1/2-inch dice (1 cup)	1/8 tsp salt
2 turnips, cut in 1/2-inch dice (1 cup)	1/8 tsp pepper
	1 lb broccoli
<C 2 small parsnips, cut in 1/2-inch dice (1/2 cup)	2 1/2 cups cooked turkey (2/3 dark and 1/3 white meat)

Sauce

<C 3/4 lb parsnips, peeled, roughly chopped, and steamed until tender

<C 1 cup evaporated skim milk
1/4 tsp salt

Cheese Biscuits (*adapted from* Eating Well: Secrets of Low-Fat Cooking)

<C 1 cup all-purpose flour	3/4 cup buttermilk
<C 1 cup cake flour	1 Tbsp non-aromatic olive oil
<C 1 Tbsp sugar	1/4 cup grated low-fat sharp cheddar cheese
1 1/2 tsp baking powder	
1/2 tsp baking soda	1 Tbsp low-fat milk to brush on top
1/4 tsp salt	
1 1/2 Tbsp cold, hard, butter flavored margarine, cut in small piece	

1 Heat the oil in a chef's pan or skillet on medium high. Sauté the onions, carrots, turnips, and parsnips on medium heat 3 minutes. Pour in the stock and season with salt and pepper. Bring to a boil, reduce the heat, cover, and simmer until the vegetables are tender, about 6 minutes.

2 Whiz the steamed parsnips in a blender with a little of the evaporated milk until smooth, about 2 minutes. Add the rest of the milk and the salt and whiz until smooth and velvety, another 30 seconds.

3 Preheat the oven to 425°F. Coat a baking sheet with pan spray. Whisk together the flours, sugar, baking powder, soda, and salt in a bowl or combine in a processor.

4 Scatter the pieces of margarine over the top and cut in with 2 knives or pulse 2 or 3 times in the processor. Make a well in the center of the dry ingredients and pour in the buttermilk and oil. Stir with a fork just until blended or pulse 2 or 3 times in the processor.

5 Knead the dough very lightly on a floured board. Pat or roll out about 1/2-inch thick and cut into 4 large 3-inch biscuits. Place on the prepared baking sheet, brush with milk, dust with cheese, and bake 15 minutes or until golden.

6 While the biscuits are baking, lay the broccoli on the simmering vegetables and cook until tender, 6 minutes or until tender but still bright green. Stir in the turkey and parsnip sauce and heat through.

7 Biscuits by the nature of their chemistry are high in calories and fat. To fit into your meal plan, make a whole recipe, cut the tops off 4 to use in the recipe, and save the bottoms and extra biscuit to toast for breakfast. Spoon the turkey mixture into 4 hot soup plates and lay the biscuit halves on top.

<C **To Cut Carb**

<C Carrot: reduce to one.
<C Parsnips: remove completely, the sauce will pick up the flavor.
<C Sauce parsnips: reduce to 1/2 lb.
<C Evaporated milk: reduce to 1/2 cup.

Per serving: 485 calories, 10 g fat, 4 g saturated fat, 1% calories from saturated fat, 60 g carbohydrate, 10 g dietary fiber, 739 mg sodium, 39 g protein
Exchanges: 2 1/2 Starch, 3 Lean Meat, 3 Vegetable, 1/2 Fat-Free Milk

Low Carb
Per serving: 418 calories, 10 g fat, 4 g saturated fat, 1% calories from saturated fat, 47 g carbohydrate, 6 g dietary fiber, 689 mg sodium, 36 g protein
Exchanges: 2 1/2 Starch, 3 Lean Meat, 2 Vegetable

Field Burgers

SERVING SIZE: 1 burger, SERVES: 4

4 large Portabello mushrooms	Dijon mustard
2 Tbsp lemon juice	4 leaves Romaine lettuce
1/4 tsp salt	4 large tomato slices
1/4 tsp pepper	4 thin slices sweet onion
<C 4 whole-wheat hamburger buns	

(Continued)

1 Remove the stems from the Portabellos and clean with a dry cloth or soft brush. Spray a large skillet with olive oil pan spray and heat on medium high. Place the mushrooms in round side down. Sprinkle with lemon juice, salt, and pepper. Cook 2 minutes, turn, and cook 2 minutes more on the other side.

2 Split the buns and spread with Dijon mustard. Lay a Portabello on one half of each bun and make sandwiches with the garnishing vegetables and the other halves of the buns.

<C **To Cut Carb**

<C Serve "open faced": take the bun tops, wrap tightly, and freeze for a future use.

Per serving: 152 calories, 3 g fat, 0 g saturated fat, 0% calories from saturated fat, 27 g carbohydrate, 3 g dietary fiber, 590 mg sodium
Exchanges: 1 1/2 Starch, 1 Vegetable, 1/2 Fat

Low Carb
Per serving: 96 calories, 2 g fat, 0 g saturated fat, 0% calories from saturated fat, 17 g carbohydrate, 2 g dietary fiber, 491 mg sodium
Exchanges: 1 Starch, 1 Vegetable

Seattle Summer Halibut

SERVING SIZE: 1/4 of recipe, SERVES: 4

Crostini

1 baguette (see sidebar)	1/8 tsp salt
1/2 cup fish stock (page 468)	1/8 tsp freshly ground pepper
pinch saffron	extra virgin olive oil pan spray

Roasted Garlic Sauce

1 head garlic	tiny pinch saffron
1/2 cup nonfat yogurt cheese (see page 475)	1 tsp extra virgin olive oil
	1 Tbsp freshly squeezed lemon juice

Halibut

1 tsp extra virgin olive oil
6 cloves garlic, bashed and
   chopped (generous 2 Tbsp)
3 cups fish stock (see page 468)
1 Tbsp chopped parsley
1/4 tsp salt
1 Tbsp freshly squeezed lemon
   juice

pinch saffron
4 (6 oz) halibut fillets
4 Roma tomatoes, cut in eighths
   lengthwise then in half crosswise
1 Tbsp arrowroot mixed with 2 Tbsp
   fish stock or water (slurry)
3 Tbsp chopped parsley

1 Preheat the oven to 350°F. To make the crostini, cut the baguette in long diagonal slices starting the cuts from the top of the loaf. You will need 8 long thin slices. Heat the fish stock with the saffron, salt, and pepper until it turns bright yellow. Brush the bread on both sides with the yellow broth. Spray lightly with the extra virgin olive oil pan spray. Bake on a baking sheet with a rack 5 minutes. Turn and bake 5 minutes more or until the bread is quite crisp. Set aside.

2 Cut the root end off the head of garlic and wrap in foil. Roast for an hour in the preheated oven or until very soft. Remove and cool before pressing out the cooked flesh. You should have 2 Tbsp. Combine with the yogurt cheese, saffron, olive oil, and lemon juice. Set aside.

3 Stir the olive oil and garlic together in a small saucepan on medium heat. Cook until it starts to sizzle, about 2 minutes, then add 2 cups of the fish stock and parsley. Turn to high and reduce the liquid by half at a vigorous reducing boil, about 5 minutes. Strain into a skillet large enough to hold the fish fillets. Add the other cup of stock, salt, lemon juice, and saffron. Bring to a boil. Set the fillets in the stock and reduce the heat to medium. Cover with a sheet of waxed paper, cut to fit the pan. Simmer 5 minutes then turn and cook 2 minutes longer. Remove to 4 hot soup plates.

4 Toss the tomatoes into the boiling liquid to just heat through, about 1 minute. Stir in the slurry and parsley. It should thicken almost immediately. Spoon over the fish fillets and serve with a dollop of the garlic sauce and 2 crostini. Scatter more chopped parsley over it if you like.

Per serving: 403 calories, 6 g fat, 0 g saturated fat, 0% calories from saturated fat, 40 g carbohydrate, 2 g fiber, 699 mg sodium, 46 g protein
Exchanges: 2 1/2 Starch, 5 Very Lean Meat, 1 Vegetable, 1/2 Fat

Scottish Irish Stew

SERVING SIZE: 1/6 of recipe, SERVES: 6

Stew Base

1 tsp non-aromatic olive oil
1 medium onion, coarsely chopped

1 1/4 lb lamb necks
5 cups low-sodium chicken stock (page 463)

Stew

1/4 cup barley
4 medium carrots, peeled and cut into 1/2-inch pieces
1 lb yellow potatoes, peeled and cut into 1/2-inch pieces
18 small boiling onions, peeled

1/2 tsp black pepper
1/4 tsp salt
18 whole white mushrooms, to match onion size
1 lb fresh spinach leaves, washed and stemmed

Vegetarian Option

1 lb parsnips, peeled and cut into 2-inch pieces
2 Tbsp tamari
2 turnips peeled and cut into 1/2-inch pieces
1/4 cup barley (added to other 1/4 cup above, making 1/2 cup)
5 cups low-sodium vegetable broth (page 473)

Sprinkle the parsnips with tamari and let set for 15 minutes. Heat olive oil in a high-sided skillet and sauté the parsnips, carrots, potatoes, onions, and turnips for 2 minutes. Add barley and pepper and pour in low-sodium vegetable broth. (Leave the salt out as the tamari is very salty.) Bring to a boil, reduce the heat, and simmer 30 minutes. Stir in the mushrooms and cook 5 minutes more. Serve in spinach-lined bowls as in step 3.

---

1 To make the stew base, heat the oil in a high-sided skillet on medium. Sauté the onions 1 minute. Add 4 cups of the stock and the lamb necks and bring to a boil. Reduce the heat and simmer, covered, 2 1/2 hours or until the meat falls off the bone. When the lamb is cooked, remove from broth and take the meat off the bones. Strain the broth into a fat separator.

2 To make the stew, return the defatted broth to the pan and pour in the remaining cup of chicken broth. Now add the barley, carrots, potatoes, onions, pepper, and salt. Simmer, covered, on medium low for 30 minutes. Add the mushrooms and meat and cook 5 more minutes.

3 Line 6 bowls with raw spinach leaves, pointed end up. Ladle the stew into the lined bowls and serve.

Per serving: 277 calories, 6 g fat, 2 g saturated fat, 6% calories from saturated fat, 35 g carbohydrate, 13 g dietary fiber, 211 mg sodium, 21 g protein
Exchanges: 1 1/2 Starch, 2 Lean Meat, 2 Vegetable

Vegetarian
Per serving: 273 calories, 2 g fat, 0 g saturated fat, 0 % calories from saturated fat, 59 g carbohydrate, 18 g dietary fiber, 200 mg sodium, 5 g protein
Exchanges: 2 1/2 Starch, 3 Vegetable

Grilled Fish on a Bed of Bitter Greens

SERVING SIZE: 1/4 of recipe, SERVES: 4

4 cups arugula, radicchio, endive,
   escarole, romaine, or a mixture of these
4 tsp low-fat vinaigrette dressing
4 (4 oz) halibut fillets

1/4 tsp salt
1/4 tsp pepper
  2 Tbsp lemon juice

1 Wash the greens and spin dry. Tear into bite size pieces and toss with the vinaigrette. Divide among 4 dinner plates.

2 Season the fish with salt and pepper. Grill, skin side up, 3–5 minutes. Turn and cook 3–5 minutes more. (You can gauge the time by measuring the thickness of the fish and cooking 10 minutes per inch.)

3 Remove the skin as you take the halibut off the pan. Set the fillets on the greens and sprinkle with lemon juice. Tiny, new red potatoes go wonderfully with this.

Per serving: 147 calories, 2 g fat, 1 g saturated fat, 6% calories from saturated fat, 2 g carbohydrate, 0 g dietary fiber, 238 mg sodium, 30 g protein
Exchanges: 4 Very Lean Meat

Sea Bass

SERVING SIZE: 1 fillet, SERVES: 6

1/4 tsp salt
1/4 tsp freshly ground black pepper
1 1/2 Tbsp finely chopped fresh tarragon
1 1/2 Tbsp finely chopped fresh parsley

1 1/2 Tbsp finely chopped fresh chives
1 1/2 Tbsp finely chopped fresh basil
6 sea bass fillets, about 6 oz each

Vegetarian Option: Broiled Artichoke Bottoms

12 artichoke bottoms

Substitute 2 artichoke bottoms for each serving of fish. Season the artichoke bottoms with the mixed herbs and broil, just until heated through and slightly browned, about 4 minutes. Serve over couscous, as you would the fish, and top with the chutney. Garnish with the chopped herbs.

---

1 Preheat the broiler. Sprinkle the salt and pepper on a large plate, then spray the plate with cooking spray. Mix the tarragon, parsley, chives, and basil in a small bowl and sprinkle a third of this mixture over the plate.

2 Drag the fish fillets one at a time across the plate to pick up the seasonings, then place on a broiler pan, herbed side down. Sprinkle the fillets with another third of the herb mixture, then spray the tops of the fish lightly with cooking spray. (Save the rest of the herbs for garnish.)

3 Broil the fillets for 4 minutes on each side, or until the flesh is no longer translucent, but white throughout.

4 Serve the fish on top of a bed of couscous. Heap a spoonful of Mango Chutney (page 472) on top of each fillet and sprinkle the reserved herb mixture over all.

Per serving (fish only): 166 calories, 3 g fat, 0 g saturated fat, 0% calories from saturated fat, 0 g carbohydrate, 0 g dietary fiber, 215 mg sodium, 32 g protein
Exchanges: 5 Very Lean Meat

Vegetarian
Per serving: 32 calories, 0 g fat, 0 g saturated fat, 0% calories from saturated fat, 6 g carbohydrate, 1 g dietary fiber, 338 mg sodium, 2 g protein
Exchanges: 1 Vegetable

Packed Pita Pocket

SERVING SIZE: 1 pita pocket, SERVES: 2

8 1/2-inch slices eggplant
  2 small zucchini, sliced lengthwise into 8 slices
  4 1/2-inch slices sweet onions
  1 red bell pepper, sliced in rings
  olive oil pan spray
1/4 tsp salt

1/4 tsp pepper
1/2 tsp dried oregano
1/2 tsp dried basil
  1 tsp extra virgin olive oil
  1 Tbsp balsamic vinegar
<c 2 whole-wheat pitas

1 Preheat your broiler. Set the oven rack so the vegetables will be about 6 inches from the heat.

2 Lay the vegetables on a broiler pan in a single layer. If you want more servings, use 2 pans and cook them separately. Spray lightly with the pan spray and season with salt and pepper. Scatter oregano and basil over the top. Broil until they brown, turn, then brown the other side.

3 Tip into a bowl and toss with the oil and vinegar. Cut the pitas in half and fill each half with broiled vegetables. Serve warm or at room temperature. If you want to carry the sandwiches to work or on a picnic, carry the vegetables in one zip-top plastic bag and the pita in another.

<c To Cut Carb

<c Whole-wheat pitas: reduce to one only, serve the vegetables "cornucopia style," literally overflowing. (I love this as a snack.)

Per serving: 277 calories, 5 g fat, 0 g saturated fat, 0% calories from saturated fat, 58 g carbohydrate, 11 g dietary fiber, 431 mg sodium
Exchanges: 2 Starch, 5 Vegetable

Low Carb
Per serving: 207 calories, 4 g fat, 0 g saturated fat, 0% calories from saturated fat, 43 g carbohydrate, 10 g dietary fiber, 366 mg sodium
Exchanges: 1 Starch, 5 Vegetable

Roasted Vegetable Lasagna

SERVING SIZE: 1 piece, SERVES: 8

<C 1/2 pound dried lasagna, cooked according to package directions

Sauce (for all reason)

1/2 tsp non-aromatic olive oil
 2 cups chopped onions
 3 cloves garlic, bashed and chopped
 1 tsp dried basil
 1 tsp dried oregano

1 cup nonalcoholic red wine
 2 (10 1/2 oz) cans tomato puree
1/4 tsp salt
1/4 tsp pepper

Filling

 1 cup low-fat ricotta cheese
 2 Tbsp grated Parmesan cheese
1/4 cup chopped fresh basil

1/4 tsp salt
1/4 tsp pepper

Vegetables

1 large eggplant, cut in 1/2-inch slices
6 large Roma tomatoes, halved, cored,
   seeded

<C 1 bunch fresh spinach, stemmed
   and lightly steamed

Topping

4 slices non-fat mozzarella cheese
2 Tbsp Parmesan

2 Tbsp chopped fresh basil

1 Heat the oil in a chef's pan on medium. Sauté the onions with the basil and oregano until soft, about 5 minutes. Add the garlic and cook 1 minute more. Pour in the wine, tomato puree, salt, and pepper and bring to a boil. Cover and simmer until you are ready to use it, but not more than 15 minutes.

2 Heat the oven to 450°F. Lay the eggplant slices and tomato halves skin side down on a greased baking sheet with sides. Spray lightly with olive oil pan spray and sprinkle lightly with salt and pepper. Roast 20 minutes in the pre-heated oven. Set aside. Reduce the oven heat to 375°F. Press the water out of the steamed spinach.

3 Combine the ricotta, Parmesan, salt, pepper, and basil in a bowl.

4 Spoon enough sauce into the bottom of a chef's pan or baking dish to cover thinly. Lay noodles, cut to fit, in the bottom of the pan and cover them with another thin layer of sauce. Make a layer of eggplant slices and cover with

the steamed spinach. Lay the slices of nonfat cheese on top of the spinach. Cover with noodles, then more sauce, then the ricotta filling. Lay more noodles over the filling and spread with more sauce. Layer in the tomato halves. Cover with the remaining noodles and sauce.

5 Bake in the preheated oven until heated through. Because of the density of the dish, this may take as long as 40 minutes. When the sauce is bubbling up around the sides, it's hot. Let set for at least 10 minutes before cutting into 8 pieces to serve. Combine the Parmesan cheese and chopped basil and sprinkle over the top.

<c **To Cut Carb**

<c Dried lasagna noodles: reduce to only 1/4 pound.

<c Spinach: replace entirely with Bok Choy (dark green leaves on heavy white stalks). Strip the leafy green from broad stems and use for spinach. Gently simmer whole stems to *just* soften and use for the inner layer of Lasagna noodle (see step 4). It makes a good substitute.

Per serving: 261 calories, 3 g fat, 1 g saturated fat, 4% calories from saturated fat, 43 g carbohydrate, 6 g dietary fiber, 666 mg sodium
Exchanges: 1 1/2 Starch, 1 Lean Meat, 4 Vegetable

Low Carb
Per serving: 205 calories, 3 g fat, 1 g saturated fat, 4% calories from saturated fat, 32 g carbohydrate, 5 g dietary fiber, 664 mg sodium
Exchanges: 1/2 Starch, 1 Lean Meat, 4 Vegetable

Cauliflower Vegetable Curry

SERVING SIZE: 1/4 of recipe, SERVES: 4

1 tsp non-aromatic olive oil	<c 1 cup orange juice
1 cup chopped onions	<c 2 cup petit peas, thawed
1 Tbsp curry powder	1/4 tsp salt
4 cups cauliflower florets	1/4 cup cashew nuts
<c 2 cup thinly sliced carrots	<c 2 cups cooked brown rice
<c 1/2 cup raisins	

Heat the oil in a high-sided skillet on medium high. Sauté the onions 1 minute. Add the curry powder, and cook 2 minutes more. Stir in the cauliflower, carrots, and raisins, and toss to coat with curry. Pour in the orange juice, cover, and cook on medium 10 minutes or until the vegetables are tender.

(Continued)

2 Stir in the peas and salt, and heat through. Serve over rice, and scatter the cashews over the top.

<c **To Cut Carb**

<c Carrots: reduce to 1 cup.
<c Raisins: reduce to 2 Tbsp.
<c Orange juice: delete.
<c Peas: reduce to 1 cup.

<c Brown rice: reduce to 1 1/2 cups.
+> Add 2 cups of vegetables of your choice and 1 cup vegetable stock.

Per serving: 383 calories, 7 g fat, 1 g saturated fat, 3% calories from saturated fat, 73 g carbohydrate, 13 g dietary fiber, 331 mg sodium
Exchanges: 2 1/2 Starch, 2 Vegetable, 1 1/2 Fruit, 1 Fat

Low Carb

Per serving: 262 calories, 7 g fat, 1 g saturated fat, 3% calories from saturated fat, 45 g carbohydrate, 10 g dietary fiber, 377 mg sodium
Exchanges: 2 Starch, 3 Vegetable, 1 Fat

Israeli Beef Stew

SERVING SIZE: 1/4 of recipe, SERVES: 4

1 tsp non-aromatic olive oil
12 oz beef shank meat cut in 8 large pieces
1/4 tsp freshly ground black pepper
1 onion, roughly chopped
2 cloves garlic, bashed and chopped
2 large carrots, peeled and cut into 1-inch slices

<c 1/2 cup dry red kidney beans, soaked over night or quick soaked
<c 1/2 cup barley, rinsed
2 Turkish bay leaves
6 cups water
1/2 tsp salt
<c 1 cup frozen peas, thawed
<c Matzo Dumplings (see page 132)

Vegetarian Option

3/4 lb Jerusalem artichokes, peeled and cut in 1-inch chunks
1 (27 oz) can low-sodium kidney beans
1 Tbsp low-sodium tamari

This is a faster version of the stew. It cooks in half the time because there is no meat to tenderize. Note the use of canned kidney beans and tamari

---

and changes in the amounts of salt and water. Heat all the oil in the skillet and sauté the onions as in step 1. When the onions have gotten some color and begun to wilt, add the garlic and Jerusalem artichokes and cook, stirring, another minute. Add the carrots, kidney beans, barley, bay leaves, 4 cups water, and 1/4 tsp salt. Pour in tamari for flavor and cook, covered, in the preheated oven for 30 minutes. Add the dumplings as in step 3 and cook, uncovered, 30 minutes more. Stir in the peas and serve.

1 Preheat the oven to 350°F. Heat 1/2 tsp of the oil in a high-sided skillet on high. Drop the meat in to brown on one side, about 3 minutes. Remove the meat to a plate and set aside. Reduce the heat to medium high, add the remaining 1/2 tsp of the oil to the pan and toss in the onions. Sauté 3 minutes, turning often. After 2 or 3 minutes, add the garlic and cook 1 minute more.

2 Return the meat to the pan. Add the carrots, kidney beans, barley, bay leaves, water, and salt. Bring to a boil, skimming off any foam that rises as it heats. Cover and cook in the preheated oven for 1 hour.

3 When the stew has cooked for an hour, add Matzo Dumplings. Spoon the stew over the top and return the pan, uncovered, to the oven for 1 more hour.

4 Stir in the peas and serve.

<C **To Cut Carb**

<C Kidney beans: reduce to 1/4 cup.
<C Barley: reduce to 1/4 cup.

<C Peas: reduce to 1/2 cup.
<C Dumplings: delete.

Per serving: 377 calories, 5 g fat, 1 g saturated fat, 3% calories from saturated fat, 57 g carbohydrate, 12 g dietary fiber, 611 mg sodium, 26 g protein
Exchanges: 3 Starch, 1 Lean Meat, 2 Vegetable, 1/2 Fat

Low Carb
Per serving: 196 calories, 4 g fat, 1 g saturated fat, 3% calories from saturated fat, 25 g carbohydrate, 7 g dietary fiber, 343 mg sodium, 17 g protein
Exchanges: 1 Starch, 1 Lean Meat, 2 Vegetable

Vegetarian
Per serving: 442 calories, 4 g fat, 1 g saturated fat, 1% calories from saturated fat, 82 g carbohydrate, 18 g dietary fiber, 592 mg sodium, 22 g protein
Exchanges: 5 Starch, 2 Vegetable

Spaghetti Carbonara

SERVING SIZE: 1/4 of recipe, SERVES: 4

<C 8 oz uncooked spaghetti
    1 tsp salt
    1/2 tsp non-aromatic olive oil
    3 oz Canadian bacon, cut in
      thin 1-inch strips
    2 Tbsp pine nuts
    4 sun-dried tomato halves, cut
      in thin strips

1/2 cup egg substitute
  2 Tbsp chopped parsley
  2 Tbsp chopped chives or
    1 finely chopped green onion
1/4 tsp freshly ground black pepper
1/8 tsp salt
1/4 cup grated Parmesan cheese

Vegetarian Option

3 oz soy bacon bits

Simply replace the Canadian bacon with soy bacon bits found at the health food store or food co-op.

1 Bring a large pan of water to a boil and drop in the spaghetti and salt. Stir and time it for 10 minutes when it comes back to the boil.

2 While you wait for the spaghetti to cook, heat the oil in a medium sized skillet and add the Canadian bacon, pine nuts and sun-dried tomatoes. Fry, stirring, until the pine nuts are golden and the bacon lightly browned. Set aside.

3 Set a colander over a large heatproof bowl. Pour the spaghetti, water and all, into the colander. Take the colander out of the water to drain on a plate and pour the hot water out of the bowl. Now the bowl is hot enough to finish the dish.

4 Tip the spaghetti into the hot bowl. Add the bacon mixture, egg substitute, parsley, chives, pepper, salt, and cheese. Toss to mix and watch as the hot pasta cooks the egg substitute. Serve immediately on preheated plates.

<C To Cut Carb
<C Pasta: reduce to 6 oz of whole-wheat spaghetti.

Per serving: 324 calories, 8 g fat, 2 g saturated fat, 5% calories from saturated fat, 46 g carbohydrate, 2 g dietary fiber, 526 mg sodium
Exchanges: 3 Starch, 1 Lean Meat, 1/2 Fat

Low Carb
Per serving: 269 calories, 8 g fat, 2 g saturated fat, 7% calories from saturated fat, 35 g carbohydrate, 3 g dietary fiber, 525 mg sodium
Exchanges: 2 1/2 Starch, 1 Lean Meat, 1/2 Fat

Vegetarian
Per serving: 386 calories, 11 g fat, 2 g saturated fat, 6% calories from saturated fat, 52 g carbohydrate, 4 g dietary fiber, 630 mg sodium
Exchanges: 3 1/2 Starch, 2 Lean Meat, 1/2 Fat

Sugar Snaps with Penne Pasta and Roasted Peppers

SERVING SIZE: 1/4 of recipe, SERVES: 4

1 lb sugar snap peas
<C 8 oz uncooked penne pasta
1 cup reduced-sodium vegetable broth (page 473)
1 Tbsp extra virgin olive oil

2 tsp arrowroot or cornstarch
+> 1/2 cup roasted red bell peppers, cut in 2-inch strips
1/4 cup Parmesan cheese

1 Remove the strings from each side of the peas. Steam 5 minutes or until crisp but tender and still bright green. Chill under cold water and set aside. Cook the pasta according to package directions, drain, chill with cold water, and set aside.

2 Combine the vegetable broth, oil, and arrowroot and heat until it thickens and turns glossy. Stir in the pasta, peas, and roasted peppers to heat through.

3 Divide among 4 hot plates and scatter Parmesan over the top.

<C **To Cut Carb**
<C Pasta: reduce to 4 oz.   +> Peppers: increase to 1 cup.

Per serving: 333 calories, 7 g fat, 2 g saturated fat, 5% calories from saturated fat, 55 g carbohydrate, 5 g dietary fiber, 191 mg sodium
Exchanges: 3 Starch, 2 Vegetable, 1 Fat

Low Carb
Per serving: 233 calories, 6 g fat, 2 g saturated fat, 6% calories from saturated fat, 35 g carbohydrate, 4 g dietary fiber, 228 mg sodium
Exchanges: 1 1/2 Starch, 3 Vegetable, 1 Fat

Chiliquiles

SERVING SIZE: 1/4 of recipe, SERVES: 4

<C 10 medium corn tortillas
1 (28 oz) can diced tomatoes
in juice
2 canned chipotle chilis,
rinsed and seeded
1/2 tsp non-aromatic olive oil
<C 1 large sweet onion,
cut in 1/4-inch dice
(save 1/2 cup for garnish)

3 cloves garlic, bashed and chopped
2 cups low-sodium chicken stock
1/4 tsp salt
1/2 cup low-fat yogurt
1 1/2 cups shredded chicken
1/4 cup grated Parmesan cheese
1/2 cup chopped cilantro

Vegetarian Option

2 cups vegetable stock or water
2 chayote squash

Use vegetable stock or water in place of chicken stock. Slice and steam the squash until tender to substitute for the chicken.

---

1 Preheat oven to 350°F. Stack tortillas and cut into eighths. Coat 2 baking sheets with spray and lay tortilla wedges on them in one layer. Lightly spray the tops and bake 20 to 30 minutes, until crisp.

2 Drain tomatoes, reserving the liquid. Blend tomatoes with the chipotles on puree but with some texture.

3 Heat oil in a large chef's pan or skillet. Sauté half of the chopped onion until golden, about 7 minutes. Stir in garlic and cook 1 minute. Turn to medium high and pour in tomato puree. Cook, stirring often, until sauce thickens and starts to spatter the stove, 5 minutes. Pour the reserved tomato juice into a measuring cup and add stock to make 2 1/2 cups. Add to the tomato mixture with the salt and bring to a boil (should be 4 1/2 cups). Stir in the tortilla chips, coating each with sauce. Bring back to boil, then remove from heat. Cover and set 5 minutes. No more!

4 Divide among 4 hot plates, topping with onions, yogurt, chicken, cheese, and cilantro. Or serve from the dish it was cooked in topped with the garnish.

<C Corn tortillas: reduce to 6.
<C Onion: reduce to 1 cup *total*, 1/4 cup garnish.

Per serving: 421 calories, 10 g fat, 3 g saturated fat, 7% calories from saturated fat, 58 g carbohydrate, 8 g dietary fiber, 933 mg sodium
Exchanges: 3 Starch, 2 Lean Meat, 2 Vegetable, 1/2 Fat

Low Carb
Per serving: 359 calories, 9 g fat, 3 g saturated fat, 7% calories from saturated fat, 45 g carbohydrate, 6 g dietary fiber, 892 mg sodium
Exchanges: 2 Starch, 2 Lean Meat, 3 Vegetable, 1/2 Fat

Vegetarian
Per serving: 331 calories, 6 g fat, 2 g saturated fat, 6% calories from saturated fat, 62 g carbohydrate, 11 g dietary fiber, 833 mg sodium
Exchanges: 3 Starch, 3 Vegetable, 1/2 Fat

Mediterranean Roasted Eggplant

SERVING SIZE: 1/4 of recipe, SERVES: 4

2 small eggplants
1 cup low-sodium pizza sauce

1/4 cup low-fat plain yogurt
1 clove garlic, finely chopped

> This recipe also works great as a side dish. Just cut the serving size in half and make 8 servings instead of four!

1 Preheat the oven to 350°F. Remove the stem end and slice the eggplants into 3/4-inch slices. Spray a baking pan with olive oil and lay the eggplant on it in a single layer. Spoon pizza sauce on each slice. Bake 30 minutes in the preheated oven.

2 Stir the yogurt and garlic together. Drizzle the sauce in thin lines on each of the eggplant slices before serving. (You can do this easily by putting the sauce in a plastic squirt bottle.) Serve as an entrée or side dish.

Per serving (main dish): 86 calories, 1 g fat, 0 g saturated fat, 0% calories from saturated fat, 19 g carbohydrate, 5 g dietary fiber, 210 mg sodium
Exchanges: 3 Vegetable

Pea Sea Pie

SERVING SIZE: 1 slice, SERVES: 4

<C 2 lb medium red potatoes
14 oz fresh salmon fillet
1 generous Tbsp chopped fresh basil
1 generous Tbsp chopped fresh dill
1 generous Tbsp chopped fresh parsley
1 tsp non-aromatic olive oil
1/2 large sweet onion, sliced (generous cup)

3 cloves garlic, bashed and chopped (1 Tbsp)
2 1/2 cups low-sodium fish or chicken stock (pages 468, 463), divided
1/2 tsp salt
1/4 tsp freshly ground black pepper
3 Tbsp freshly grated Parmesan cheese
1 lb frozen petite peas, thawed
2 Tbsp arrowroot mixed with 1/4 cup stock or water (slurry)

1 Steam the potatoes whole for 25 minutes or until tender but not mushy. Cool, peel, and slice about 1/8-inch thick. Cut thin slices of the salmon across the fillet on the diagonal from the top down to the skin. Discard the skin. Combine the chopped herbs and divide in half. Coat a 9-inch pie dish with pan spray. Preheat the oven to 350°F.

2 Heat the oil in a chef's pan on medium high. Sauté the onions until they start to turn translucent, about 3 minutes. Add the garlic and cook 2 minutes more. Pour in 2 cups of the stock and the salt and bring to a boil to reduce while you assemble the dish.

3 Lay half of the potato slices (use the uneven end pieces here) on the bottom of the baking dish. (You will use half the herbs assembling the dish.) Sprinkle with herbs and pepper then lay half the salmon slices on top of the potatoes. Add a little more herbs and pepper. Now layer the rest of the salmon on top and scatter with more herbs, pepper, and the onions from the sauce. Top with the remaining potatoes in an attractive pattern and a little more of the mixed herbs. Pour the hot stock and onion mixture over the top. Sprinkle with the cheese and bake in the preheated oven for 15 minutes.

4 Reserve 1 cup of the peas for garnish. Whiz the rest with the remaining stock in a blender until very smooth, about 2 minutes. Press the puree through a sieve into a saucepan and set aside. When the pie is done, strain the remaining juice into the pureed peas. (A suitably sized plate, held firmly in place with cloth, will help you do this.) Add the remaining fresh herbs, whole peas, and slurry. Heat just until it thickens to preserve the bright color of the peas, which will turn yellow if heated too long. Pour the sauce in a puddle to cover each plate. Cut the pie in 4 pieces and serve your potato islands on the pea green sea!

<C Potatoes: reduce to 1 lb. Use only the top layer (at the end of step 3).

Per serving: 504 calories, 12 g fat, 3 g saturated fat, 4% calories from saturated fat, 66 g carbohydrate, 11 g dietary fiber, 474 mg sodium
Exchanges: 4 Starch, 3 Lean Meat, 1 Vegetable

Low Carb
Per serving: 410 calories, 12 g fat, 2 g saturated fat, 4% calories from saturated fat, 44 g carbohydrate, 9 g dietary fiber, 470 mg sodium
Exchanges: 2 1/2 Starch, 3 Lean Meat, 1 Vegetable, 1/2 Fat

Tsimmes

SERVING SIZE: 1/6 of recipe, SERVES: 6

<C 2 lb orange sweet potatoes
<C 2 large carrots, sliced
    1 heaping cup shopped onions
<C 20 large pitted prunes
       juice of 1 lemon

1/2 tsp salt
<C 2/3 cup orange juice
<C 1/4 cup matzo meal
    2 Tbsp butter flavored margarine
       or butter

1 Preheat the oven to 350°F. Peel and chop the sweet potatoes into small pieces. Combine with the carrots, apple, onion, prunes, lemon juice, salt, cinnamon, and orange juice in a casserole. Scatter the matzo meal over the top. Dot with the butter.

2 Bake in the preheated oven, covered, for 1 hour. Uncover and bake another hour.

<C **To Cut Carb**
<C Sweet potatoes: reduce to 1 1/2 lb.   <C Orange juice: reduce to 1/3 cup.
<C Large carrots: reduce to one only.   <C Matzo meal: reduce to 2 Tbsp.
<C Prunes: reduce to 10.

Per serving: 275 calories, 4 g fat, 1 g saturated fat, 3% calories from saturated fat, 58 g carbohydrate, 6 g dietary fiber, 268 mg sodium
Exchanges: 2 Starch, 1 Vegetable, 1 1/2 Fruit, 1/2 Fat

Low Carb
Per serving: 189 calories, 4 g fat, 1 g saturated fat, 4% calories from saturated fat, 37 g carbohydrate, 4 g dietary fiber, 258 mg sodium
Exchanges: 1 1/2 Starch, 1 Vegetable, 1/2 Fruit, 1/2 Fat

Kheema: Minced Lamb Curry

SERVING SIZE: 1/4 of recipe, SERVES: 4

2 tsp non-aromatic olive oil
<C   2 onions, roughly chopped
      (3 cups)
6 cloves chopped garlic
2 tsp grated ginger
1 tsp ground cumin
1/4 tsp ground red pepper
1/4 tsp turmeric
1 tsp ground coriander
1/2 tsp salt
12 oz lean lamb, ground in a
    food processor
2 carrots, peeled and thinly
    sliced (1 cup)

<C 3 medium unpeeled red potatoes,
    cut in 1-inch pieces
4 Roma tomatoes, cored and
    chopped (2 cups)
1 serrano chile, seeded and
    chopped
2 Tbsp lemon juice
<C 1 cup frozen peas, thawed
1 Tbsp arrowroot mixed with
2 Tbsp water (slurry)
1 tsp garam masala (see box)
1 Tbsp chopped fresh cilantro
1 Tbsp chopped fresh spearmint

Vegetarian Option

To make this recipe without meat, follow the directions in step 1 but leave the onions in the pan. Add 1 cup lentils, carrots, potatoes, 1 1/2 cups tomatoes, chile, and 2 cups vegetable stock. Bring to a boil, reduce heat, and cook 35–40 minutes or until lentils and vegetables are tender. Follow steps 3 and 4.

---

1 Heat 1 tsp oil in a high-sided skillet. Sauté onions for 3 minutes, add garlic, ginger, cumin, red pepper, turmeric, coriander, and salt. Cook until onions are soft and golden, 5 minutes. Put in a bowl.

2 Without washing the pan, heat remaining oil. Crumble lamb into hot pan, and brown on one side 3 minutes without stirring. Stir in carrots, potatoes, 1 1/2 cups tomatoes, chile, and sautéed onions. Cover, and simmer 30 minutes.

3 Add lemon juice, peas, and 1 cup water. When boiling, stir in the slurry. Add garam masala to taste.

4 Serve in preheated bowls with remaining tomatoes and herbs on top.

<C **To Cut Carb**

<C Onions: reduce to 2 cups.

<C Potatoes: replace with 1/2 cup lentils.

<C Peas: reduce to 1/4 cup, as a garnish.

Garam Masala

1/2 tsp whole allspice

1/2 tsp whole cloves

1-inch cinnamon stick

1/4 tsp ground nutmeg

Grind all ingredients together in a designated coffee grinder.

Per serving: 351 calories, 8 g fat, 2 g saturated fat, 5% calories from saturated fat, 46 g carbohydrate, 9 g dietary fiber, 415 mg sodium
Exchanges: 1 1/2 Starch, 2 Lean Meat, 4 Vegetable, 1/2 Fat

Low Carb
Per serving: 311 calories, 8 g fat, 2 g saturated fat, 5% calories from saturated fat, 34 g carbohydrate, 10 g dietary fiber, 385 mg sodium
Exchanges: 1 Starch, 2 Lean Meat, 4 Vegetable, 1/2 Fat

Vegetarian
Per serving: 375 calories, 4 g fat, 0 g saturated fat, 0% calories from saturated fat, 72 g carbohydrate, 18 g dietary fiber, 538 mg sodium
Exchanges: 3 1/2 Starch, 4 Vegetables

Vegetable Burritos

SERVING SIZE: 1/4 of recipe, SERVES: 4

1 tsp olive oil

1 sweet onion (2 cups)

3 cloves garlic

1 red bell pepper (1 1/2 cups)

2 cups sliced mushrooms

1 (15 oz) can no-sodium-added black beans

<C 4 flour tortillas

1/2 cup chopped cilantro

(Continued)

1 | Preheat the oven to 350°F. Heat the oil in a high-sided skillet. Fry the onions until soft and just slightly golden, about 5 minutes. Add the garlic, bell pepper, and mushrooms and cook until the vegetables are tender, about 5 minutes. Stir in the black beans with a little of their liquid and heat through.

2 | Heat the tortillas in a paper bag in the microwave about 1 minute. Lay the warm tortillas on the counter and divide the filling among them. Roll, turning in the sides, into a neat package. Lay in a baking dish covered lightly with aluminum foil and warm through in the oven, 10 minutes (20–30 minutes if they have been made earlier and chilled).

<c **To Cut Carb**

<c Tortillas: delete. It's hard to imagine a burrito without its tortilla wrapping, but getting rid of it is really the only way to bring the dish into line. You could try a couple of Wonton Wrappers—if that doesn't cause too much cultural confusion!

Per serving: 247 calories, 4 g fat, 1 g saturated fat, 3% calories from saturated fat, 44 g carbohydrate, 9 g dietary fiber, 162 mg sodium
Exchanges: 2 Starch, 3 Vegetable, 1/2 Fat

Low Carb
Per serving: 150 calories, 2 g fat, 0 g saturated fat, 0% calories from saturated fat, 28 g carbohydrate, 8 g dietary fiber, 19 mg sodium
Exchanges: 1 Starch, 3 Vegetable

Red, Yellow, and Green Pasta

SERVING SIZE: <c 1/4 of recipe, SERVES: 4

8 oz orzo or other small pasta shape
1 tsp extra virgin olive oil
1 cup chopped onion
2 cloves garlic, bashed and
   chopped
1 red bell pepper, chopped
1 yellow bell pepper, chopped

4 cups chopped fresh spinach or
   1 (10 oz) package frozen chopped
   spinach, thawed and squeezed dry
1/4 tsp salt
1/4 tsp black pepper
1/4 cup grated Parmesan cheese

1 | Cook the pasta according to package directions, drain, and cool under cold water. Set aside.

2 Heat the oil in a high-sided skillet large enough to hold the whole dish, on medium high. Sauté the onion 2 minutes; add the garlic and cook 1 minute longer. Toss in the red and yellow peppers and cook until tender, 3–5 minutes.

3 Add the fresh spinach just to wilt or in the case of the thawed spinach, to heat through. Stir in the reserved pasta and the salt and pepper. Scatter cheese over each serving.

<c To Cut Carb

<c Serving size: simply cut in half and serve as a side dish.

Per serving: 283 calories, 4 g fat, 1 g saturated fat, 3% calories from saturated fat, 51 g carbohydrate, 4 g dietary fiber, 144 mg sodium, 11 g protein
Exchanges: 2 1/2 Starch, 3 Vegetable, 1/2 Fat

Low Carb
Per serving: 142 calories, 2 g fat, 0 g saturated fat, 0% calories from saturated fat, 25 g carbohydrate, 2 g dietary fiber, 72 mg sodium, 5 g protein
Exchanges: 1 1/2 Starch, 1 Vegetable

Broiled Salmon with Beans

SERVING SIZE: 1 fillet, SERVES: 4

4 (4 oz) salmon fillets   2 tsp winter savory
<c 2 (15 oz) cans white navy beans

1 Preheat broiler. Drain and rinse beans. Add winter savory to the beans and pour into a flameproof dish. Heat the beans and then place the salmon fillets on top of the beans. Broil for 6 to 8 minutes.

<c To Cut Carb

<c White Navy Beans: reduce to 1 can.
+> Serve with your favorite green leaf vegetable.

Per serving: 397 calories, 11 g fat, 2 g saturated fat, 4% calories from saturated fat, 369 mg sodium, 38 g carb, 9 g dietary fiber, 37 g protein, 77 mg cholesterol
Exchanges: 2 1/2 Starch, 4 Lean Meat

Low Carb
Per serving: 294 calories, 10 g fat, 2 g saturated fat, 5% calories from saturated fat, 213 mg sodium, 19 g carbohydrate, 5 g dietary fiber, 30 g protein, 77 mg cholesterol
Exchanges: 1 Starch, 4 Lean Meat

Chicken A La King

SERVING SIZE: 1/6 of recipe, SERVES: 6

Chicken

1 whole frying chicken, about 3 1/2 lb
8 cups water or to cover chicken
   Bouquet garni (page 467)
3 cups chicken broth (from cooked chicken)

1/2 cup wild rice
1/2 cup long-grain white rice
1/4 tsp salt

Sauce

3 cups chicken broth
  (from cooked chicken)
1 large red bell pepper, chopped
  into 1-inch dice
12 medium mushrooms, quartered
1/8 tsp ground nutmeg
1/4 tsp salt
1/4 tsp pepper

1/8 tsp cayenne
3 Tbsp cornstarch mixed with
6 Tbsp water (slurry)
1 cup nonfat yogurt cheese
  (page 475)
  chopped parsley
  chopped fresh tarragon
  (optional)

1. Rinse the chicken and place in a large pan. Cover the chicken with water, and add the bouquet garni. Bring to a boil, and then simmer 1 hour or until tender. Skim off scum as it rises. Place the chicken on a plate, and strain the broth. Pour 3 cups of the de-fatted broth into a saucepan and 3 cups into a 10-inch chef's pan. Save leftover broth for other uses. When chicken cools, remove skin and bones. Pull the meat into bite-size pieces.

2. Bring broth in saucepan to a boil; add wild rice and salt. Cover and cook for 30 minutes. Add white rice, and continue cooking 15 minutes or until tender.

3. Bring broth in chef's pan to a boil, and reduce to 2 cups, about 10 minutes. Add peppers, mushrooms, nutmeg, salt, pepper, and cayenne, and simmer 2 minutes. Add the chicken. Stir in the slurry, and boil 30 seconds to cook the cornstarch. Place the yogurt cheese in a bowl. Stir 1 cup of the thickened sauce into the yogurt, to temper; then stir yogurt into sauce. Pour into the chicken mixture.

4. Serve with a 3/4-cup mound of rice and steamed snow peas or sugar snaps. Garnish with parsley or tarragon.

Per serving: 336 calories, 6 g fat, 2 g saturated fat, 4% calories from saturated fat, 34 g carbohydrate, 2 g dietary fiber, 387 mg sodium
Exchanges: 2 Starch, 4 Very Lean Meat, 1 Vegetable, 1/2 Fat

Petite Coq au Vin

SERVING SIZE: 1/6 of recipe, SERVES: 6

1/2 tsp olive oil
2 Rock Cornish game hens (24 oz each), cut in half
10 oz pearl onions, peeled
3 oz Canadian bacon, cut in 1/2-inch pieces
2 medium turnips, peeled and cut in 1-inch pieces
12 medium mushrooms, whole
1 lb tiny new potatoes, whole with skin
1/2 tsp dried thyme

1/4 tsp salt
1/4 tsp pepper
3 bay leaves
1 1/2 cups low-sodium canned or homemade chicken stock (page 463)
1 1/2 cups nonalcoholic red wine
2 Tbsp arrowroot mixed with 4 Tbsp water (slurry)
1 lb spinach leaves, washed and stemmed
2 Tbsp chopped fresh parsley

1 Preheat the oven to 350°F. Heat the oil in a 10 1/2-inch chef's pan on medium. Brown the hens skin side down, turning once, about 5 minutes (it will be a tight squeeze). Remove from the pan and set aside.

2 Place the onions, Canadian bacon, turnips, mushrooms, potatoes, and thyme into the pan and cook, stirring, 2 or 3 minutes. Add the salt, pepper, bay leaves and pour in the stock and wine. Return the browned hens to the pan, cover, and bring to a boil. Bake in the preheated oven for 40 minutes.

3 Remove the chicken to a plate to cool slightly, before removing the skin and bones. Leave the flesh in the largest pieces possible. Discard the skin, bones, and bay leaves. Carefully strain the liquid into a fat strainer then pour back into the pan (through a sieve) without the fat. Bring to a boil and let it boil, uncovered, 10 minutes to reduce the liquid and finish the vegetables.

4 Stir in the slurry and return the cooked chicken. Place a handful of raw spinach leaves into each of 6 bowls and ladle the stew over the top. Sprinkle parsley on each serving.

Per serving: 316 calories, 7 g fat, 2 g saturated fat, 6% calories from saturated fat, 31 g carbohydrate, 9 g dietary fiber, 707 mg sodium, 32 g protein
Exchanges: 1 Starch, 3 Lean Meat, 3 Vegetable

Chicken Enchiladas

SERVING SIZE: 1/4 of recipe, SERVES: 4

Sauce

1/2 tsp non-aromatic olive oil
1/2 cup roughly chopped onions
  1 clove garlic, bashed and chopped
  1 jalapeño chili, seeded and chopped
1/4 tsp cayenne pepper, (optional)
  1 tsp ground cumin

  1 lb Roma tomatoes, peeled and
    roughly chopped
  1 (10 3/4 oz) can tomato puree
  1 tsp dried oregano
1 1/2 cups low-sodium chicken stock

Filling

8 oz boned, skin-on chicken breast
  1 cup low-sodium chicken stock
    (page 463)
1/2 cup low-fat cottage cheese
1/4 cup low-fat yogurt
  2 Tbsp chopped cilantro
  2 tsp cornstarch

  4 whole canned mild green chilies,
    cut in 1/2-inch strips
1/4 cup finely chopped onion
  8 5-inch flour tortillas
    (cut larger ones to size)
1/2 cup low-fat Monterey
    jack cheese

Vegetarian Enchiladas

1 cup low-sodium vegetable stock
2 Tbsp canned or homemade vegetarian refried beans

Replace chicken stock with low-sodium vegetable broth. Instead of chicken, spread refried beans on the cottage cheese mixture and make enchiladas as shown.

---

1 Preheat oven to 350°F. Heat oil in a pan, sauté onion 2 minutes. Add garlic, jalapeño, cayenne, and cumin, and cook 2 minutes. Stir in tomatoes, tomato puree, and oregano. Whip in blender or processor, return to pan, and add chicken stock. Bring to a boil; then simmer 20 minutes.

2 Place chicken breast, skin side up, in small skillet. Add stock and cover with a piece of waxed paper cut to size. Bring to a boil, reduce heat, and poach gently 20 minutes. Cool, remove skin, and cut across the grain in thin slices. It may still be a little pink but will finish cooking with the enchiladas.

3 Blend or process cottage cheese until smooth. Add yogurt, cilantro, and cornstarch and pulse to mix.

4 Spoon a little sauce into a 9-inch × 13-inch baking dish. Dip a tortilla in the sauce and lay on a plate. Spread a tablespoon of the cottage cheese mixture down the center. Lay pieces of chicken and green chilies on top and sprinkle with onion. Roll and lay in the baking dish. Repeat for all tortillas. Cover with remaining sauce, scatter cheese on top, and bake 20 minutes or until heated through.

Per serving: 361 calories, 9 g fat, 3 g saturated fat, 7% calories from saturated fat, 45 g carbohydrate, 6 g dietary fiber, 970 mg sodium
Exchanges: 2 Starch, 2 Lean Meat, 3 Vegetable, 1/2 Fat

Vegetarian
Per serving: 236 calories, 6 g fat, 3 g saturated fat, 9% calories from saturated fat, 33 g carbohydrates, 5 g fiber, 869 mg sodium
Exchanges: 1 Starch, 3 Vegetables, 1 Lean Meat, 1/2 Fat

Great Northern Bean and Salmon Bake

SERVING SIZE: 1/4 of recipe, SERVES: 4

2 cups canned Great Northern beans, drained and rinsed
1 tsp dried or 1 Tbsp fresh savory
2 cloves garlic, bashed and chopped

4 (5 oz) skinless salmon fillets
1/4 tsp salt
1/4 tsp freshly ground pepper

1 Preheat the oven to 450°F. Combine the beans with the savory and garlic. Coat a 9-inch × 13-inch baking pan with pan spray. Spoon 4 mounds of beans into the baking dish. Season the salmon with the salt and lay a fillet on top of each mound of beans. Spray lightly with olive oil pan spray.

2 Bake for 10 minutes or until the salmon flakes with a fork. Top with a few grinds of black pepper and serve.

Per serving: 276 calories, 9 g fat, 1 g saturated fat, 3% calories from saturated fat, 18 g carbohydrate, 6 g dietary fiber, 698 mg sodium, 31 g protein
Exchanges: 1 Starch, 4 Lean Meat

Pacific Paella

SERVING SIZE: 1/6 of recipe, SERVES: 6

2 chicken thighs
1 1/2 tsp reserved chicken fat
1/2 lb tuna cut in 1-inch cubes <C
1/2 lb medium shrimp, peeled and deveined
1 onion, finely diced
1 clove garlic, bashed and chopped
1 jalapeño pepper, seeded and chopped (leave the seeds in if you like it hot)
1 1/2 cups frozen or canned corn niblets

1 red bell pepper, seeded and cut in 1-inch pieces
1 cup medium grain rice
1/8 tsp pepper
1/2 tsp salt
1/8 tsp saffron threads
2 cups canned or homemade low-sodium chicken stock (page 463)
1 1/2 lbs Roma tomatoes, peeled, seeded and cut in 1-inch pieces
1 recipe Graham's coconut cream (page 465)
6 Tbsp chopped cilantro (optional)

1 Heat a chef's pan or high-sided skillet on medium high. Drop the chicken in, skin side down, and cook 7 minutes, turning several times to cook through. Remove to a plate and cover. Drain off the accumulated fat and put 1 tsp back into the hot pan. Cook the tuna and shrimp 2 minutes. Tip onto the plate with the chicken.

2 Pour 1/2 tsp of the accumulated chicken fat into the hot pan still on medium high. Sauté the onion, garlic, and jalapeno chili, 3 minutes or until the onion wilts. Add the corn and cook, stirring to caramelize the corn, 2 minutes. Stir in the bell pepper and rice. Season with 1/4 tsp salt, 1/8 tsp pepper and 1/8 tsp saffron. Pour in the stock, bring to a boil, cover, and reduce the heat to medium. Cook 20 minutes, shaking once or twice.

3 Remove and discard the skin and bones from the chicken and add the meat, fish, and tomatoes to the rice. Stir in the coconut cream. Heat through and serve from the pan or tip into a 3 quart bowl and pat down. Top with a large serving platter and turn up side down to mold. Scatter the cilantro over the molded rice and serve in wedges.

<C To Cut Carb

<C Rice: replace with 1/2 cup brown rice, cook for 35 minutes at step 2.

Per serving: 346 calories, 8 g fat, 3 g saturated fat, 8% calories from saturated fat, 47 g carbohydrate, 4 g dietary fiber, 347 mg sodium
Exchanges: 2 1/2 Starch, 2 Lean Meat, 2 Vegetable

Low Carb
Per serving: 296 calories, 8 g fat, 3 g saturated fat, 9% calories from saturated fat, 33 g carbohydrate, 4 g dietary fiber, 347 mg sodium
Exchanges: 1 1/2 Starch, 2 Lean Meat, 2 Vegetable

Lentil and Rice Pilaf

SERVING SIZE: 1/4 of recipe, SERVES: 4

1 Tbsp extra virgin olive oil	<C 1/2 cup long-grain white rice
<C 2 large onions, peeled and sliced	1/4 tsp salt
4 cups low-sodium chicken or vegetable broth	1/4 tsp pepper
<C 1 cup lentils, washed	2 Tbsp chopped cilantro

1 Heat broth in saucepan. Add lentils, and simmer 20 minutes.

2 While lentils are cooking, heat oil in large high-sided skillet on medium high. Fry onions until golden brown. Take half the onions out of the pan, and set aside.

3 Add remaining onions, rice, salt, and pepper to lentils. Cover, and bring to a boil. Reduce heat, and cook slowly about 20 minutes or until lentils and rice are tender.

4 Serve in a bowl topped with reserved onions and chopped cilantro.

<C To Cut Carb

<C Onions: reduce to 1 only.
<C Lentils: reduce to 1/2 cup.
<C Celery: add 1 cup (chopped) at step 3.

<C Rice: reduce to 1/4 cup brown rice and simmer 35 minutes. You may need 1/2 cup extra stock.

Per serving: 334 calories, 6 g fat, 1 g saturated fat, 3% calories from saturated fat, 55 carbohydrate, 12 g dietary fiber, 265 mg sodium
Exchanges: 3 Starch, 2 Vegetable, 1 Fat

Low Carb
Per serving: 208 calories, 6 g fat, 1 g saturated fat, 4% calories from saturated fat, 29 g carbohydrate, 7 g dietary fiber, 303 mg sodium
Exchanges: 1 1/2 Starch, 2 Vegetable, 1 Fat

Pasta with Mushrooms, Ham, and Peas

SERVING SIZE: 1/4 of recipe, SERVES: 4

<C 1/2 lb dry butterfly (or another shape you like) pasta
1 tsp non-aromatic olive oil
1/2 cup chopped onions
1/4 lb lean smoky ham, cut in 1/2-inch cubes
+> 1/2 lb cremini or white button mushrooms, quartered

<C 2 cups thawed petit peas
1/4 tsp salt
1/4 tsp pepper
1 tsp arrowroot or cornstarch
1/2 cup chicken broth
1/4 cup grated Parmesan cheese

1 Cook the pasta according to package directions. Drain and keep warm in a covered colander over hot water.

2 While the pasta is cooking, heat the oil in a high-sided skillet on medium-high. Cook the onion, without browning, until it starts to wilt and turn translucent. Stir in the ham and mushrooms and cook until the mushrooms are done, about 5 minutes.

3 Add the peas and reserved pasta and cook, stirring, just until heated through. Season with salt and pepper. Combine the arrowroot with the broth and pour into the hot pasta. Stir until it thickens and gets glossy. Divide among 4 hot plates, sprinkle with Parmesan, and serve with a nice green salad.

<C **To Cut Carb**
<C Pasta: reduce to 1 oz per serving.   +> Mushrooms: increase to 3/4 lb.
<C Pears: reduce to 1 1/2 cups.

Per serving: 379 calories, 6 g fat, 2 g saturated fat, 5% calories from saturated fat, 59 g carbohydrate, 7 g dietary fiber, 720 mg sodium
Exchanges: 3 1/2 Starch, 1 Lean Meat, 1 Vegetable, 1/2 Fat

Low Carb
Per serving: 264 calories, 6 g fat, 2 g saturated fat, 7% calories from saturated fat, 36 g carbohydrate, 5 g dietary fiber, 705 mg sodium
Exchanges: 2 Starch, 1 Lean Meat, 1 Vegetable, 1/2 Fat

Vegetable Beef Stew with Radishes

SERVING SIZE: 1/4 of recipe, SERVES: 4

1/2 lb lean beef, cut in 1-inch chunks
1 1/2 tsp non-aromatic olive oil
1 cup chopped onions
2 cloves garlic, bashed and chopped
3 Tbsp tomato paste
3 cups low-sodium beef stock (page 466)
4 medium carrots, peeled and cut in 1-inch chunks

<C 8 small new potatoes, cut in half
12 radishes, scrubbed and trimmed (or 3 turnips, peeled and cut in quarters)
<C 1 cup frozen peas
2 Tbsp cornstarch or arrowroot mixed with 1/4 cup broth or water (slurry)
1/4 tsp salt
1/4 tsp pepper
2 Tbsp chopped fresh parsley

1 Pat the meat dry with paper towels. Heat 1 tsp of the oil in a large high-sided skillet over medium-high heat and brown the meat on one side, about 3 minutes. Remove the meat and set aside.

2 Heat the remaining oil in the same skillet and cook the onions 2 minutes. Add the garlic and tomato paste and cook, stirring often, until the tomato paste darkens. Return the meat to the pan and pour in the broth. Cover, bring to a boil, reduce the heat, and simmer 30 minutes or until the meat is almost tender.

3 Add the carrots, potatoes, and radishes and cook 20 minutes or until tender. Stir in the peas, slurry, salt, and pepper and heat until thick and glossy. Garnish with parsley and serve.

<C **To Cut Carb**

<C New Potatoes: reduce to 4.   <C Pears: reduce to 1/2 cup.

Per serving: 281 calories, 5 g fat, 1 g saturated fat, 4% calories from saturated fat, 44 g carbohydrate, 8 g dietary fiber, 331 mg sodium, 17 g protein
Exchanges: 2 Starch, 1 Lean Meat, 3 Vegetable

Low Carb

Per serving: 223 calories, 5 g fat, 1 g saturated fat, 3% calories from saturated fat, 31 g carbohydrate, 6 g dietary fiber, 312 mg sodium, 15 g protein
Exchanges: 1 Starch, 1 Lean Meat, 3 Vegetable

Pork Tenderloin with Tomato Garlic Sauce

SERVING SIZE: 1/4 of recipe, SERVES: 4

1 1/2 tsp olive oil
1 lb pork tenderloin, trimmed
2 red bell peppers, chopped
1/2 lb mushrooms, quartered
3 cloves garlic, peeled, bashed, and chopped
1/2 tsp dried thyme

1/2 tsp dried oregano
2 bay leaves
6 Tbsp tomato puree
1/2 cup nonalcoholic red wine
4 slices polenta, 1-inch thick
1 Tbsp arrowroot mixed with 2 Tbsp water (slurry)

Vegetarian Option

2 cups fresh or canned fava beans

Replace the pork tenderloin with the fava beans. Sauté the peppers and mushrooms in 1 tsp of the olive oil and continue to follow step 2. Stir in the beans with the thyme, oregano, and bay. Proceed through steps 3 and 4 ignoring the meat. Remove the polenta to hot plates, thicken the sauce with all the vegetables, and spoon over the polenta.

---

1 Preheat the oven to 350°F. Heat 1 tsp of the oil in a large high-sided skillet on medium high. Drop the tenderloin into the hot pan and brown on all sides, 4 minutes. Remove the meat to a plate and set aside.

2 Add the peppers, mushrooms, and garlic to the same pan and cook for 2 minutes. Add the thyme, oregano, and bay leaves. Stir in the tomato puree and keep stirring while it darkens in color, 2 minutes. Pour in the wine.

3 Replace the meat in the pan and cover with sauce and vegetables. Lay the polenta slices around the pan and spoon vegetables and sauce over them. Cover and bake in the preheated oven for 30 minutes.

4 Remove the meat, slice on the diagonal, and divide among 4 hot plates. Set a polenta slice on each plate. Stir the slurry into the sauce and heat until thick and glossy, less than 30 seconds. Spoon over the meat and polenta. A good serving of just steamed baby leaf spinach makes a great side dish.

Per serving: 269 calories, 8 g fat, 2 g saturated fat, 6% calories from saturated fat, 20 g carbohydrate, 4 g dietary fiber, 247 mg sodium, 29 g protein
Exchanges: 1 Starch, 3 Lean Meat, 1 Vegetable

Vegetarian
Per serving: 213 calories, 4 g fat, 1 g saturated fat, 4% calories from saturated fat, 36 g carbohydrate, 8 g dietary fiber, 369 mg sodium
Exchanges: 2 Starch, 1 Lean Meat

Roasted Eggplant and Red Pepper Sandwich

SERVING SIZE: 1 sandwich, SERVES: 4

<C 8 slices French or Italian bread, toasted
  2 cloves garlic, peeled and cut in half
  1 medium eggplant, cut in
     1/2-inch slices

1/4 tsp salt
1/4 tsp pepper
  1 cup roasted red pepper, cut
     in strips

1 Preheat the broiler. Lay the bread on the broiler pan, spray with extra virgin olive oil spray, and toast lightly on both sides. Rub the top of each with the garlic and set aside.

2 Reduce the oven heat to 450°F. Lay the eggplant slices on a greased baking sheet and coat lightly with olive oil pan spray. Season with salt and pepper. Roast 20 minutes or until tender and caramelized.

3 Cover each slice of bread with the roasted eggplant and lay the red pepper strips over the top. Give each one a quick spray of extra virgin olive oil and serve.

<C To Cut Carb
<C French or Italian bread: reduce to one slice per serving. It should be loaded!

Per serving: 171 calories, 0 g fat, 0 g saturated fat, 0% calories from saturated fat, 36 g carbohydrate, 4 g dietary fiber, 546 mg sodium
Exchanges: 2 Starch, 1 Vegetable

Low Carb
Per serving: 103 calories, 0 g fat, 0 g saturated fat, 0% calories from saturated fat, 22 g carbohydrate, 3 g dietary fiber, 395 mg sodium
Exchanges: 1 Starch, 1 Vegetable

Minestrone

SERVING SIZE: 1/6 of recipe, SERVES: 6

Basil Pesto

2 Tbsp chopped fresh basil leaves

2 Tbsp pine nuts

1 clove garlic, bashed and chopped

1 Tbsp Pecorino Romano cheese

Soup

    1 tsp non-aromatic olive oil

    1 medium onion, chopped in 1/2-inch pieces

    3 ribs celery, chopped in 1/2-inch pieces

    4 carrots, peeled and chopped in 1/2-inch pieces

\<C 1/2 lb red potatoes, chopped in 1/2-inch pieces

    7 cups hot water

 1 1/2 tsp salt

\<C 1/4 lb small shell pasta

\<C 1 (15 oz) can cannellini or other white beans, rinsed and drained

    1 lb Roma tomatoes, peeled and diced or 1 (14.5 oz) can diced tomatoes in juice

    1 bunch spinach, washed, stemmed and cut into 1/4-inch × 1-inch pieces

    1 tsp extra virgin olive oil

    6 Tbsp grated Pecorino Romano cheese

    6 leaves fresh basil, finely sliced

Parsley Pesto

If fresh basil is hard to find, try this fresh parsley pesto made with dried basil.

  2 Tbsp chopped fresh parsley

  1 Tbsp dried basil

1/8 tsp extra virgin olive oil

2 Tbsp pine nuts or walnuts

1 clove garlic, bashed and chopped

1 Tbsp grated Pecorino Romano cheese

Combine parsley, basil, olive oil, nuts, garlic, and cheese in a small processor and whiz to a paste.

Place the basil, pine nuts, garlic, and cheese in a small processor and whiz to a paste. Scrape into a small bowl, spray the top with olive oil and lay a small piece of plastic wrap directly on top of the pesto to keep it from turning black.

2 Heat the oil in a high-sided skillet or small Dutch oven. Sauté the onion on medium high until it starts to get soft, about 2 minutes. Add the celery, carrots, and potatoes and continue cooking 3 minutes. Pour in the hot water, cover, and bring to a boil. Stir in the salt and pasta and boil, uncovered, 6 minutes.

3 Add the pesto, beans, tomatoes, spinach, and extra virgin olive oil. Bring back to a boil and it's ready to serve. Sprinkle grated cheese and chopped basil on each serving.

<C **To Cut Carb**

<C Red potatoes: delete completely. <C Beans: reduce to 10 oz total.
<C Pasta: reduce to 2 oz raw weight.

Per serving: 287 calories, 7 g fat, 2 g saturated fat, 6 % calories from saturated fat, 46 g carbohydrate, 9 g dietary fiber, 818 mg sodium
Exchanges: 2 Starch, 3 Vegetable, 1 Fat

Low Carb
Per serving: 220 calories, 6 g fat, 2 g saturated fat, 8% calories from saturated fat, 32 g carbohydrate, 8 g dietary fiber, 818 mg sodium
Exchanges: 1 Starch, 3 Vegetable, 1 Fat

Stuffed Mild Chilis

SERVING SIZE: 1 chili, SERVES: 2

2 mild chili peppers such as poblano or Anaheim	2 cups chopped Swiss chard or spinach
1/2 tsp olive oil	1/2 cup low-sodium salsa
1/2 cup chopped onion	1/3 cup reduced fat Monterey jack cheese
1/4 tsp cumin	
1 clove garlic, chopped	1 Tbsp grated Parmesan cheese
1/2 cup fresh or frozen corn kernels	2 Tbsp breadcrumbs

1 Preheat the oven to 375°F. Cut the chilis in half lengthwise and remove the seeds and content.

2 Heat the oil in a skillet and sauté the onions with the cumin until soft and translucent but not brown, 5 minutes. Add the garlic and cook 1 minute more. Stir in the corn, Swiss chard, and salsa. Stir in the reduced fat Monterey jack cheese off the heat.

(Continued)

3 Combine the Parmesan cheese and breadcrumbs. Divide the filling among the chilis and top with the Parmesan bread mixture. Bake on a greased baking sheet 20 minutes or until the vegetables are tender and the top golden.

Per serving: 216 calories, 7 g fat, 3 g saturated fat, 14% calories from saturated fat, 30 g carbohydrate, 4 g dietary fiber, 263 mg sodium
Exchanges: 1 Starch, 1 Medium Fat Meat, 3 Vegetable

Duck Breasts in Plum Sauce

SERVING SIZE: 1/6 recipe, SERVES: 6

6 boned duck breasts or 3 whole ducks, about 4 lb each

Marinade

1/2 tsp light olive oil
  3 cloves garlic, peeled, bashed, and chopped
1/2 cup dry white wine (I prefer nonalcoholic chardonnay)

1/2 cup fresh orange juice
1/8 tsp salt
1/8 tsp freshly ground black pepper

Plum Sauce

1/2 tsp light olive oil
3/4 cup sliced onion
  6 red plums, quartered and pitted
  1 tsp dried oregano

1/3 cup dry red wine (I prefer nonalcoholic cabernet sauvignon)
<C 1 Tbsp brown sugar
1/2 cup fresh orange juice

1 If you start with whole ducks, see carving instructions.

2 Lay duck breasts skin side down in a glass baking dish.

3 Warm oil in small saucepan. Sauté garlic for 1 minute, then stir in white wine, orange juice, salt, and pepper. Bring mixture to a boil, then simmer gently for 20 minutes.

4 Strain marinade through a sieve, and pour into a flavor injector. Inject as much marinade as possible into each breast. Set aside leftover marinade

to use in the sauce. If you don't have a flavor injector, pour marinade over the breasts, cover, and refrigerate for at least 8 hours.

5   Warm oil in large saucepan. Sauté onion until soft and lightly brown, about 6 minutes. Add plums, oregano, red wine, and sugar. Cover and bring to a boil, then simmer for 25 minutes.

6   Strain sauce through a sieve over a saucepan, discarding the pulp. Stir in orange juice.

7   Heat large frying pan over medium-high heat. Dry breasts, and lay them in the pan, skin side down. (I leave skin on the breasts to preserve moisture and make the meat tender. The fat will be drained before serving.) Sprinkle meat with salt and pepper. Brown for 2 minutes to render some fat into the pan. Turn the breasts, and cook 2 minutes. Turn back on the skin side for 4 minutes.

8   Transfer the breasts to a plate, and remove the skin, being careful to save juices that drain onto the plate. Return breasts to frying pan and brown the skinned side, then remove to a warmed plate and cover.

9   Pour fat out of the frying pan, but do not clean it. Add remaining marinade to pan with reserved duck juices and bring to a boil, scraping flavorful bits from the bottom with a wooden spoon. Remove from heat, and strain through a sieve into the pan with the plum sauce. Stir, then pour sauce into large frying pan.

10   Add the duck breasts to the sauce, and warm over medium heat. Remove as soon as they are heated through, and carve in thin diagonal slices across the grain.

11   Spoon a puddle of hot plum sauce onto a warmed plate, and arrange a few slices of duck on top of the sauce. Serve with a scoop of Celery Root and Potato Purée (page 243) and a serving of Mesclun Salad with Fruit (page 181).

<C **To Cut Carb**

<C Brown sugar: reduce to 1 tsp and add 2 tsp Splenda.

Per serving: 229 calories, 8 g fat, 2 g saturated fat, 8% calories from saturated fat, 14 g carbohydrate, 1 g dietary fiber, 143 mg sodium
Exchanges: 3 Lean Meat, 1 Fruit

Low Carb
Per serving: 224 calories, 8 g fat, 2 g saturated fat, 8% calories from saturated fat, 13 g carbohydrate, 1 g dietary fiber, 142 mg sodium
Exchanges:3 Lean Meat, 1 Fruit

Rabbit Pie

SERVING SIZE: 1 piece, SERVES: 8

Filling

2 fennel bulbs, trimmed and cut in thick slices
1 Tbsp freshly squeezed lemon juice
1/2 lb medium mushrooms, halved
2 tsp dried mushroom powder
1 1/2 tsp non-aromatic olive oil, divided
1/2 cup flour
1/4 tsp salt
1/4 tsp pepper

1 rabbit, cut into pieces
1 onion, cut in 1/4-inch dice (2 cups)
3 cloves garlic, bashed and chopped
2 carrots, peeled and cut on the diagonal in 1/2-inch pieces (1 1/2 cups)
2 ribs celery, cut in 1/2-inch slices (generous cup)
2 Tbsp tomato paste
2 cups nonalcoholic red wine

Tie the next 4 herbs in cheesecloth or place in an herb ball:

8 big fresh sage leaves or 2 Tbsp powdered sage
4 4-inch sprigs rosemary or 1 Tbsp dried

1/4 tsp salt
1/4 tsp pepper

Pie Crust

1 recipe Graham's Basic Pie Crust (see page 479)

1. Steam the fennel slices for 10 minutes. Preheat oven to 350°F. Lay the slices of steamed fennel in the bottom of a greased 9-inch × 13-inch baking dish or large oval baker. Heat the oil in a skillet on medium high. Pour the lemon juice into the hot pan and add the mushrooms. Cook until browned and tender, stirring often. Stir in the mushroom powder and scatter over the fennel in the baking dish.

2. Reheat the pan on medium and add 1 tsp of the oil. Combine the flour, salt, and pepper in a bag. Shake the rabbit pieces in the flour until covered and tap off excess. Brown on both sides in the hot pan. Remove to a plate and set aside.

3. Sauté the onions in the same pan for 2 minutes then add the garlic, carrots, and celery and cook 2 or 3 minutes more. Pull the vegetables to the side and add the tomato paste. Cook, mixing with the vegetables until the tomato paste darkens and coats all the vegetables. Pour in the wine and season with the salt, sage, and rosemary. Lay the browned rabbit on top, cover, and

bring to a boil. Place in the preheated oven and bake 30–40 minutes or until the rabbit is tender but not falling off the bone.

4 Remove the rabbit to a plate to cool a bit. Increase the oven heat to 425°F. Take the meat off the bones in large pieces and lay on top of the mushrooms in the baking dish. Pour the baking liquid and vegetables over the top. Roll out the piecrust to fit the pan. Pinch the crust around the edges and prick the center with a fork. Brush the tip with a little whole or 2% milk. Bake 15 or 20 minutes or until golden. Cut into 8 pieces and serve. Steamed broccoli and carrots would make up a really attractive plate.

Per serving: 355 calories, 13 g fat, 3 g saturated fat, 8% calories from saturated fat, 28 g carbohydrate, 2 g dietary fiber, 280 mg sodium, 32 g protein
Exchanges: 1/2 Starch, 3 Lean Meat, 4 Vegetable, 1 Fat

Spaghetti with a Secret

SERVING SIZE: 1/6 of recipe, SERVES: 6

<C 12 oz dry spaghetti
   2 cups steamed broccoli or carrots
     or 1 cup of each

4 cups of your favorite low-sodium
   spaghetti sauce
6 Tbsp grated Parmesan cheese

1 Cook the spaghetti according to package directions, drain, rinse with cold water, and set aside.

2 Whiz the steamed vegetables with the spaghetti sauce in a blender until the broccoli is no longer visible. Heat.

3 Toss the spaghetti with the sauce and heat through. Divide among 6 hot plates and scatter the cheese over the top.

<C **To Cut Carb** ══════════════════
<C Pasta: reduce to 6 oz dry spaghetti.

Per serving: 309 calories, 3 g fat, 1 g saturated fat, 3% calories from saturated fat, 59 g carbohydrate, 4 g dietary fiber, 99 mg sodium
Exchanges: 3 Starch, 3 Vegetable

Low Carb
Per serving: 203 calories, 2 g fat, 1 g saturated fat, 4% calories from saturated fat, 38 g carbohydrate, 3 g dietary fiber, 97 mg sodium
Exchanges: 1 1/2 Starch, 3 Vegetable, 1/2 Fat

Cannery Scallops Claudia

SERVING SIZE: 1/4 of recipe, SERVES: 4

Barley

1/2 tsp non-aromatic olive oil	1 Tbsp Thai fish sauce
1 heaped Tbsp chopped lemon grass	1/2 cup pearl barley
1 Tbsp chopped fresh ginger	1 cup corn kernels
1 1/2 cups water	2 Tbsp chopped fresh parsley

Seafood

1 1/2 tsp non-aromatic olive oil, divided	1/2 lb medium shrimp, peeled
1 stalk lemongrass, trimmed and finely sliced	8 medium sea scallops
1/4 cup finely chopped shallots	1/8 tsp cayenne pepper
1/4 cup chopped fresh basil, divided	1/8 tsp toasted sesame oil
1 kafir lime leaf, finely sliced, or 1 strip lime zest	1/2 tsp Thai fish sauce
1 lb mussels, scrubbed and bearded	2 tsp arrowroot with 1/4 cup nonalcoholic white wine (slurry)
1 cup nonalcoholic chardonnay	2 tsp freshly squeezed lime juice

1 Heat the oil in a saucepan on medium high. Add the lemon grass and ginger and cook 1 minute to release the flavors. Add the water and fish sauce and bring to a boil. Cover and set off the heat 4 minutes. Strain, add the barley, bring back to a boil, reduce the heat cover and simmer 20 minutes. Add the corn and cook 5 more minutes. Set aside and keep warm until ready to serve.

2 Heat 1/2 tsp of the oil in a large skillet or chef's pan on medium high. Add the lemongrass, shallots, 2 Tbsp of the basil, and the lime leaf or zest. Sauté 2 minutes to break out the flavors. Drop in the mussels and pour in the wine. Cover and cook 2 1/2 minutes or until the mussels open. Strain, reserving the liquid and place the mussels on a plate to cool. Remove the meats and set aside.

3 Add the cayenne, sesame oil and fish sauce to the liquid in the pan and simmer 10 minutes. Strain the liquid and reserve.

4 Reheat the pan. Add another 1/2 tsp oil. Drop the scallops into the pan to brown, about 2 minutes per side. Remove to a hot plate and cover to finish cooking. Heat the remaining oil. Add the shrimp and cook until the first one

turns pink, adding a little of the reserved liquid if the pan is too dry. Turn and cook 1 minute more. Pour in the remaining reserved liquid. Stir in the slurry and heat to thicken. Add the rest of the basil, reserved mussel meats and scallops. Add the lime juice to brighten the flavors.

5 Divide the barley and corn mixture among 4 hot plates. Arrange the seafood attractively on top and spoon just a little of the sauce over the shellfish. Scatter more chopped basil or parsley over the top. Lightly steamed sugar snap peas are a lovely addition to this dish.

Per serving: 399 calories, 7 g fat, 1 g saturated fat, 2% calories from saturated fat, 54 g carbohydrate, 4 g dietary fiber, 848 mg sodium
Exchanges: 3 1/2 Starch, 3 Very Lean Meat, 1/2 Fat

Spaghetti Squash

SERVING SIZE: 1/4 of recipe, SERVES: 4

1 spaghetti squash (3 cups)
2 cups prepared low-sodium spaghetti sauce
1 cup sliced mushrooms

2 Tbsp chopped parsley
2 Tbsp Parmesan cheese

1 Preheat the over to 400°F. Wash the outside of the squash and pierce it a few times with a fork. Set on a baking sheet and bake 1 hour or until very tender when tested with a fork. Cool.

2 Cut the cooked squash in half lengthwise and remove the seeds. Take the spaghetti-like threads out with a fork and place in a baking dish. Toss with the low-sodium spaghetti sauce and mushrooms. Cover lightly with aluminum foil. Return to the oven for 20–30 minutes or until well heated through.

3 Scatter with parsley and Parmesan cheese and serve with a piece of bread and a salad for a hearty meal. It also makes a very tasty side dish with fish or chicken.

Per serving: 125 calories, 4 g fat, 1 g saturated fat, 7% calories from saturated fat, 21 g carbohydrate, 4 g dietary fiber, 358 mg sodium
Exchanges: 4 Vegetable, 1/2 Fat

Palusamis

SERVING SIZE: 1/6 of recipe, SERVES: 6

Coconut Cream

3/4 cup plus 2 Tbsp 2% milk
1/2 tsp sugar
2 Tbsp desiccated coconut

1 Tbsp cornstarch
1/2 tsp coconut essence

Palusamis

6 taro roots or red potatoes, about 2 oz each
1/3 to 1/2 fresh pineapple, about 6 oz, peeled and cored
18 large collard leaves (2 bunches)
1 1/2 tsp light olive oil
6 oz Canadian bacon, cut into 1/4-inch × 2-inch julienne
2 green onions, white parts only, cut into 1/4-inch slices
2 Tbsp plus 1 1/2 tsp fresh lime juice
1/4 tsp dried crushed red pepper flakes
18 oz fresh tuna, cut into 6 pieces

Garnish

2 fresh tomatoes, cut into 12 thin slices

Vegetarian Option (per serving)

1/2 tsp light olive oil
1/2 plantain, peeled and sliced
1 oz pineapple, cut into 1/4-inch
  matchsticks
2 green onions, white parts only,
  cut into 1/4-inch (3/4-cm) slices
1 taro root, about 2 oz, peeled
  and boiled

1/4 tsp fresh lime juice
1/16 tsp salt
1/16 tsp chipotle sauce
3 collard leaves, trimmed
  and blanched
2 Tbsp coconut cream

Warm the oil in a large frying pan over medium-high heat. Add the
plantain, pineapple, onions, taro, salt, and chipotle sauce. Cook for
2 minutes, stirring to keep from burning. Pour the mixture into the
center of a collard leaf or leaves, sprinkle the lime juice over the top,
and add a dollop of the coconut cream. Wrap and tie as in steps 11-12.
Serve with the remaining coconut cream.

To Prepare the Coconut Cream

1 Combine the milk, sugar, and coconut in a small saucepan and simmer over medium heat for 10 minutes. Strain the coconut and return the liquid to the pan.

2 Combine the cornstarch with the remaining 2 Tbsp of milk to make a slurry. Add the slurry to the warm milk and stir over medium heat until it thickens. Add the coconut essence and pour the mixture into a flat metal pan. Put in the refrigerator to cool.

To Prepare the Filling

3 Place the taro roots in a large steamer, cover, and steam for 30 minutes, or until tender. Rinse under cold water until cool enough to handle, then peel with a paring knife. Cut the roots into 1/4-inch × 2-inch julienne.

4 Cut the fresh pineapple into julienne the same size as the taro root.

5 Cut out and discard the heavy stems from the collard leaves. Boil the leaves in a large pan of water for 1 minute, or until they are pliable but still a nice dark green. Drain and plunge into very cold water, then drain again and set aside.

6 Warm 1/2 tsp of the oil in a large frying pan over medium-high heat. Sauté the Canadian bacon and green onions for 1 minute and remove to a large bowl.

7 Heat another 1/2 tsp of oil in the same frying pan and add the taro strips. Spray lightly with cooking spray and sauté for 2 minutes. Sprinkle 2 Tbsp of the lime juice over the top and add the pineapple strips. Continue cooking for another minute.

8 Transfer the taro and pineapple to the bowl with the Canadian bacon. Stir to combine and sprinkle with the crushed pepper flakes and the remaining 1 1/2 tsp of lime juice.

9 Preheat the oven to 350°F.

(Continued)

10 Warm the frying pan over high heat and add the remaining 1/2 tsp of oil. Lay the tuna in the hot pan, dust with salt and pepper, and sear each side for 30 seconds. Remove to a plate.

To Assemble the Palusamis

11 Arrange the collard leaves, coconut cream, pineapple-taro filling, and tuna close at hand. You may have to play with the collard leaves a little to get them to wrap up into neat little packages. The trick I have found is to lay one leaf flat on the counter, its tip pointing at 12 o'clock. Lay 2 more leaves perpendicular to the first, their tips pointing to 3 o'clock and 9 o'clock and their bases meeting at the bottom of the first leaf. The leaves should form an upside-down T or three-pointed fan shape.

12 Spoon 1/4 cup of the filling onto the center of the leaf arrangement. Top with a piece of tuna, another 1/4 cup of filling, and 1 Tbsp of the chilled coconut cream. Fold the ends of the leaves over the filling into a little packet and secure with string. There is no set way to do this and a lot depends on the size of the collard leaves, so do what works for you. Repeat for the remaining 5 packages.

13 Lay the palusamis in a 9-inch × 13-inch baking dish. Cover loosely with foil and bake in the preheated oven for 20 minutes.

To Serve

14 Place one palusami on each warmed dinner plate. Remove the string and spoon some of the remaining coconut cream over the top. Garnish with two tomato slices and serve a scoop of Green Bean Rice Pilau (page 256) alongside.

Per serving: 327 calories, 8 g fat, 3 g saturated fat, 8% of calories from saturated fat, 34 g carbohydrate, 3 g dietary fiber, 30 g protein
Exchanges: 1 Starch, 3 Lean Meat, 2 Vegetable, 1/2 Fruit

Vegetarian
Per serving: 271 calories, 5 g fat, 2 g saturated fat, 6% of calories from saturated fat, 58 g carbohydrate, 7 g dietary fiber
Exchanges: 3 Starch, 1/2 Fruit, 1 Vegetable

Cottage Pie

SERVING SIZE: 1/6 recipe, SERVES: 6

3 cups canned or homemade low-sodium beef stock
1/4 cup bulgur wheat
1 tsp non-aromatic olive oil
12 oz extra lean (9%) ground beef
3 Tbsp tomato paste
<C 1 1/2 cups chopped onion
2 cloves garlic
<C 1 cup finely chopped carrots

1/4 cup finely chopped celery
1 tsp dried thyme
1 Tbsp Worcestershire sauce
1/4 tsp salt
4 tsp arrowroot or cornstarch mixed with 2 Tbsp beef stock (slurry)
<C 1 recipe mashed potatoes (page 210)
1 Tbsp chopped fresh parsley

1 Preheat oven to 350°F. Heat beef stock, and pour 2 cups over bulgur wheat. Set aside for at least 10 minutes to soften.

2 Heat a large skillet until very hot. Add 1/2 tsp oil, break the beef into small pieces, and add to the pan to brown. Mash the meat so it crumbles after it has browned. Reduce heat, stir in tomato paste, and cook until the paste turns dark red. Pour in the remaining cup of beef stock, and stir up flavorful bits on the bottom of the pan. Pour into a bowl.

3 Without washing the pan, heat remaining 1/2 tsp oil, and sauté onions. After 2 minutes, add garlic, carrots, celery, and thyme. Cook for 2 more minutes. Add Worcestershire sauce, bulgur with its stock, and cooked meat. Simmer 10 minutes, or until the carrots are tender. Stir in slurry to thicken.

4 Cover filling with mashed potatoes, one spoonful at a time. Make designs on top with a fork. Bake for 20 minutes to heat through. Broil for 2 to 3 minutes to brown the top. Sprinkle with parsley and cut into 6 wedges. A classic side dish would be peas with mint and a broiled tomato.

<C To Cut Carb

<C Onions: reduce to 1 cup.
<C Carrots: reduce to 3/4 cup.

<C Mashed potatoes: reduce to 1/4 cup.

Per serving: 265 calories, 7 g fat, 3 g saturated fat, 9% calories from saturated fat, 34 g carbohydrate, 5 g dietary fiber, 478 mg sodium
Exchanges: 1 1/2 Starch, 2 Lean Meat, 2 Vegetable

Low Carb
Per serving: 212 calories, 7 g fat, 3 g saturated fat, 9% calories from saturated fat, 22 g carbohydrate, 3 g dietary fiber, 404 mg sodium
Exchanges: 1 Starch, 2 Lean Meat, 1 Vegetable

Steamed Swiss Chard

SERVING SIZE: 1/4 of recipe, SERVES: 4

2 bunches Swiss chard
1 Tbsp balsamic vinegar or lemon juice

1 tsp extra virgin olive oil

1   Wash the chard leaves in a sink full of cold water. Cut the stems off and slice crosswise into 1/2-inch pieces. Cut the leaves, also crosswise into, 1/2-inch strips.

2   Toss the stems into a steamer and steam, covered, 2 minutes. Add the leaves and cook until tender, 4 to 6 minutes. Toss with the vinegar and oil and serve.

Per serving: 30 calories, 1 g fat, 0 g saturated fat, 0% calories from saturated fat, 4 g carbohydrate, 2 g dietary fiber, 157 mg sodium
Exchanges: 1 Vegetable

Ensenada Seafood Stew with Roasted Tomato Salsa

SERVING SIZE: 1/6 of recipe, SERVES: 6

Stew

  8 oz squid "steaks" free of cartilage and tentacles
12 small clams in the shell
12 oz large prawns
  6 oz orange roughy fillet
  2 tsp light olive oil
  1 large sweet onion, roughly chopped
  3 cloves garlic, peeled, bashed, and chopped
  3 carrots, peeled and cut on the diagonal into 1/4-inch slices (1 cup)

  3 stalks celery, cut on the diagonal into 1/2-inch slices (1 cup)
  1 red bell pepper, cored and cut into 1-inch strips
  1 cup quartered mushrooms
1/2 cup dry white wine (I prefer nonalcoholic chardonnay)
1/2 cup low-sodium fish or vegetable stock (pages 468, 473)
1/4 tsp salt
1/4 tsp freshly ground black pepper

Sauce

1 cup yogurt cheese (page 475)
1/4 cup arrowroot
1/2 cup dry white wine
   (I prefer nonalcoholic chardonnay)

2 cups low-sodium fish or
   vegetable stock (pages 468, 473)
3 Tbsp Roasted Tomato Salsa
   (page 478), or to taste

Garnish

1/4 cup chopped cilantro

Vegetarian Option

2   small cooked artichoke hearts, fresh, or canned, cut in half
2   canned hearts of palm, cut diagonally into 3 pieces

Delete the squid, clams, prawns, and orange roughy. When almost ready to serve, heat the reserved vegetable mixture in a small saucepan. Add the artichoke hearts and hearts of palm and heat through. Pour the reserved yogurt cheese sauce over the heated vegetables and season with salsa to taste. Heat very gently, not allowing it to boil.

To Prepare the Stew

1 Cut the squid into 1-inch squares. Cover with water in a small saucepan and cook over low heat for 25 minutes. If the squid has been tenderized (it will be full of tiny holes made by tenderizing needles), it will cook tender in about 5 minutes. Strain and place the chopped squid in a pile on a large plate.

2 Scrub the clams and place in a frying pan with 1/4 cup water. Cover and bring to a boil. Remove from the heat as soon as the clams open, 3 to 5 minutes. When cool enough to handle, remove the meat from the shells. Place the clams in a separate pile on the plate with the squid.

3 Peel the prawns, leaving on the last bit of shell and the tail. If they haven't been previously deveined, make a shallow cut down the back of each prawn and remove the gritty digestive tract. Place the prawns on the plate with the squid and clams.

4 Cut the orange roughy fillet into 1-inch squares. Add to the plate with the other fish, cover, and refrigerate until ready to cook.

(Continued)

5 Warm 1 tsp of the oil in a large high-sided skillet over medium-high heat. Sauté the onion for 2 minutes to release its flavorful oils. Toss in the garlic and cook for 1 more minute. Add the carrots, celery, pepper, and mushrooms. Stir for a minute or two, then add the wine.

6 Boil, uncovered, over medium-high heat until the carrots are tender, 10 to 12 minutes. Add up to 1/2 cup of the fish or vegetable stock as the liquid evaporates. (Vegetarian Option: Use vegetable stock here. Set aside 1/6 of this mixture for each vegetarian serving before proceeding to the next step.)

7 Heat the remaining 1 tsp of oil in a large saucepan or small Dutch oven. Add the prawns and orange roughy, sprinkle with the salt and pepper, and cook for 30 seconds. Gently stir in the cooked vegetables, clams, and squid. Remove from the heat while you prepare the sauce.

To Prepare the Sauce

8 Spoon the yogurt cheese into a 4-cup measuring glass.

9 Mix the arrowroot with the wine to make a slurry. Combine the stock and the slurry in a saucepan and stir over medium heat until thick and glossy. (Vegetarian Option: Use vegetable stock here. Set aside 1/4 cup of sauce at the end of this step.) Pour a little of the hot, thickened stock into the yogurt cheese and mix well to temper the yogurt. Add the rest of the stock to the yogurt cheese and whisk until no pure white remains.

10 Pour the sauce over the fish and vegetables. Add salsa to your taste and heat very gently, not allowing the stew to boil.

To Serve

11 Place a scoop of saffron rice in the center of a warmed dinner plate and surround the rice with a ring of stew. Garnish with the chopped cilantro and pass the remaining salsa for those, like Treena, who like it hot.

Per serving (without rice): 246 calories, 4 g fat, 1 g saturated fat, 4% of calories from saturated fat, 22 g carbohydrate, 3 g dietary fiber, 33 g protein
Exchanges: 1/2 Starch, 3 Very Lean Meat, 2 Vegetable, 1/2 Fat-Free Milk, 1/2 Fat

Vegetarian
Per serving: 126 calories, 2 g fat, 0 g saturated fat, 0% of calories from saturated fat, 22 g carbohydrate, 3 g dietary fiber
Exchanges: 1/2 Starch, 1/2 Fat-Free Milk, 2 Vegetable, 1/2 Fat

St. Augustine Perlow

SERVING SIZE: 1/6 of recipe, SERVES: 6

1 tsp non-aromatic olive oil	1 tsp salt
1 cup finely chopped onion	<C 1 cup washed long-grain white rice
1 clove garlic, bashed and chopped	
1/4 lb Canadian bacon, cut in 1/2-inch dice	+> 2 cups low-sodium chicken stock (page 463)
1 large red bell pepper, cut in 1/2-inch dice	1/2 cooked chicken breast (4 oz), bone and skin removed, cut in large pieces
3/4 cup celery, cut in 1/2-inch dice	
4 Roma tomatoes, cut in 1/2-inch dice	2 cooked chicken thighs, bone and skin removed, cut in large pieces
1 tsp mild chili powder	
1/4 tsp thyme	
pinch cloves	15 large black pitted olives, halved
1/4 tsp datil chili powder or cayenne pepper	

1 Preheat the oven to 450°F. Heat the oil in a large skillet or chef's pan on medium high. Saute the onion 2 minutes or until it starts to wilt. Add the garlic and cook 1 minute more. Stir in the bacon, red pepper, tomatoes, celery, chili powder, thyme, cloves, datil or cayenne, and salt. Cook, stirring, 5 minutes more. Stir in the rice and pour the stock over all. Bake, uncovered, in the preheated oven 20 minutes or until the rice is tender and fluffy.

2 Add the chicken and olives, mix, and return to the oven for 6 more minutes to heat through. Serve on hot plates scattered with fresh parsley.

<C To Cut Carb

<C Rice: reduce to 2/3 cup and convert to long-grain brown rice and bake for 40 minutes.

+> Chicken stock: add an extra 1/2 cup stock.

Per serving: 275 calories, 7 g fat, 2 g saturated fat, 7% calories from saturated fat, 33 g carbohydrates, 3 g fiber, 812 mg sodium
Exchanges: 1 1/2 Starch, 2 Lean Meat, 2 Vegetable

Low Carb

Per serving: 239 calories, 7 g fat, 2 g saturated fat, 7% calories from saturated fat, 25 g carbohydrate, 3 g dietary fiber, 822 mg sodium
Exchanges: 1 Starch, 2 Lean Meat, 2 Vegetable

Savory Stew with Tomato Paste

SERVING SIZE: 1/4 of recipe, SERVES: 4

1 tsp non-aromatic olive oil
1 onion, sliced
4 Tbsp tomato paste
4 cups cubed vegetable (carrots, celery, potatoes, turnips, or any other mixture)

12 oz cubed lean beef stew meat
5 cups beef stock (page 466), or enough to cover meat and vegetables
3 Tbsp arrowroot or cornstarch dissolved in 6 Tbsp water

In large saucepan, heat oil over medium-high heat. Sauté onion slices until softened and beginning to brown. Add the tomato paste, stirring well, and allow it to slowly brown. Be sure that the paste does not burn. Add vegetables, beef, and stock to cover. Stir and cover pan. Lower heat and simmer until beef is fork-tender, about 1 hour or longer. Slowly add arrowroot or cornstarch mixture to thicken sauce until desired consistency is achieved. Serve.

Per serving: 318 calories, 8 g fat, 2 g saturated fat, 6% calories from saturated fat, 22 g carbohydrate, 5 g dietary fiber, 329 mg sodium, 36 g protein, 53 mg cholesterol
Exchanges: 1/2 Starch, 4 Lean Meat, 3 Vegetable

Curried Chicken, Sweet Potatoes, and Bananas Wakaya

SERVING SIZE: 1/6 of recipe, SERVES: 6

Tamarind Sauce

1 1/2 oz (about 15 inches) peeled tamarind pods
1 tsp light olive oil
1/4 tsp yellow mustard seeds
1 tsp cumin seeds

1/4 tsp garam masala (page 335)
1/8 tsp cayenne pepper (optional)
5 quarter-size slices fresh ginger root
<C 3 oz pitted dates (about 12)
<C 1 mango, peeled and cubed

Chicken

3/4 tsp India Ethmix (page 477) or good Madras curry powder
3 boneless chicken breasts, skin on, about 6 oz each
2 tsp light olive oil

Curry

        2 heads bok choy
<C   3 bananas
      1/3 cup fresh lemon juice
<C   12 oz steamed sweet potato, peeled, halved, and cut into 1-inch pieces
        1 tsp arrowroot
      1/2 cup low-sodium chicken or vegetable stock (pages 463, 473)
        2 cloves garlic, peeled, bashed, and chopped
        2 tsp India Ethmix or good Madras curry powder
      1/2 cup yogurt cheese (page 475)
        4 green onions, white and green parts, cut into 1/4-inch slices
+>   9 oz pineapple wedges
        1 mango, peeled and sliced
      1/2 English cucumber, unpeeled, cut into very thin strips
       12 small radishes

Vegetarian Option: Tofu and Bananas Wakaya

    4 oz extra-firm light tofu
1/2 tsp light olive oil
1/2 tsp India Ethmix or good Madras curry powder
1/4 cup low-sodium vegetable stock

Cut tofu into 1-inch cubes and dry with a paper towel. Warm the oil in a frying pan. Add tofu and sprinkle with India Ethmix. Pour 1 Tbsp tamarind sauce or chutney over tofu, and cook for 2 minutes. Add vegetable stock, and simmer until reduced to a thick syrup. Combine with bananas and sweet potatoes. Garnish.

---

1 Cut peeled tamarind pods into small pieces, and soak in 1/2 cup warm water for 15 minutes. Strain, reserving liquid and pulp, and discard the seeds.

2 Warm oil in a small frying pan. Add mustard and cumin seeds, and cook for 2 minutes. Transfer to a blender or food processor.

3 Add garam masala, cayenne, ginger, and tamarind pulp and liquid. Process at high speed for 1 minute. Add dates and mango, and blend for 1 minute. Press the sauce through a strainer with a large spoon.

(Continued)

4 Rub 1/2 tsp India Ethmix or curry powder into the skinless side of each chicken breast.

5 Warm oil in a large frying pan. Sauté chicken, skin side down, for 2 minutes. Turn and cook another 3 minutes. Turn twice more, cooking for a total of 9 minutes, or until cooked through. Remove from the pan, and set aside. Do not wash the pan.

6 Cut leaves off the bok choy stems, and wash well. Steam leaves for 1 minute, and cool immediately under cold running water. Drain well, and pat dry; set aside to use as a bed for the curry.

7 Cut off and discard tough bottoms of the bok choy stems. Slice the tender parts of the stems into 1/2-inch strips. Set aside for garnish.

8 Peel bananas; cut into 1-inch pieces. Coat pieces with lemon juice to keep them from turning brown. Gently toss sweet potato pieces with bananas, and transfer to a large steamer. Cover, and steam for 5 minutes. (Vegetarian: Set aside 1/6 of this mixture per serving before proceeding to the next step.)

9 Combine arrowroot with stock to make a slurry.

10 Reheat oil and chicken juices in the large frying pan. Add garlic and India Ethmix, and stir until heated through. Deglaze pan with arrowroot slurry, loosening the flavorful bits from the bottom.

11 Spoon yogurt cheese into a 2-cup glass measure. Add a little hot stock, and mix to temper the yogurt. Whisk in the rest of stock to make a smooth, creamy sauce.

12 Combine curry sauce with hot bananas and sweet potatoes in a skillet. Keep warm but do not boil.

13 Remove and discard skin from chicken, and cut meat into 1-inch pieces. Gently stir chicken and onions into banana mixture over medium-high heat.

14 Arrange two or three bok choy leaves on each plate. Place a serving of curry on bok choy and garnish with bok choy strips, mango slices, cucumber strips, and radishes. A dollop of tamarind sauce or mango chutney goes on the side.

<C **To Cut Carb**

<C Dates: remove entirely.   <C Sweet potatoes: reduce to 6 oz.

<C Bananas: replace with 9 oz pineapple.

Per serving: 382 calories, 6 g fat, 1 g saturated fat, 2% calories from saturated fat, 66 g carbohydrate, 7 g dietary fiber, 125 mg sodium
Exchanges: 1 Starch, 2 Very Lean Meat, 1 Vegetable, 3 Fruit, 1/2 Fat

Low Carb

Per serving: 277 calories, 5 g fat, 1 g saturated fat, 3% calories from saturated fat, 39 g carbohydrate, 5 g dietary fiber, 121 mg sodium
Exchanges: 1/2 Starch, 2 Very Lean Meat, 1 Vegetable, 2 Fruit, 1/2 Fat

Vegetarian

Per serving: 306 calories, 4 g fat, 1 g saturated fat, 3% calories from saturated fat, 66 g carbohydrate, 7 g dietary fiber, 143 sodium
Exchanges: 1 Starch, 1 Vegetable, 3 Fruit, 1/2 Fat

Italian Pasta Vegetable Toss

SERVING SIZE: 1/4 of recipe, SERVES: 4

1 tsp olive oil
1 cup chopped onion
1 cup chopped red bell pepper
2 cloves garlic, chopped
1 cup sliced fresh mushrooms
1 (15 oz) can no-salt-added
  tomato sauce

1 tsp dried basil
1 tsp dried oregano
1/2 tsp salt
1 cup cooked macaroni or
  other small pasta
4 cups spinach leaves
3 Tbsp grated Parmesan cheese

1 Heat the oil in a high-sided skillet on medium high. Fry the onions 2 minutes. Add the bell pepper, garlic, and mushrooms and cook 3 or 4 minutes.

2 Pour in the tomato sauce, basil, oregano, and salt and bring to a boil. Reduce the heat and simmer 5 minutes.

3 Stir in the pasta and spinach and cook until the spinach wilts and the pasta is heated through, about 3 minutes. Top with Parmesan cheese.

Per serving: 130 calories, 4 g fat, 1 g saturated fat, 7% calories from saturated fat, 19 g carbohydrate, 7 g dietary fiber, 433 mg sodium, 5 g protein
Exchanges: 1/2 Starch, 2 Vegetable, 1 Fat

Indian Ocean Gumbo

SERVING SIZE: 1/4 of recipe, SERVES: 4

<C 1/4 cup all-purpose flour
  1/8 tsp ground cinnamon
    1 lb small shrimp
      (51 to 60 shrimp per lb)
<C 1 cup long-grain white rice
 1/16 tsp saffron powder
  1/2 tsp salt
    2 tsp non-aromatic olive oil
    1 large onion, finely chopped
    2 cloves garlic, peeled, bashed, and chopped
    1 red bell pepper, cut in 1-inch squares

    1 green bell pepper, cut in 1-inch squares
  1/4 cup tomato paste
    1 tsp dried thyme
  1/2 tsp cayenne pepper
    2 Turkish bay leaves
    4 cups low-sodium chicken stock (page 463)
<C 1 can (15 oz) palm hearts, cut in 1-inch lengths
  1/4 cup coconut cream (optional)
    2 small green onions, chopped
    1 Tbsp chopped fresh parsley

1. Preheat the oven to 400°F. Combine the flour and cinnamon, place in a glass pie plate, and bake 8 minutes. Set aside. Shell the shrimp reserving the shells. Bring the shells to a boil in a saucepan with 2 cups water and simmer 2 minutes. Strain, reserving the water in a saucepan, add the rice, saffron, and 1/4 tsp of the salt and bring to a boil. Reduce the heat to simmer and cook, uncovered, 15 minutes. Cover and keep warm.

2. Heat 1 tsp oil in a high-sided skillet on medium high. Sauté the onion 8 minutes or until golden brown. Add the garlic and roasted flour and sauté 2 minutes more. Remove to a bowl and set aside.

3. Add the remaining 1 tsp oil to the pan and fry the peppers 1 minute. Add the tomato paste and continue cooking until it darkens, about 2 minutes. Stir in the onion flour mixture and add the thyme, cayenne, and bay. Continue cooking for 5 minutes, stirring so the flour won't burn. Pour the stock in slowly, stirring constantly to prevent any lumps from forming. When it comes to a boil, add the palm hearts, shrimp, and salt and simmer 3 minutes.

4. Place 1/2 cup rice in each of four preheated bowls. Spoon the gumbo over the rice and add a dollop of the coconut cream. Scatter the onions and parsley on top.

<C To Cut Carb

<C Flour: reduce to 2 Tbsp.
<C Rice: change to brown rice and reduce to 1/4 cup (as a garnish). Simmer uncovered for 35 minutes. You may need to increase the water by 1 cup.
<C Palm hearts: delete altogether.

Per serving: 405 calories, 6 g fat, 1 g saturated fat, 1% calories from saturated fat, 62 g carbohydrate, 6 g dietary fiber, 790 mg sodium, 27 g protein
Exchanges: 3 Starch, 2 Very Lean Meat, 3 Vegetable, 1/2 Fat

Low Carb
Per serving: 246 calories, 6 g fat, 1 g saturated fat, 3% calories from saturated fat, 28 g carbohydrate, 4 g dietary fiber, 588 mg sodium, 22 g protein
Exchanges: 1 Starch, 2 Very Lean Meat, 3 Vegetable, 1/2 Fat

Pasta Primavera

SERVING SIZE: 1/4 of recipe, SERVES: 4

<C 8 oz penne pasta
1 Tbsp extra virgin olive oil
2 large cloves garlic, bashed and chopped
1 package frozen artichoke hearts, thawed
3 cups fresh or 1 package frozen chopped spinach

4 Roma tomatoes, seeded and chopped
1/4 tsp salt
1/4 tsp freshly ground black pepper
1/4 cup freshly grated Parmesan cheese

1 Cook the pasta according to package directions and set aside.

2 Heat the oil in a high-sided skillet on medium. Add the garlic and cook 30 seconds. Toss in the artichoke hearts and mushrooms. Cook until they begin to brown, about 3 minutes. Stir in the spinach, tomatoes, salt, pepper, and reserved pasta. Cook until heated through.

3 Serve on hot plates garnished with the Parmesan cheese.

<C **To Cut Carb** ══════════════════════
<C Pasta: reduce pasta to 1 oz dry weight per serving.

Per serving: 314 calories, 7 g fat, 2 g saturated fat, 6% calories from saturated fat, 53 g carbohydrate, 6 g dietary fiber, 249 mg sodium
Exchanges: 3 Starch, 2 Vegetable, 1 Fat

Low Carb
Per serving: 209 calories, 6 g fat, 2 g saturated fat, 6% calories from saturated fat, 31 g carbohydrate, 5 g dietary fiber, 247 mg sodium
Exchanges: 1 1/2 Starch, 2 Vegetable, 1 Fat

Boston Baked Beans

SERVING SIZE: 1/6 of recipe, SERVES: 6

<C 1 lb navy beans, soaked overnight
    1/2 tsp baking soda
    1 medium onion, peeled
<C 1/4 cup brown sugar
<C 1/4 cup molasses
    1 tsp dry mustard

1 1/2 tsp salt
1/4 tsp black pepper
1/2 tsp non-aromatic olive oil
1/4 lb Canadian bacon cut in
    1/2-inch chunks

Vegetarian Option

You can leave out the Canadian bacon if you prefer to cook this dish with no meat.

---

1 Bring a large pot of water to a boil. Drain the soaked beans and add to the boiling water with the soda. Boil 15 minutes. Place the onion in the bottom of a bean pot or other baking dish with a small opening. You can also put a collar of foil over a small basin and wrap it tightly, leaving a 2-inch diameter hole in the middle. Drain the beans and return to the pan.

2 Preheat the oven to 300°F. Combine the brown sugar, molasses, mustard, salt, and pepper in a small bowl. Heat the oil in a small skillet on medium high. Sauté the bacon 2 minutes to release the flavors. Add a tsp of the molasses mixture and stir while cooking 1 more minute. Stir into the drained beans with the rest of the molasses mixture and pour over the onion in the bean pot. Deglaze the pan with a little water and pour over the beans.

3 Cover with boiling water and bake in the preheated oven 6 hours or until the beans are tender and the sauce, syrupy. Stir every once in a while but don't add water unless it gets really dry. Serve with Boston Brown Bread (page 187), but remember your *total* carbs!

<C **To Cut Carbs**

<C Navy beans: reduce to 12 oz (dry).
<C Brown sugar: reduce to 2 Tbsp and add 1 Tbsp Splenda.
<C Molasses: reduce to 1 Tbsp and add 1 Tbsp Splenda.

Per serving: 371 calories, 3 g fat, 1 g saturated fat, 2% calories from saturated fat, 68 g carbohydrates, 12 g dietary fiber, 830 mg sodium
Exchanges: 3 Starch, 1 Lean Meat, 1 1/2 Carbohydrate

Low Carb
Per serving: 265 calories, 3 g fat, 1 g saturated fat, 2% calories from saturated fat, 46 g carbohydrate, 9 g dietary fiber, 825 mg sodium
Exchanges: 2 1/2 Starch, 1 Lean Meat, 1/2 Carbohydrate

Vegetarian
Per serving: 343 calories, 2 g fat, 0 g saturated fat, 0% calories from saturated fat, 68 g carbohydrate, 12 g dietary fiber, 592 mg sodium
Exchanges: 3 Starch, 1 1/2 Carbohydrate

Super-Charged Sandwich

SERVING SIZE: 1 sandwich, SERVES:1

<C 2 slices whole-wheat bread
  2 tsp Dijon mustard
  1 oz reduced-fat low-sodium
    cheddar cheese
  4 slices cucumber, zucchini, or
    crookneck squash

2 slices tomato
1/2 cup red bell pepper strips
1 thin slice onion (optional)
4 leaves fresh spinach or
  2 romaine leaves

Open the bread slices on a plate. Spread both sides thinly with mustard. Lay the cheese, cucumber, tomato, bell pepper, onion, and lettuce on one side and top with the second slice of bread. Cut in half on the diagonal and enjoy!

<C To Cut Carb
<C Bread: this sandwich almost clears the 30 g carb limit, but not quite. Trim the crusts off and you should be fine (and they make great croutons).

Per serving: 249 calories, 9 g fat, 4 g saturated fat, 13% calories from saturated fat, 37 g carbohydrate, 7 g dietary fiber, 813 mg sodium
Exchanges: 1 1/2 Starch, 1 Medium Fat Meat, 2 Vegetable, 1/2 Fat

Low Carb
Per serving: 199 calories, 8 g fat, 4 g saturated fat, 14% calories from saturated fat, 28 g carbohydrate, 6 g dietary fiber, 708 mg sodium
Exchanges: 1 Starch, 1 Medium Fat Meat, 2 Vegetable

Baked Falafel and Pita

SERVING SIZE: 2 falafels (1/2 pita apiece), SERVES: 4

Falafel

<C 1 cup uncooked garbanzo beans soaked over night, or 2 cups canned reduced-sodium garbanzo beans rinsed and drained
4 green onions, trimmed and sliced
2 cloves garlic, bashed and chopped
1/2 cup chopped fresh parsley
1/4 tsp salt
1/4 tsp freshly ground black pepper

1 tsp baking powder
1/4 tsp baking soda,
1 tsp ground coriander
1 tsp ground cumin
1/4 tsp ground red pepper
<C 5 pieces whole-wheat pita bread,1 torn into pieces, the rest left whole

Relish

3 Roma tomatoes, seeded and cut into 1/2-inch pieces
1 cup chopped unpeeled English cucumber

1/4 cup chopped green onion
1 serrano chile, minced with seeds
1 Tbsp chopped fresh parsley
1 Tbsp lemon juice

Sauce

2 oz soft goat cheese
1 cup plain low fat yogurt

1/8 tsp chopped garlic
1/8 tsp salt

1 Pulse the beans, onions, garlic, parsley, salt, pepper, baking powder, soda, coriander, cumin, cayenne, and torn pita in a food processor or blender until they hold together. The paste should have texture. Set aside to rest for 15 minutes.

2 While the mix is resting, combine the tomatoes, cucumber, onion, chile, parsley, and lemon juice and set aside. Mash the goat cheese into the yogurt with the back of a spoon until smooth. Stir in the garlic and salt and refrigerate until you're ready to use it.

3 Preheat the oven to 350°F. Make the bean mixture into 16 equal patties. Bake on a greased cookie sheet 10 minutes.

4 Cut the pitas in half; place 2 patties in each and spoon in the relish and sauce. If you're in a hurry, you can use sliced tomatoes and cucumbers instead of the relish and plain low-fat yogurt instead of the sauce.

<C Garbanzo: reduce beans to 3/4 cup before soaking.
<C Pita: reduce to 2 1/2, use the 1/2 piece torn into pieces at step 1.

Per serving: 470 calories, 9 g fat, 3 g saturated fat, 6% calories from saturated fat, 81 g carbohydrate, 13 g dietary fiber, 692 mg sodium
Exchanges: 4 1/2 Starch, 1 Lean Meat, 2 Vegetable, 1/2 Fat

Low Carb
Per serving: 337 calories, 8 g fat, 3 g saturated fat, 8% calories from saturated fat, 54 g carbohydrate, 10 g dietary fiber, 608 mg sodium
Exchanges: 3 Starch, 1 Lean Meat, 1 Vegetable, 1/2 Fat

Nonsuch Poele

SERVING SIZE: 1/4 of recipe, SERVES: 4

1 tsp olive oil
1 cup chopped sweet onion
1 Tbsp finely chopped ginger
2 cloves garlic, bashed and chopped
1 parsnip (1/2 cup)
1 carrot (1/2 cup)
1 turnip (1/2 cup)
1/2 cup sliced celery
1/2 cup chopped peeled orange
   sweet potato

1 tsp Southern France Ethmix
   (page 476) or herbs de provence
1 cup low-sodium chicken (page 463)
   or vegetable broth (page 473)
8 tiny cherry tomatoes
1/2 cup diagonally cut snow peas
2 tsp arrowroot or cornstarch mixed
   with 2 Tbsp water (slurry)
1 Tbsp Parmesan cheese
1 Tbsp chopped parsley

1 Heat the oil in a high-sided skillet on medium high. Fry the onion and ginger 3 minutes or until the onion begins to turn translucent. Add the garlic and cook 1 more minute.

2 Add the parsnip, carrot, turnip, celery, sweet potato, and herb mixture. Pour in the broth, cover, and bring to a boil. Reduce the heat and simmer 10 minutes or until the vegetables are tender.

3 Add the tomatoes and snow peas. Stir in the slurry and heat to thicken. Serve topped with Parmesan and parsley.

Per serving: 114 calories, 2 g fat, 1 g saturated fat, 8% calories from saturated fat, 22 g carbohydrate, 4 g dietary fiber, 222 mg sodium, 2 g protein
Exchanges: 4 Vegetable, 1/2 Fat

Greek Chicken Pie

SERVING SIZE: 1 piece, SERVES: 4

 1 tsp olive oil
 1 bunch green onions, sliced in
   1/2-inch rounds
1/2 lb mushrooms, quartered (2 cups)
 1 tsp lemon juice
 1 medium zucchini, cut in chunks
1/8 tsp white pepper
1/4 tsp salt
 1 tsp dried oregano
1/2 cup low-sodium chicken stock
   (page 463)

1/2 cup nonalcoholic dry
   white wine (optional)
 8 oz chicken breast meat,
   cut in large chunks
 2 Tbsp grated Parmesan cheese
 1 Tbsp arrowroot
 1 cup egg substitute
 8 sheets phyllo dough
 1 (10 oz) package frozen, chopped
   spinach, thawed and pressed dry

Vegetarian Option

1/2 cup vegetable stock (page 473)
1 (15 oz) can fava or cannellini beans, drained and rinsed

To make a Phyllo Vegetable Pie, replace the chicken stock with
vegetable stock and use the fava or cannellini beans instead of chicken.

---

1 Preheat the oven to 350°F. Heat the oil in a high-sided skillet on medium high. Cook the onions for 1 minute then toss in the mushrooms and lemon juice and cook 3 minutes more. Stir in the zucchini, pepper, salt, and oregano and cook, stirring, for 1 minute more.

2 Pour in the stock (if you're not using wine, use 1 cup of stock) and wine and bring to a vigorous boil to reduce by half. Pull off the heat and stir in the chicken and Parmesan cheese. Combine the arrowroot with the egg substitute and pour over the mixture in the pan. Stir and let cool while you work on the crust.

3 Spray an 8-inch square baking dish with pan spray. Lay the stack of phyllo leaves on the counter. Spray the top leaf, peel it off, and lay it in the pan allowing it to overlap the edges. Spray the second sheet and set it on top of the first one. Do the same thing to the third and fourth leaves but lay them the other direction. Cover the phyllo with plastic while you fill the pie.

4 Scatter half the spinach on the bottom and spread half the chicken mixture over it evenly. Make another layer of spinach and chicken and fold in the overlapping phyllo leaves. Spray another leaf of phyllo, fold, and lay on top. Spray, fold, and stack 3 more leaves. Trim the edges, cut through the top layer of phyllo, making 4 pieces, and bake for 35 to 40 minutes or until golden on top. Cut all the way through the bottom and serve on hot plates.

Per serving: 352 calories, 13 g fat, 2 g saturated fat, 5% calories from saturated fat, 30 g carbohydrate, 3 g dietary fiber, 525 mg sodium
Exchanges: 1 1/2 Starch, 3 Lean Meat, 2 Vegetable, 1/2 Fat

Vegetarian
Per serving: 330 calories, 11 g fat, 1 g saturated fat, 2% calories from saturated fat, 43 g carbohydrate, 6 g dietary fiber, 636 mg sodium
Exchanges: 2 Starch, 1 Very Lean Meat, 2 Vegetable, 2 Fat

Spinach Ricotta Quiche

SERVING SIZE: 1/6 of recipe, SERVES: 6

12 cups well washed fresh spinach or 2 packages frozen spinach, thawed	1/2 tsp dried dill weed
2 tsp olive oil	1/4 tsp pepper
1/2 cup finely chopped onions	pinch nutmeg
1 cup low-fat ricotta cheese	3 plum tomatoes, seeds and juice removed, chopped (1 cup)
1/2 cup egg substitute or 2 whole eggs, beaten	1 Tbsp grated Parmesan cheese

1 Preheat the oven to 350°F. Grease a 9-inch pie dish. Steam the fresh spinach until just wilted. (Frozen spinach won't need to be cooked, just thawed.) Press the water out of the cooked or thawed spinach and set aside.

2 Heat the oil in a small skillet and cook the onions until soft but not brown. Combine the ricotta cheese, egg substitute, dill, pepper, and nutmeg in a large bow. Add the prepared spinach, tomatoes, and onions. Mix thoroughly and tip into the pie pan.

3 Sprinkle Parmesan cheese over the top and bake until set, about 30 minutes. Let the quiche cool for 5 or 10 minutes before serving.

Per serving (with egg substitute): 115 calories, 3 g fat, 1 g saturated fat, 8% calories from saturated fat, 9 g carbohydrate, 6 g dietary fiber, 234 mg sodium
Exchanges: 1 Lean Meat, 2 Vegetable

Pickled Green-Lipped Mussels

SERVING SIZE: 1/6 of recipe, SERVES: 6

Court Bouillon (Poaching Liquid)

1/2 tsp light olive oil
1 medium sweet onion, finely chopped
4 cloves garlic, peeled, bashed, and chopped
1 Tbsp dried basil

4 cups dry white wine (I prefer nonalcoholic Ariel Chardonnay)
2 bay leaves
3 broad sprigs fresh parsley, bashed
1 tsp salt
1/2 lemon

Mussels

2 dozen New Zealand Green-Lipped Mussels or 3 dozen blue mussels, fresh or frozen

Pickling Liquid

1/2 lemon, thinly sliced
1 cup rice vinegar
1 bay leaf
1 tsp whole cloves

1 tsp whole allspice
1/2 red bell pepper, cored, seeded, and cut into thin strips
2 sprigs fresh dill weed

Garnish

Belgian endive

12 slices dark rye cocktail bread

Vegetarian Option

Replace the mussels with 4 marinated artichoke heart quarters, or halves if they are small.

To Prepare the Court Bouillon

1 Warm the oil in a large frying pan over medium heat. Sauté the onion, garlic, and basil for 2 minutes, or until softened. Add the wine, bay leaves, parsley, and salt. Squeeze the lemon juice into the pan and add the rind as well. Simmer for 10 minutes.

2 Strain the bouillon, returning the liquid to the frying pan and discarding the seasonings.

To Cook the Mussels

3 Scrub and debeard the mussels. Discard any that are no longer alive (if you have bought mussels frozen on the half shell, this step isn't necessary).

4 Bring the court bouillon to a boil and add the mussels. Cover the pan and poach for 3 minutes. Strain, reserving 4 cups of the liquid. Scoop the meat out of the shells into a small bowl. Carefully wash the shells and remove the "foot" from the inside. Set the shells aside to use at serving time.

To Prepare the Pickling Liquid

5 Add the lemon slices to the reserved court bouillon. Stir in the rice vinegar, bay leaf, cloves, allspice berries, and red pepper strips.

6 Place the mussels in a jar and cover with the seasoned pickling liquid. Top with the dill. Cover and store in the refrigerator overnight, or up to 3 days. This is a light pickle not suited to storage.

To Serve

7 Place four mussel shells on each plate. Lay an endive leaf in each shell and top with mussels and pepper strips. Serve the bread on the side.

Per serving: 179 calories, 3 g fat, 1 g saturated fat, 5% of calories from saturated fat, 21 g carbohydrate, 3 g dietary fiber, 17 g protein
Exchanges: 1 1/2 Starch, 2 Very Lean Meat

Vegetarian
Per serving: 127 calories, 5 g fat, 0 g saturated fat, 0% calories from saturated fat, 20 g carbohydrate, 5 g dietary fiber
Exchanges: 1 Carbohydrate, 1 Vegetable, 1 Fat

Upside Down Lamb Pie

SERVING SIZE: 1/4 of recipe, SERVES: 4

1/16 tsp saffron powder	1/16 tsp ground cloves
1/4 cup water	3/4 tsp salt
<C 1 cup long-grain white rice	1/2 tsp freshly ground black pepper
1 tsp non-aromatic olive oil	12 oz lean lamb leg or shoulder,
1 onion, chopped fine (1 cup)	ground in a processor
2 cloves garlic, bashed and	1/2 tsp almond extract
chopped	<C 1/2 cup cooked or canned
1 small eggplant, cut in	garbanzo beans
3/4-inch pieces	2 Tbsp lemon juice
3/4 tsp ground cumin	2 cups low sodium chicken
1/2 tsp ground allspice	broth
1 tsp ground cardamom	1 Tbsp chopped fresh parsley
1/16 tsp ground cinnamon	1 Tbsp chopped fresh spearmint

Vegetarian Option

1/2 cup almonds
2 cups low-sodium vegetable broth

1 (15 1/2 oz) can garbanzo beans

Make the recipe through step 2 but leave the vegetables in the pan. Pull them aside to roast the almonds. Stir in a whole can of drained and rinsed garbanzo beans and the lemon juice. Place the mixture in a 10-inch skillet and spread the rice over the top. Replace the chicken broth with vegetable broth and cook and serve as in steps 4 and 5.

---

1 Stir the saffron into the water to dissolve. Add the rice, mix well, and set aside.

2 Heat 1/2 tsp of the oil in a high-sided skillet on medium high. Sauté the onion for 5 minutes then stir in the garlic and eggplant. Add the cumin, all-spice, cardamom, cinnamon, cloves, salt, and pepper. Continue cooking for 3 more minutes. Tip out of the pan into a bowl and set aside.

3 Heat the remaining oil in the same pan without washing it. When it's nice and hot, crumble the meat and drop it in. Brown on one side without stir-ring, about 3 minutes. When browned add the eggplant mixture, garbanzo beans, and lemon juice and cook for 5 minutes. Stir in the almond extract.

4 Spread the meat mixture evenly in a greased 10-inch non-stick skillet. Cover with the saffron rice and pour 1 1/2 cups broth over the top. Bring to a boil, reduce the heat to low, cover and cook for 30 minutes. Remove the cover and shake the pan to make sure it's not sticking. Press the uncooked rice down into the liquid, adding more stock as you need it. Place the lid back on and cook 15 more minutes or until the rice is tender and the liquid is gone.

5 Cover the pan with a serving plate and turn it over carefully. The pie should slip right out. Combine the parsley and mint and scatter over the top. Cut into 4 wedges and serve on hot plates.

<C **To Cut Carb**

<C Rice: reduce to 1/2 cup of brown rice and cook for 30 minutes longer at step 4.

<C Garbanzo beans: reduce to 1/4 cup. Add 1/2 cup diced celery at step 2.

Per serving: 413 calories, 9 g fat, 3 g saturated fat, 9% calories from saturated fat, 53 g carbohydrate, 5 g dietary fiber, 553 mg sodium
Exchanges: 3 Starch, 2 Lean Meat, 2 Vegetable, 1/2 Fat

Low Carb

Per serving: 316 calories, 9 g fat, 3 g saturated fat, 11% calories from saturated fat, 32 g carbohydrate, 5 g dietary fiber, 565 mg sodium
Exchanges: 1 1/2 Starch, 2 Lean Meat, 2 Vegetable, 1/2 Fat

Vegetarian

Per serving: 363 calories, 7 g fat, 1 g saturated fat, 3% calories from saturated fat, 65 g carbohydrate, 9 g fiber, 556 mg sodium
Exchanges: 3 1/2 Starch, 2 Vegetable, 1 Fat

Lentil Minestrone

SERVING SIZE: 1/4 of recipe, SERVES: 4

	1 tsp extra virgin olive oil
	1 cup chopped onions
	2 cloves garlic, bashed and chopped
	1 Tbsp tomato paste
+>	1 cup chopped carrots
+>	1/2 cup chopped celery
<C	1 cup dried brown lentils

5 cups low-sodium chicken or
    vegetable broth
1 bunch spinach, washed and
    chopped or 1 package
    frozen chopped spinach
<C 1 cup cooked pasta shells
1/4 cup grated Parmesan cheese

(Continued)

1 Heat oil in large saucepan on medium high. Sauté onions 2 minutes or until wilting. Add garlic, and cook 1 minute. Stir in tomato paste, carrots, celery, and lentils and cook, stirring, until tomato paste starts to darken.

2 Pour in broth, bring to a boil, reduce heat and simmer, uncovered, 30 minutes or until lentils and carrots are tender. Stir in spinach and pasta, and heat through. Serve with a scattering of Parmesan cheese and a piece of crusty bread.

<C **To Cut Carb**

<C Brown lentils: reduce by 1/2 cup.
<C Pasta shells: reduce by 1/2 cup.
+> Carrots and celery or your favorite vegetable: increase.

Per serving: 328 calories, 6 g fat, 2 g saturated fat, 5% calories from saturated fat, 49 g carbohydrate, 14 g dietary fiber, 285 mg sodium
Exchanges: 2 1/2 Starch, 1 Very Lean Meat, 2 Vegetable, 1 Fat

Low Carb
Per serving: 238 calories, 6 g fat, 2 g saturated fat, 7% calories from saturated fat, 33 g carbohydrate, 10 g dietary fiber, 303 mg sodium
Exchanges: 1 Starch, 1 Very Lean Meat, 3 Vegetable, 1 Fat

Moussaka

SERVING SIZE: 1 wedge, SERVES: 6

1 tsp olive oil	2 cups nonalcoholic red wine
1 cup chopped onion	1/8 tsp cinnamon
3 cloves garlic, chopped	1/8 tsp salt
12 oz very lean ground lamb	1/4 tsp freshly ground pepper
3 Tbsp tomato paste	8 oz eggplant, peeled and sliced
1 tsp dried oregano	1/4 cup plus 2 Tbsp grated Parmesan
1/4 cup bulgur wheat	

Topping

1 cup 1% milk	1/8 tsp nutmeg
2 Tbsp cornstarch mixed with 4 Tbsp water (slurry)	2 Tbsp egg substitute

Vegetarian Option

1 1/2	lb mushrooms, chopped	1	cup nonalcoholic red wine
	in a processor	1	Tbsp Worcestershire sauce
1/2	cup bulgur wheat		

Replace the lamb with the mushrooms. Sauté the onion and garlic as in step 1, but after 3 minutes, toss in the chopped mushrooms. Raise the heat to high and cook until you start to see a lot of liquid bubbling up. Stir in bulgur wheat, and continue cooking until the liquid is gone, about 10 minutes all together. Add the oregano and tomato paste and cook for 2 minutes more. Pour in 1 cup nonalcoholic red wine, the cinnamon, salt, pepper, and Worcestershire sauce and cook 2 more minutes. The rest is just like the version with meat; broil the eggplant, make the topping, assemble, and bake. This one turned out so well, I think I like it more than the one with meat!

1 Preheat the oven broiler. Heat the oil in a high-sided skillet and sauté the onions for 3 minutes on medium high. Add the garlic and cook another minute. Remove the onions to a plate and reheat the pan.

2 When the pan is good and hot, crumble in the ground lamb and fry until brown. Add the tomato paste and stir until it starts to darken, 2 minutes.

3 Return the cooked onions to the pan with the lamb and stir in the oregano and bulgar wheat. Pour in the wine and season with the cinnamon, salt, and pepper. Bring to a boil and simmer 5 minutes.

4 Lay the eggplant slices on a broiler pan and sprinkle with 1/4 cup of the grated Parmesan cheese. Broil for 5 minutes 3 to 5 inches from the broiler element. Remove, set aside and turn the oven down to 350°F.

5 Combine the milk, slurry, and nutmeg in a small saucepan. Bring to a boil, and cook stirring, until thick. Pull it off the heat and add the egg substitute.

6 Tip the meat mixture out of the pan into a bowl. Cover the bottom of the pan with a layer of eggplant slices. Spread a cup of the meat sauce over the broiled eggplant, sprinkle with a third of the Parmesan cheese. Make a second and third layer the same way with the meat sauce on the top. Make an indentation in the top layer of meat sauce to hold the liquid topping.

7 Pour the custard sauce topping into the indentation without letting too much spill over. Sprinkle with the remaining Parmesan cheese and bake in the preheated oven for 25 minutes or until the topping is solid and the eggplant tender. Place under the broiler for five minutes or until golden brown on top. Cut into 6 wedges and serve.

(Continued)

Per serving: 239 calories, 9 g fat, 4 g saturated fat, 15% calories from saturated fat, 17 g carbohydrate, 3 g dietary fiber, 211 mg sodium
Exchanges: 1/2 Starch, 3 Lean Meat, 2 Vegetable

Vegetarian
Per serving: 167 calories, 4 g fat, 2 g saturated fat, 10 % calories from saturated fat, 27 g carbohydrate, 6 g dietary fiber, 196 mg sodium
Exchanges: 1/2 Starch, 4 Vegetable, 1/2 Fat

Cuban Black Beans

SERVING SIZE: 1/4 of recipe, SERVES: 4

	1 tsp non-aromatic olive oil	<c	2 (15 oz) cans black beans
+>	1 cup chopped onions		1 bay leaf
	2 cloves garlic, bashed and chopped	<c	3/4 cup long-grain white rice
	1 red bell pepper, cut in 1/2-inch dice		2 Tbsp chopped cilantro

1 Heat the oil in a high-sided skillet and cook the onions until they start to wilt and turn translucent, 3 minutes. Add the garlic and pepper and cook 1 minute more.

2 Pour in the black beans with their liquid, add the bay leaf and simmer 20 minutes. Combine the rice with 1 1/2 cups water and bring to a boil. Reduce the heat to the lowest possible temperature and cook, covered, 15 minutes. Turn the heat off and set aside.

3 Discard the bay leaf, divide the rice among 4 bowls and spoon the beans over the top. Garnish with the chopped cilantro.

<c **To Cut Carb**

+> Onions: increase to 2 cups.
<c Black beans: reduce to 1 (15 oz) can.
<c White rice: change to 1/2 cup brown rice (cook covered in 1 1/2 cup water for 35–40 minutes.)

Per serving: 332 calories, 2 g fat, 0 g saturated fat, 0% calories from saturated fat, 63 g carbohydrate, 10 g dietary fiber, 595 mg sodium
Exchanges: 4 Starch, 1 Vegetable

Low Carb
Per serving: 221 calories, 2 g fat, 0 g saturated fat, 0% calories from saturated fat, 43 g carbohydrate, 8 g dietary fiber, 300 mg sodium
Exchanges: 2 Starch, 2 Vegetable

Hearty Vegetable Stew Seasoned with Beef

SERVING SIZE: 1/6 of recipe, SERVES: 6

8 oz beef bottom round, cut into 1/2-inch pieces
1 1/2 tsp non-aromatic olive oil
1 large onion, sliced
1/3 cup tomato paste
2 cloves garlic, bashed and chopped
1/4 cup nonalcoholic red wine
3 cups low-sodium beef broth
1 lb carrots, peeled and cut in 1-inch chunks

<C 12 tiny red potatoes, scrubbed
12 medium mushrooms, quartered
<C 2 cups frozen peas, thawed
2 Tbsp arrowroot or cornstarch mixed with 1/4 cup nonalcoholic red wine (slurry)
1/4 tsp salt
1/4 tsp pepper
2 Tbsp chopped parsley plus extra for garnish

1 Heat 1 tsp of the oil in a large skillet on medium-high. Brown the meat on one side then remove from the pan and set aside. Pour the remaining oil into the same skillet and cook the onions and tomato paste until the onions begin to soften and the tomato paste darkens. Stir in the garlic and set aside.

2 Pour in the wine and stock, bring to a boil, reduce the heat and simmer, covered, for 30 minutes. Add the carrots and potatoes and simmer 30 minutes more. Toss in the mushrooms to cook 5 minutes.

3 Remove from the heat, stir in the slurry and peas and return to the heat. Heat, stirring, until thick and glossy. Add the salt, pepper, and parsley. Ladle into bowls and scatter more fresh parsley over the top.

<C To Cut Carb

<C Potatoes: reduce to 6.
<C Peas: reduce to 1 1/2 cups.
+> Add 1 cup of your favorite non-root vegetable.

Per serving: 223 calories, 3 g fat, 0 g saturated fat, 0% calories from saturated fat, 36 g carbohydrate, 8 g dietary fiber, 258 mg sodium, 14 g protein
Exchanges: 1 1/2 Starch, 1 Lean Meat, 3 Vegetable

Low Carb
Per serving: 193 calories, 3 g fat, 1 g saturated fat, 3% calories from saturated fat, 30 g carbohydrate, 7 g dietary fiber, 248 mg sodium, 14 g protein
Exchanges: 1 Starch, 1 Lean Meat, 3 Vegetable

Fill-Up-Those "Souper Bowls" Chili

SERVING SIZE: 1/4 of recipe, SERVES: 4

1 tsp non-aromatic olive oil	1/2 cup chopped celery
<C 1 cup chopped onion	1/2 cup chopped carrots
1 Tbsp (or more to taste) mild chili powder	1 cup diced eggplant
	<C 1 (15 1/2 oz) can kidney beans, drained and rinsed
1 tsp cumin	
1 tsp dried oregano	1 (28 oz) can chopped tomatoes in juice
3 cloves garlic, peeled and chopped	1/4 tsp pepper
1 red bell pepper, cut in 1/2-inch pieces	1/2 lb lean ground turkey (optional)

1 Heat the oil in a large high-sided skillet. Cook the onions until they start to wilt, about 2 minutes. If using meat, cook the turkey, onion, and garlic in a large pot on medium-high heat until meat is brown. With either option, add the chili powder, cumin, oregano, and garlic, and cook 1 minute more.

2 Stir in the bell pepper, celery, carrots, and eggplant and continue to cook until the vegetables are coated with the spices, about 2 minutes. Add the beans, tomatoes, and pepper. Bring to a boil, reduce the heat, and simmer for 30 minutes or until all the vegetables are tender.

<C To Cut Carb
<C Onion: reduce to 1/2 cup.
<C Kidney beans: reduce to 2/3 cup.

Per serving (without meat): 189 calories, 2 g fat, 0 g saturated fat, 0% calories from saturated fat, 36 g carbohydrate, 10 g dietary fiber, 540 mg sodium, 10 g protein
Exchanges: 1 Starch, 4 Vegetable, 1/2 Fat
Per serving (with meat): 253 calories, 3 g fat, 0 g saturated fat, 0% calories from saturated fat, 37 g carbohydrate, 9 g dietary fiber, 568 mg sodium, 24 g protein
Exchanges: 1 Starch, 2 Very Lean Meat, 4 Vegetable

Low Carb
Per serving (without meat): 124 calories, 2 g fat, 0 g saturated fat, 0% calories from saturated fat, 24 g carbohydrate, 7 g dietary fiber, 465 mg sodium, 6 g protein
Exchanges: 1/2 Starch, 3 Vegetable, 1/2 Fat

Low Carb

Per serving (with meat): 187 calories, 2 g fat, 0 g saturated fat. 0% calories from saturated fat, 24 g carbohydrate, 7 g dietary fiber, 492 mg sodium, 20 g protein
Exchanges: 1/2 Starch, 2 Very Lean Meat, 3 Vegetable

Sweet Potato Pasta Sauce

SERVING SIZE: 1/4 of recipe, SERVES: 4

<C   1 lb orange sweet potatoes
<C   1 (12 oz) can nonfat evaporated milk
    1/4 tsp salt
    1/4 tsp pepper

<C 8 oz dry pasta
    4 Tbsp grated Parmesan cheese
    2 Tbsp chopped fresh parsley

1 Peel and slice the sweet potatoes. Steam 14 minutes or until soft. Toss into a blender with the milk, salt, and pepper and whiz 7 minutes. This will seem like a long time but lovely changes happen in the process and they become a wonderful glossy rich color.

2 While the sweet potatoes are steaming, cook the pasta according to package directions. Drain and keep warm in a covered colander over hot water.

3 Divide the pasta among 4 hot plates and pour the sauce over the top. Scatter Parmesan cheese and parsley on each serving

<C **To Cut Carb** ━━━━━━━━━━━━━━━━━━

<C Sweet potatoes: reduce to 8 oz.   <C Dry pasta: reduce to 4 oz.
<C Evaporated milk: reduce to 2/3 cup.

Per serving: 398 calories, 3 g fat, 1 g saturated fat, 2% calories from saturated fat, 74 g carbohydrate, 4 g dietary fiber, 326 mg sodium
Exchanges: 4 Starch, 1 Fat-Free Milk

Low Carb

Per serving: 208 calories, 3 g fat, 1 g saturated fat, 5% calories from saturated fat, 36 g carbohydrate, 2 g dietary fiber, 252 mg sodium
Exchanges: 2 Starch, 1/2 Fat-Free Milk

Hoppin' John

SERVING SIZE: 1/6 of recipe, SERVES: 6

Hoppin' John

<C 1 cup dry black-eyed peas
   2 lb ham hocks
   5 cups water
   1 tsp non-aromatic olive oil
<C 1 large sweet onion, chopped
    (2 cups)
   3 cloves garlic, bashed and
    chopped
   1 rib celery, chopped (1/2 cup)

1/2 tsp dried thyme
   4 cups stock from the ham hocks
   2 bay leaves
<C 1 cup raw long grain white rice
1/8 tsp ground cloves
1/8 tsp cayenne pepper
1/4 tsp salt (optional)
   3 heaping Tbsp chopped parsley

Collards

1/2 tsp non-aromatic olive oil
   1 dried red pepper or 1/8 tsp
    cayenne pepper
1/2 lemon sliced
   1 tsp lemon zest

   8 cups washed and stemmed
    collard greens
   2 cups ham stock
1/8 tsp salt
   1 Tbsp lemon juice

1. Cover the black-eyed peas with 3 or 4 cups of water and soak over night. To quick soak, bring to a boil, turn off the heat, and let set for 1 hour. Rinse the ham hocks and cover with 8 cups water. This step can be done in a pressure cooker by cooking 30 minutes under high pressure or the old simmering way by covering and simmering 1 hour or until tender. Remove the hocks to a plate to cool and pour the stock into a fat strainer. Set aside to use later. When the hocks are cool enough, remove and discard the skin and fat and save the meat to add at the end.

2. Heat 1 tsp oil in a 10 1/2-inch chef's pan on medium high. Sauté the onion 3 minutes then add the garlic to cook for 1 minute more. Stir in the celery, stock, thyme, bay leaves, rice, soaked peas, cloves, and cayenne. Bring to a boil then reduce to simmer. Add ham hock meat and cook for 20 minutes or until the rice and peas are tender but not mushy.

3. While the beans are cooking, start the collard greens. Heat the oil in a chef's pan on medium high. Lay the lemon slices and chili pepper in the pan and cook 2 minutes. Pour in 2 cups of the defatted ham stock and collards, torn in roughly 2-inch pieces, and boil gently 10 minutes. Stir in the zest, salt, and lemon juice and set aside until you are ready to serve.

4 When the peas are done, taste for salt and add if need be. Stir in the chopped parsley and you are ready to serve. Divide the collards among 6 hot bowls. Pour the juice left in the pan into the rice and pea mixture. Ladle the Hoppin' John onto the collards and you are ready for a real down home treat!

<C **To Cut Carb**

<C Onion: reduce to 1 cup.

<C Rice: convert to brown rice and reduce to 1/2 cup. You will need to cook the rice at step 2 for a total 35 minutes or until tender.

Per serving: 344 calories, 7 g fat, 2 g saturated fat, 6% calories from saturated fat, 48 g carbohydrate, 6 g dietary fiber, 93 mg sodium, 23 g protein
Exchanges: 2 1/2 Starch, 2 Lean Meat, 2 Vegetable

Low Carb

Per serving: 278 calories, 7 g fat, 2.2 g saturated fat, 7% calories from saturated fat, 33 g carbohydrate, 8 g dietary fiber, 92 mg sodium, 22 g protein
Exchanges: 2 Starch, 2 Lean Meat, 1 Vegetable

Roast Chicken

SERVING SIZE: 1/4 of recipe, SERVES: 4

Vegetables

2 Tbsp freshly squeezed lemon juice
1/2 tsp ground ginger
1/2 tsp salt
1/2 tsp paprika
1/4 tsp freshly ground black pepper
1 tsp fresh or dried rosemary, chopped

1/2 cup fresh parsley, chopped
<C 4 medium carrots, peeled and cut in half lengthwise and again across
<C 4 (6 inch) parsnips, peeled and cut like the carrots
<C 3/4 lb Yellow Finn or Yukon Gold potatoes, quartered

Chicken

1 (3 lb) whole chicken
1 good size knob fresh ginger root, thinly sliced, peel on
1/2 lemon, thinly sliced
2 Tbsp freshly squeezed lemon juice

1/4 tsp paprika, divided
1 tsp arrowroot mixed with 2 tsp water (slurry)
1 Tbsp chopped parsley

(Continued)

1 Preheat the oven to 350°F. Combine 2 Tbsp of the lemon juice, ginger, salt, paprika, pepper, and rosemary and toss together in a large bowl with the cut vegetables. Tip out into a baking pan and spray lightly with olive oil pan spray and roast 25 minutes.

2 Cut the chicken along both sides of the breastbone. Separate and discard the bone. Now cut through the ribs along the backbone and save for stocks later on. You will now have two separate halves of chicken ready to roast. Cut through the skin around the thigh and slide 3 thin slices of ginger under the skin of the breast, thigh, and leg of each half. Turn over and place 3 more slices of ginger, followed by 3 slices of lemon in the cavity on the bony side. Set each chicken half, skin side up on a piece of foil and pinch the foil up around the edges leaving the skin exposed. This will hold the seasonings close to the meat and catch the flavorful juice. Place on a rack in a baking pan and start roasting after the vegetables have cooked 25 minutes. Roast 35 minutes, leaving the vegetables in for a total of 1 hour.

3 Remove the vegetables from the oven and keep warm. Pour the juice accumulated in the foil into a fat strainer. Discard the skin, ginger, and lemon slices from the chicken halves, leaving the skin on the wings. Bone the breasts and lay them with the wings in a skillet large enough for all the pieces. Separate the legs from the thighs. Lay in the skillet with the breasts. Cut the ends off the legs, leaving the bone in and arrange in the pan with the rest of the chicken. Pour in the defatted juice. Coat with the remaining lemon juice, sprinkle evenly with 1/8 tsp of the paprika, and set under the broiler 5 minutes or until golden brown.

4 Arrange the chicken and vegetables on a large hot platter. Bring the juice in the pan to a boil, add the remaining paprika, and thicken with the slurry. Stir in the parsley. Pour over the chicken and vegetables and serve to a hungry family.

<C To Cut Carb

<C Carrots: reduce to 2.   <C Potatoes: reduce to 1/2 lb.
<C Parsnips: reduce to 2.

Because of these reductions I would add 2 cups of your favorite lower carbohydrate green vegetable.

Per serving: 349 calories, 9 g fat, 2 g saturated fat, 6% calories from saturated fat, 33 g carbohydrate, 6 g dietary fiber, 423 mg sodium, 35 g protein
Exchanges: 1 1/2 Starch, 4 Very Lean Meat, 2 Vegetable, 1 Fat

Low Carb
Per serving: 295 calories, 8 g fat, 2 g saturated fat, 6% calories from saturated fat, 21 g carbohydrate, 3 g dietary fiber, 407 mg sodium
Exchanges: 1 Starch, 4 Very Lean Meat, 1 Vegetable, 1 Fat

Kedgeree: Smoked Fish and Rice

SERVING SIZE: 1/4 of recipe, SERVES: 4

<C 1 cup long-grain white rice
   Pinch of saffron
2 cups 1% milk
1/2 cup nonalcoholic white wine
1/8 tsp white pepper
1 bay leaf
1 lb Finnan Haddie (smoked haddock or halibut or other local smoked white fish)

1 Tbsp butter flavored margarine (soft tub)
1 Tbsp dry mustard
2 tsp arrowroot mixed with 1 Tbsp water
2 Tbsp chopped fresh chives
   Whites of 2 hard cooked eggs, chopped (discard yolks)
1/8 tsp ground red pepper

1 Please soak the fish in plain milk for half an hour to reduce about 30% of the sodium.

2 Cook rice according to package directions with the saffron.

3 Combine milk, wine, white pepper, and bay leaf in a high-sided skillet, and simmer. Lay pieces of Finnan Haddie in milk mixture, cover with grease-proof paper, and simmer 8 minutes. Remove fish to a plate. Strain, and reserve the milk.

4 Flake the fish, removing bones and bits of connective tissue. Stir margarine and mustard into the milk, and reheat in the skillet. Add fish and rice, and simmer 5 minutes. Stir in the slurry. Add egg whites, chives, and red pepper.

<C To Cut Carb

<C White rice: replace with brown rice and reduce to 1/2 cup.

Per serving: 388 calories, 4 g fat, 1 g saturated fat, 2 % calories from saturated fat, 46 g carbohydrate, 1 g dietary fiber, 721 mg sodium
Exchanges: 2 1/2 Starch, 4 Very Lean Meat, 1/2 Fat-free Milk

Low Carb
Per serving: 305 calories, 5 g fat, 1 g saturated fat, 2 % calories from saturated fat, 27 g carbohydrate, 1 g dietary fiber, 721 mg sodium
Exchanges: 1 1/2 Starch, 4 Very Lean Meat, 1/2 Fat-free Milk

Lamb Greystone

SERVING SIZE: 1/6 of recipe, SERVES: 6

Polenta

2 cups low-sodium chicken stock	1/4 cup grated Parmesan
<C 2 cups 1% milk	1/4 tsp salt
1 cup cornmeal or polenta	

Filling

2 tsp non-aromatic olive oil, divided

8 oz lean ground lamb

<C 1 onion cut in 1/4-inch dice (1 1/2 cups)

1 red bell pepper, cut in 1/2-inch dice (1 cup)

1 yellow bell pepper, cut in 1/2-inch dice (1 cup)

3 large cloves garlic, bashed and chopped

2 Tbsp tomato paste

1 small eggplant cut in 1/2-inch dice (3 cups)

1 medium zucchini, cut in 1/2-inch chunks (1 cup)

1 yellow summer squash, cut in 1/2-inch chunks (1 cup)

6 Roma tomatoes, cored, seeded and cut in 1/2-inch dice

4 Tbsp + 1 tsp balsamic vinegar

1/2 cup chopped fresh basil

3 Tbsp chopped fresh oregano

1/4 tsp salt

1/4 tsp pepper

2 Tbsp grated Parmesan cheese

1 tsp arrowroot mixed with 2 tsp water

1 Combine chicken stock and milk in a 4-quart saucepan. Bring to a boil. Rain cornmeal into the hot liquid, whisking constantly. Cook on low heat, stirring often, 30 minutes. Stir in Parmesan cheese and salt, and set aside.

2 Heat 1 tsp oil in large skillet on medium high. Brown ground lamb, and tip onto a plate. Heat remaining oil and sauté onion 2 minutes or until it wilts. Add peppers and garlic, and cook 3 minutes. Stir in tomato paste and cook, stirring, until it darkens. Add eggplant and stir to coat with tomato paste. Toss in squash, meat, 1/4 cup balsamic vinegar, basil, oregano, salt, and pepper. Simmer 15 to 20 minutes or until vegetables are tender. Stir in tomatoes and heat through.

3 Grease a baking sheet. Lay 6 flan rings on the pan and spray. Divide the polenta among the rings, and press flat with the back of an oiled spoon. Squeeze liquid out of the filling, and reserve it in the pan as you pack vegetables into a 1-cup measure, and turn out onto each tart. Scatter Parmesan over filling, and bake 15 to 20 minutes or until heated through.

4 Stir slurry into reserved liquid with remaining balsamic vinegar to make a finishing sauce and heat to thicken. Slide tarts to dinner plates and drizzle sauce over each.

<C To Cut Carb

<C Milk: reduce to 1 1/2 cups. <C Onion: reduce to 1 cup.
<C Cornmeal: reduce to 2/3 cup.

Per serving: 295 calories, 8 g fat, 3 g saturated fat, 8% calories from saturated fat, 40 g carbohydrate, 6 g dietary fiber, 356 mg sodium
Exchanges: 1 1/2 Starch, 1 Lean Meat, 3 Vegetable, 1 Fat

Low Carb
Per serving: 317 calories, 9 g fat, 3 g saturated fat, 9% calories from saturated fat, 40 g carbohydrate, 6 g dietary fiber, 374 mg sodium
Exchanges:1 Starch, 1 Lean Meat, 3 Vegetable, 1 Fat

Black Bean and Bacon Pizza

SERVING SIZE: 2 pieces, SERVES: 4

<C 1 10-inch pizza crust
3/4 cup pizza sauce
1/2 cup thinly sliced sweet onions
1/2 cup chopped bell pepper
1/2 cup sliced mushrooms
3/4 cup cooked or canned (rinsed and drained) black beans

1 cup grated reduced fat mozzarella cheese
2 oz pizza cut Canadian bacon
1 tsp crushed dried chilis (optional)

1 Preheat oven to 400°F. Bake the pizza crust 10 minutes.

2 Spread the sauce over the cooked crust. Scatter onions, peppers, mushrooms, and beans over the sauce. Sprinkle on the cheese and place the Canadian bacon around the edge. Top with crushed chilis and bake 15 minutes or until the crust is brown and the cheese bubbly.

3 Cut into 8 wedges and serve.

(Continued)

<c Pizza Crust: Substitute a Greek style Pita (thicker crust) and cut it in half carefully (horizontally), spray the inside surface lightly and bake briefly to only *just* crisp.

Per serving: 375 calories, 11 g fat, 4 g saturated fat, 10% calories from saturated fat, 47 g carbohydrate, 5 g dietary fiber, 1127 mg sodium
Exchanges: 2 1/2 Starch,1 Lean Meat,2 Vegetable,1 1/2 Fat

Low Carb

Per serving: 228 calories, 6 g fat, 3 g saturated fat, 12% calories from saturated fat, 26 g carbohydrate, 4 g dietary fiber, 832 mg sodium
Exchanges: 1 Starch,1 Lean Meat,2 Vegetable,1/2 Fat

Cioppino

SERVING SIZE: 1/6 of recipe, SERVES: 6

2 tsp non-aromatic olive oil
1 large sweet onion, chopped in
  1-inch dice
6 cloves garlic, bashed and
  chopped (2 Tbsp)
1 large red bell pepper, cut in
  1-inch dice
1 (12 oz) can tomato puree
6 Roma tomatoes, peeled, seeded,
  and chopped
2 cups nonalcoholic white wine
5 parsley stems, left whole

1 tsp dried oregano
1 tsp dried thyme
18 small clams, scrubbed
18 small mussels, scrubbed,
  and bearded
1 Dungeness crab, cooked
1 lb halibut steaks, cut in
  1 1/2-inch chunks
18 medium shrimp
  (21–30 per lb), peeled
  and deveined
1/2 cup chopped parsley

1 Heat oil in a 10-inch chef's pan. Sauté onion for 3 minutes until clear but not browned. Add garlic and red pepper, and sauté 3 minutes. Stir in tomato puree, chopped tomatoes, and white wine. Season with parsley stems, oregano, basil, and thyme. Simmer 25 minutes.

2 Bring 1/2 cup water to a boil in a chef's skillet with a lid. Toss in the clams and mussels. Cover and cook 3 minutes or until they open, discarding the ones that remain closed. Drain and set aside. Break the crab in half through the thin part of the body. You will have 2 body halves with the legs and claws attached. Separate the legs and claws so each one has a body segment attached.

3　Gently stir halibut into the sauce, and simmer 4 minutes. Add shrimp, crab, clams, and mussels, and simmer 8 minutes. Remove parsley stems. Stir in chopped parsley, and serve in bowls with a slice of good hearty Italian bread.

Per serving: 271 calories, 5 g fat, 1 g saturated fat, 3% calories from saturated fat, 20 g carbohydrate, 4 g dietary fiber, 496 mg sodium
Exchanges: 4 Very Lean Meat, 4 Vegetables, 1 Fat

Halibut with Mango Chutney

SERVING SIZE: 1 fillet, SERVES: 6

Mango Chutney

　1　fresh mango, peeled, pitted, and chopped (1 cup)
　2　green onions, white parts only, chopped (1/2 cup)
　1　Tbsp peeled, grated fresh ginger root
1/2　cup fruity white wine (I prefer nonalcoholic blanc)
1/4　tsp cayenne pepper

Halibut

1/4　tsp salt
1/4　tsp freshly ground black pepper
　6　(6 oz) halibut fillets

　6　cups arugula leaves, washed and spun dry
　2　Tbsp chopped parsley

1　Combine the mango, onion, ginger, wine, and cayenne in a small saucepan. Bring to a boil over medium heat, then reduce the heat and simmer for 10 minutes. Remove from the heat and set aside until ready to serve. You can make this ahead if you like.

2　Preheat the broiler. Season the fish with the salt and pepper then spray lightly with cooking oil spray. Place the fish on a broiler pan and spray lightly with cooking spray.

3　Broil the fillets for 4 minutes on each side, or until the flesh is no longer translucent and flakes easily.

4　Divide the arugula among 6 plates and lay a fish fillet on top of each. Heap a spoonful of mango chutney on the fish and sprinkle a little chopped parsley over all.

Per serving: 219 calories, 4 g fat, 1 g saturated fat, 4% calories from saturated fat, 8 g carbohydrate, 1 g dietary fiber, 194 mg sodium, 38 g protein
Exchanges: 5 Very Lean Meat, 1/2 Fruit, 1/2 Fat

Cabbage Rolls

SERVING SIZE: 2 cabbage rolls, SERVES: 6

Rolls

1 large green cabbage
1 tsp non-aromatic olive oil
2 cups finely chopped sweet onions
4 cloves garlic, bashed and chopped
6 oz leanest ground beef
6 oz ground white meat turkey
1/4 cup raw long-grain white rice

2 Tbsp tomato puree
1/4 cup beef broth
1/4 tsp dried dill weed
1/4 tsp salt
1/4 tsp freshly ground black pepper
2 Tbsp chopped parsley

Sauce

1 1/2 cups tomato puree
1 1/2 cups beef broth
1/4 cup packed brown sugar
1/2 cup cider vinegar
1/4 tsp freshly ground black pepper

1/4 tsp dried dill weed
1/4 tsp caraway seed
3 bay leaves
2 tsp arrowroot mixed with
 2 Tbsp water (slurry)

1. Preheat oven to 350°F. Spray 9-inch × 13-inch baking pan. Fill large pan with water, cover, and bring to a boil. Cut the core out of the cabbage and place head in boiling water to cook, covered for 10 minutes. Remove and plunge into a bowl of cold water to cool.

2. Heat oil in a skillet on medium high. Sauté onions 3 minutes or until translucent. Add garlic and cook 1 more minute. Place half of this mixture in a large bowl. Leave half in the pan to make the sauce. Combine ground beef, turkey, rice, tomato puree, broth, dill weed, salt, pepper, and parsley with the onion mixture in the bowl.

3. For sauce, pour tomato puree, broth, brown sugar, vinegar, pepper, dill weed, caraway, and bay leaves into the pan with the onion mixture, and simmer, about 15 minutes.

4. Drain cabbage and take off 12 large leaves. Cut out the center rib on each leaf with a v shape. Place a heaping Tbsp of filling on each leaf. Overlap the v, fold the sides in, and roll up to enclose the filling.

5. Set rolls side by side in the pan and pour sauce over all. Lay a piece of foil on top. Bake, covered, for 1 hour. Remove foil, and bake 1/2 hour longer.

6 Place cabbage rolls on 6 warm plates. Pour sauce from baking pan into a saucepan and thicken with arrowroot slurry. Spoon over rolls. Classically a broad buttered noodle would be served, but I prefer a mashed potato spiked with horseradish and a broiled half beefsteak tomato.

Per serving: 249 calories, 7 g fat, 2 g saturated fat, 7% of calories from saturated fat, 32 g carbohydrate, 6 g dietary fiber, 291 mg sodium
Exchanges: 1 Starch, 1 Lean Meat, 3 Vegetable, 1 Fat

Braised Rabbit with Pasta

SERVING SIZE: 1/6 of recipe, SERVES: 6

1 tsp non-aromatic olive oil
1 (3 lb) rabbit cut in 8 pieces, or 3/4 lb boneless, skinless chicken thighs
3 oz Canadian bacon, chopped
1 onion, finely chopped
2 cloves garlic, chopped
2 ribs celery, chopped
<C 3 carrots, peeled and chopped
1 fennel bulb, trimmed and chopped
1 red bell pepper, chopped
1/2 cup pitted, chopped Greek olives

1 (14 1/2 oz) can diced tomatoes in juice
2/3 cup plus 2 Tbsp nonalcoholic white wine
12 fresh sage leaves, chopped or 2 tsp dried sage
2 bay leaves
1/2 tsp salt
1 Tbsp arrowroot
2 Tbsp chopped fennel fronds
2 Tbsp grated Parmesan cheese
<C 12 oz dried fettucine pasta

1 Heat 1/2 tsp of the oil in a chef's pan on medium high. Brown the rabbit pieces on both sides, turning regularly. When golden brown, 5 to 10 minutes, remove to a plate.

2 Pour the remaining oil into the unwashed pan, add the bacon and cook 1 minute. Add the onions, cook another minute, then add the garlic, celery, carrots, fennel, and bell pepper and cook, stirring, 3 minutes. Stir in the olives, tomatoes, 2/3 cup of the wine, sage, bay, and salt and bring to a boil.

3 Lay the rabbit or chicken pieces on top of the vegetables cover and simmer 45 minutes. Remove the rabbit to a plate to cool slightly. Pull the meat off the bones, shredding it as you go. Combine the remaining wine with the arrowroot and stir into the vegetable sauce. Heat to thicken, add the rabbit and serve over pasta. Garnish with the chopped fennel and Parmesan cheese.

(*Continued*)

<C Carrots: reduce by two.
<C Pasta: reduce to 1 oz raw weight per serving. The pasta therefore becomes
   a garnish.

Per serving: 541 calories, 14 g fat, 3 g saturated fat, 5% calories from saturated
fat, 60 g carbohydrate, 6 g dietary fiber, 706 mg sodium
Exchanges: 3 Starch, 4 Lean Meat, 3 Vegetable

Low Carb

Per serving: 425 calories, 13 g fat, 3 g saturated fat, 7% calories from saturated
fat, 37 g carbohydrate, 5 g dietary fiber, 695 mg sodium
Exchanges: 1 1/2 Starch, 4 Lean Meat, 3 Vegetable

Orange Ginger Sauce for Broiled Fish

SERVING SIZE: 1 fillet, SERVES: 4

1 tsp non-aromatic olive oil
6 quarter-size slices fresh ginger
6 green onions, chopped
2 cloves garlic, bashed and chopped
1 cup orange juice
1 Tbsp cornstarch mixed with
2 Tbsp orange juice (slurry)

4 (6 oz) fillets white fish
   such as tilapia, cod, or halibut
1/4 tsp salt
1/4 tsp pepper
   olive oil pan spray
1 Tbsp chopped cilantro (optional)

1 Heat the oil in a skillet on medium high. Drop in the ginger and green
onions and sauté 2 minutes. Add the garlic and cook about 30 seconds to
release the flavorful oils, but don't allow to brown. Pour in the orange juice
and simmer 5 minutes. Strain into a small saucepan. Add the slurry and
bring to a boil to thicken and turn glossy.

2 Season the fish fillets with salt and pepper. Spray lightly with olive oil pan
spray and broil until the fish flakes. Different fish will require different
times, just watch it carefully so it doesn't overcook; 2 minutes per side for
thin fillets, 4 to 6 minutes for thicker ones.

3 Spoon the hot, glossy sauce over the fish fillet and serve.

Per serving: 232 calories, 3 g fat, 0 g saturated fat, 0% calories from saturated
fat, 9 g carbohydrate, 0 g dietary fiber, 282 mg sodium, 42 g protein
Exchanges: 6 Very Lean Meat, 1/2 Carbohydrate

Family Gathering Gumbo

SERVING SIZE: 1/8 of recipe, SERVES: 8

<C 1/4 cup all-purpose flour
<C   2 cups chopped onion
   3 cloves garlic, minced
   2 cups fresh or frozen cut okra
1 1/2 cups diced green bell pepper
   1 cup diced celery
 1/4 lb turkey sausage, sliced into
     1/4-inch pieces
   1 (8 oz) bottle clam juice

1 (14 oz) can low-sodium
   chicken broth
1 (15 oz) can no-salt-added
   chopped tomatoes, undrained
1/2 tsp ground red pepper
1/2 tsp black pepper
3/4 lb (12 oz) frozen, peeled and
    deveined, cooked shrimp
<C   4 cups cooked white rice

1 Preheat oven to 350°F. Toast flour in a shallow pan until brown, about one hour.

2 Spray the bottom and sides of a large pot with cooking spray. Heat pot on medium and add carefully washed onion, garlic, okra, bell pepper, and celery. Sauté, stirring often, until vegetables soften, about 15 minutes.

3 Stir in flour. Add sausage, clam juice, broth, tomatoes, and seasonings. Bring to a boil, then reduce heat to low and simmer uncovered for 45 minutes.

4 shrimp. Simmer on low heat for 8–10 minutes, until shrimp is warmed throughout. Serve warm over 1/2 cup of rice for each person.

<C To Cut Carb

<C Flour: reduce to 2 Tbsp.   <C Rice: reduce to 2 cups brown rice.
<C Onions: reduce to 1 cup cooked.

Per serving: 234 calories, 3 g fat, 1 g saturated fat, 2% calories from saturated fat, 37 g carbohydrate, 3 g dietary fiber, 359 mg sodium, 16 g protein, 92 mg cholesterol
Exchanges: 1 1/2 Starch, 1 Lean Meat, 2 Vegetable

Low Carb
Per serving: 170 calories, 3 g fat, 1 g saturated fat, 4% calories from saturated fat, 22 g carbohydrate, 3 g dietary fiber, 345 mg sodium, 15 g protein, 94 mg cholesterol
Exchanges: 1 Starch, 1 Lean Meat, 2 Vegetable

Bishop's Lamb Stew with Rosemary Dumplings

SERVING SIZE: 1/6 of recipe, SERVES: 6

2 1/2 lb lamb shoulder steaks
  1 tsp non-aromatic olive oil
1/2 large onion, chopped (1 cup)
  2 cloves garlic, bashed and chopped
  1 fennel bulb, trimmed and cut in
    1-inch dice
1 1/2 cups celery, cut in 1-inch dice
1 1/2 cups carrots, cut in 1-inch rounds

2 Tbsp tomato paste
1 cup nonalcoholic wine
3 cups lamb (page 469) or
  low-sodium chicken stock
1/4 tsp freshly ground black pepper
1/4 tsp salt
1 Tbsp arrowroot mixed with
  1/4 cup red wine (slurry)

Rosemary Dumplings

1 cup flour
1 tsp baking powder
1/4 tsp salt

1 tsp finely chopped rosemary, fresh or dried
1 Tbsp extra virgin olive oil
1/2 cup 1% milk

1 Preheat the oven to 375°F. Trim fat and bone from the lamb steaks. You should have 1 1/4 pounds of lean meat. Cut in 2-inch chunks. There will be lots of trim from which you can make a nice rich stock. See box for instructions.

2 Heat the oil in a chef's pan or large skillet on medium high. When it's nice and hot, add the pieces of lamb in one layer on the bottom. Brown on one side, about 5 minutes. Remove to a plate and set aside.

3 Return the pan to the heat and add the onions. Cook 1 minute then stir in the garlic, fennel, celery, and carrot. Sauté for 2 minutes or until the onion starts to wilt. Pull the vegetables to the side of the pan and add the tomato paste. Stir the paste until it darkens, 2 minutes, then combine with the vegetables. Deglaze the pan with the wine, scraping the brown flavorful bits off the bottom. Add the reserved meat, pepper, and salt. Pour in the stock, bring to a boil, cover and bake in the preheated oven 1 hour.

4 Just before the stew is done, start the dumplings. Combine the flour, baking powder, rosemary, and salt in a bowl. Add the oil to the milk and pour into the flour mixture. Mix gently with a fork to make a soft dough. Divide the dough into 6 pieces. Lay the dumplings on top of the stew, cover again, and bake 15 more minutes or until the dumplings are done.

5 To finish the stew, pull the dumplings to the side of the pan on a burner set at medium high. Stir the slurry into the liquid. It will thicken almost immediately. Serve on hot plates with a green vegetable such as lightly steamed baby bok choy.

Per serving: 305 calories, 10 g. fat, 3 g. saturated fat, 9% calories from saturated fat, 29 g. carbohydrates, 3 g. fiber, 420 mg. sodium
Exchanges: 1 Starch, 2 Lean Meat, 3 Vegetable, 1 Fat

Powerhouse Pizza

SERVING SIZE: 2 slices, SERVES: 4

<C 8-oz pizza crust, homemade or store bought
3/4 cup pizza sauce
1 cup grated low-fat mozzarella cheese
1 1/2 cups sliced mushrooms

1 medium zucchini, thinly sliced lengthwise or on the diagonal
1/2 cup roasted red peppers, roughly chopped
1/2 cup thinly sliced sweet onions
2 Tbsp grated Parmesan cheese

1 Preheat the oven to 400°F. Stretch the pizza dough to make a 12-inch circle. Place on a baking sheet and bake 10 minutes in the preheated oven.

2 Spread the pizza sauce over the crust. Scatter the grated cheese over the sauce and the sliced mushrooms on top of the cheese. Arrange the zucchini around the pizza and the red peppers and onions on top. Sprinkle the Parmesan over all. Give the whole thing a very light spray of olive oil.

3 Bake for 20 minutes or until the crust is nice and brown and the center bubbly.

<C To Cut Carb

<C Pizza crust: substitute a Greek style Pita (thicker crust) and cut it in half carefully (horizontally), spray the inside surface lightly and bake briefly to only *just* crisp.

Per serving: 296 calories, 10 g fat, 4 g saturated fat, 12% calories from saturated fat, 35 g carbohydrate, 2 g dietary fiber, 938 mg sodium
Exchanges: 2 Starch, 1 Lean Meat, 1 Vegetable, 1 Fat

Low Carb
Per serving: 189 calories, 6 g fat, 3 g saturated fat, 15% calories from saturated fat, 21 g carbohydrate, 2 g dietary fiber, 723 mg sodium
Exchanges: 1 Starch, 1 Lean Meat, 1 Vegetable, 1/2 Fat

Chicken and Pineapple Adobo

SERVING SIZE: 1/4 of recipe, SERVES: 4

1 tsp non-aromatic olive oil
1 Tbsp lemon juice
4 medium chicken thighs,
   skinned and trimmed of fat
1/8 tsp and 1/4 tsp salt
1/4 tsp freshly ground black pepper
1 small red pepper, cut in 1-inch squares
1 small green pepper, cut in 1-inch
   squares
2 cloves garlic, bashed and chopped
2 cups low-sodium chicken stock
   (page 463)

2 Turkish bay leaves
<C 2 cups fresh pineapple chunks
1 (16 oz) can Great Northern
   beans, drained and rinsed
2 Roma tomatoes, peeled and
   cut in chunks
1 Tbsp chopped fresh parsley
1/4 cup lime juice
2 tsp arrowroot plus
   4 tsp water (slurry)

1 Heat the oil and lemon juice in a large skillet on medium high. Season the chicken with 1/8 tsp salt and pepper. Fry one side for 2 minutes or until browned. Reduce heat to medium low, and turn the chicken. Add the pepper pieces and garlic, and sauté 2 more minutes being careful not to brown the garlic.

2 Pour stock into the pan, cover, and simmer for 20 minutes. Add pineapple and beans, and simmer 10 minutes more. Stir in tomato chunks, parsley, 2 Tbsp lime juice, and 1/4 tsp salt and 1/8 tsp pepper. Taste, and add more lime juice if you like (3 Tbsp was right for me, and it should be slightly sour). Pour in the slurry, stirring constantly until the liquid thickens, less than 30 seconds.

<C **To Cut Carb**
<C Pineapple: reduce to 1 cup.

Per serving: 295 calories, 9 g fat, 2 g saturated fat, 7% calories from saturated fat, 33 g carbohydrate, 7 g dietary fiber, 447 mg sodium
Exchanges: 1 Starch, 2 Lean Meat, 1 Vegetable, 1 Fruit, 1/2 Fat

Low Carb
Per serving: 276 calories, 9 g fat, 2 g saturated fat, 7% calories from saturated fat, 28 g carbohydrate, 7 g dietary fiber, 447 mg sodium
Exchanges: 1 Starch, 2 Lean Meat, 1 Vegetable, 1/2 Fruit, 1/2 Fat

Pho

Cook's Illustrated, *Copyright Stephanie Lyness*

SERVING SIZE: 1/4 of recipe, SERVES: 4

Broth

3 (1 lb) cans low-sodium
   chicken broth (6 cups)
4 cloves garlic, bashed
2-inch piece ginger root, sliced and
   bruised with a knife

2 star anise pods or
   1 tsp anise seeds (optional)
3 Tbsp Thai fish sauce
1 Tbsp soy sauce
2 tsp sugar

Noodle Soup

1 recipe broth
3/4 lb boneless, skinless
   chicken thighs
1/2 lb thick rice noodles
1/2 Napa cabbage, cut in half
   lengthwise and crosswise into
   thin strips

2 scallions, sliced
12 large mint leaves, thinly sliced
12 sprigs cilantro, thinly sliced
4 large basil leaves, thinly sliced
1 large lime, cut in 6 wedges

1 Combine the broth, garlic, ginger, anise, fish sauce, soy sauce, and sugar in a chef's pan or large saucepan. Bring to a boil, reduce the heat, and let simmer, covered, 10 minutes. Drop the chicken into the simmering broth and simmer 10 minutes longer. Remove the chicken and set aside. Strain the broth and return to the pan over low heat.

2 While the broth is simmering, bring water to a boil in a large pasta pan. Pull off the heat, add the noodles and soak until tender, 10 to 15 minutes. Drain and keep warm in a colander.

3 Slice the chicken into small pieces. Add the Napa cabbage to the simmering broth and stir. Divide the noodles among 4 warm bowls. Place the chicken on top of the noodles. Ladle the broth with the barely cooked cabbage over the top. Combine the fresh herbs, scallions and scatter on each serving. Serve with a lime wedge.

Per serving: 198 calories, 6 g fat, 2 g saturated fat, 9% calories from saturated fat, 16 g carbohydrate, 1 g dietary fiber, 692 mg sodium, 20 g protein
Exchanges: 1 Starch, 2 Lean Meat

Meatloaf

SERVING SIZE: 1/10 of recipe, SERVES: 10

Meatloaf

1/2 tsp non-aromatic olive oil
1 cup finely chopped onion
2 cloves garlic, bashed and chopped
1 medium carrot, peeled and finely diced or grated (1/2 cup)
1/4 cup finely diced celery
1/2 cup finely diced red bell pepper (1/2 large pepper)
1 tsp ground cumin
1 Tbsp mild chili powder

1/2 tsp allspice
1 tsp dried thyme
1 lb extra lean (9% fat) ground beef
1 lb extra lean ground turkey
1 Tbsp cocoa powder
1/2 cup ketchup
2/3 cup dry unseasoned breadcrumbs
3/4 cup egg substitute
1/2 cup evaporated skim milk
1 tsp salt

Sauce

1/2 tsp non-aromatic olive oil
1 clove garlic, bashed and chopped
1 cup ketchup
1 heaped Tbsp chopped parsley stems

1 cup nonalcoholic dry white wine
1 Tbsp chopped parsley
1/4 cup water

1. Preheat the oven to 350°F. Coat a large loaf pan with pan spray. Heat the oil in a small skillet on medium high. Sauté the onion 2 minutes then add the garlic and continue cooking for 1 more minute. Stir in the carrot, celery, red pepper, cumin, chili powder, allspice, and thyme. Cook 4 minutes or until the vegetables are tender. Set aside to cool.

2. Place the ground beef, turkey, cocoa, ketchup, bread crumbs, egg substitute, milk, and salt in a large bowl. Add the sautéed vegetables and mix thoroughly. Tip into a large loaf pan and bake 1 hour and 15 minutes or until the internal temperature reaches 150°F. Let set 15 minutes to finish cooking before serving. As it sits the internal temperature will rise from about 10°F to 160°F.

3. For the sauce, heat the oil in a small saucepan on medium high. Sauté the garlic and parsley stems 30 seconds. Add the ketchup and cook until it darkens and gets thick. Pour in the wine, parsley, and water and simmer 5 minutes or until syrupy. Spoon over the slices of meat loaf or pass at the table.

Per serving: 263 calories, 9 g fat, 3 g saturated fat, 10% calories from saturated fat, 20 g carbohydrate, 1 g dietary fiber, 745 mg sodium, 26 g protein
Exchanges: 1 Starch, 3 Lean Meat, 1 Vegetable

Chicken Braised in Orange Juice with Tart Cherries

SERVING SIZE: 1/4 of recipe, SERVES: 4

2 chicken breasts and
    2 legs with thighs
1/4 tsp salt
<C 1 cup orange juice
2 Tbsp lemon juice
<C 2 Tbsp honey
2 Tbsp chopped jalapeño chilis
1/4 cup dried tart cherries

1 Tbsp arrowroot mixed with
    2 Tbsp water (slurry)
<C 2 navel oranges, peeled and
    cut in segments
1 Tbsp chopped parsley
<C 3 cups cooked long-grain
    white rice

1 Preheat the oven to 350°F. Lay chicken pieces in a skillet skin side down, and sprinkle with salt. Combine orange juice, lemon juice, and honey, and pour over the top. Scatter chilis over all and bake, uncovered, for 15 minutes.

2 Add dried cherries, turn the chicken pieces, and bake 30 minutes, basting 2 or 3 times.

3 Place chicken on a plate, remove and discard the skin, and cover to keep warm. Pour the cooking liquid into a fat strainer and let the fat rise to the top. Pour the liquid back into the pan leaving the fat in the strainer. Stir the slurry into the liquid and heat to thicken. Return the chicken to the pan along with orange segments and parsley. Serve over rice.

<C To Cut Carb

<C Orange juice: reduce to 1/2 cup.
<C Honey: reduce to 1 Tbsp.
<C Oranges: reduce to 1.
<C Rice: reduce to 1 cup.

Per serving: 463 calories, 6 g fat, 2 g saturated fat, 3% calories from saturated fat, 67 g carbohydrate, 3 g dietary fiber, 228 mg sodium
Exchanges: 2 1/2 Starch, 4 Very Lean Meat, 2 Fruit, 1/2 Fat

Low Carb
Per serving: 312 calories, 6 g fat, 2 g saturated fat, 3% calories from saturated fat, 32 g carbohydrate, 2 g dietary fiber, 227 mg sodium
Exchanges: 1 Starch, 4 Very Lean Meat, 1 Fruit, 1/2 Fat

Brunswick Stew

SERVING SIZE: 1/6 of recipe, SERVES: 6

3 1/2 lb frying chicken or 2 boneless skinless breasts and 2 hindquarters
  1 tsp non-aromatic olive oil, divided
  1 large sweet onion, cut in 1-inch cubes (generous 2 cups)
  3 ribs celery cut in 1/4-inch slices (1 1/2 cups)
  3 oz Canadian bacon cut the same size as the celery
  1 red bell pepper cut the same
  2 cups canned, crushed tomatoes
  1 cup low-sodium chicken stock (page 463)
  1 Tbsp Worcestershire sauce
1/4 tsp cayenne pepper
  1 cup frozen corn kernels
  1 cup frozen baby lima beans
  1 Tbsp arrowroot mixed with 2 Tbsp stock or water (slurry)
1/4 cup chopped fresh parsley
1/4 cup chopped fresh basil

1 If you are using a whole chicken, cut off the legs with the thighs and the breasts. Use the carcass and wings for stock. Remove the skin from all the pieces. Separate the legs from the thighs and bone the thigh, leaving the bone in the leg. Remove the skin and bone from the breast pieces. Bones, fat, and skin will all help to make a flavorful stock. Cut the meat into 1 1/2-inch chunks.

2 Heat 1/2 tsp of the oil in a 10 1/2-inch chef's pan on medium high. Sauté the onion 3 minutes or until starting to turn translucent. Add the celery, Canadian bacon, and red bell pepper and cook 3 more minutes. Remove to a plate and without washing the pan, add the remaining 1/2 tsp oil and heat. When the pan is nice and hot, toss in the thigh meat and legs to brown 2 minutes. Add the breast meat and brown 1 to 2 minutes more.

3 Pour in the tomatoes, stock, and Worcestershire sauce. Add the cooked vegetables and cayenne. Bring to a boil, reduce the heat, cover, and simmer 35 minutes or until the chicken is tender. Add the lima beans and corn and cook 12 minutes more or until the beans are tender. Stir in the slurry and heat to thicken. Add the parsley and basil and you are ready to serve.

Per serving: 260 calories, 6 g fat, 2 g saturated fat, 7% calories from saturated fat, 21 g carbohydrate, 3 g dietary fiber, 362 mg sodium
Exchanges: 1 Starch, 3 Lean Meat, 1 Vegetable

Bean and Vegetable Sauté

SERVING SIZE: 1/4 of recipe, SERVES: 4

> 1 tsp olive oil
>
> <C 1 1/2 cups chopped onion
>
> 3 cloves garlic
>
> 1 (1 lb) package frozen mixed vegetables
>
> seasoning of your choice (1 Tbsp curry powder, chili powder, or Italian herbs)
>
> 1 cup low-sodium chicken or vegetable broth (page 463, 473)
>
> <C 1 (15 oz) can no-salt-added beans of your choice, drained and rinsed
>
> 1 tsp arrowroot or cornstarch mixed with 1 Tbsp water (slurry)

Garnish

4 Tbsp currants with the curry or

4 Tbsp chopped cilantro with the chili powder or

4 Tbsp grated Parmesan cheese with the Italian herbs

Directions

1 Heat the oil in a high-sided skillet on medium high. Sauté the onion 3 minutes then add the garlic and continue cooking 2 minutes more. Add the frozen vegetables, seasoning, broth, and beans.

2 Bring to a boil, reduce the heat, and simmer 5 minutes. Stir in the slurry and cook 30 seconds. Serve topped with the garnish of your choice. A slice of rustic whole grain bread will complete a hearty lunch.

<C **To Cut Carb**

<C Onions: reduce to 1 cup.

<C Beans: reduce to 3/4 cup of the drained weight.

Per serving: 247 calories, 2 g fat, 0 g saturated fat, 0% calories from saturated fat, 49 g carbohydrate, 11 g dietary fiber, 103 mg sodium
Exchanges: 2 1/2 Starch, 1 Vegetable, 1/2 Fruit

Low-Carb

Per serving: 192 calories, 2 g fat, 0 g saturated fat, 0% calories from saturated fat, 38 g carbohydrate, 8 g dietary fiber, 101 mg sodium
Exchanges: 1 1/2 Starch, 1 Vegetable, 1/2 Fruit

Mexican Stuffed Peppers

SERVING SIZE: 1 pepper, SERVES: 4

4 red bell peppers
1 tsp non-aromatic olive oil
<C 1 cup chopped onions
3 cloves garlic
1 jalapeño or chipotle chili, seeds removed if you like it mild, chopped
1 Tbsp chili powder

1/2 tsp cumin
1 (15 1/4 oz) can diced tomatoes in juice
<C 1 cup cooked white rice
<C 1 cup fresh, frozen or canned corn
<C 1 cup cooked or canned pinto beans

1 Preheat oven to 350°F. Cut the tops off the peppers, core, and set aside.

2 Heat the oil in a skillet and cook the onion until it starts to wilt, 2 minutes. Add the garlic, jalapeño, chili powder, and cumin. Fry 2 more minutes. Stir in the tomatoes, rice, corn, and beans. Cook until the liquid disappears and the stuffing holds together. Spoon into the prepared peppers and set into a baking dish.

3 Bake 1 hour or until the peppers are tender.

<C To Cut Carb

<C Onions: reduce to 1/2 cup.
<C White rice: reduce to 1/2 cup.
<C Corn: reduce to 1/2 cup.
<C Pinto beans: reduce to 1/2 cup.

+> Mushrooms: small white, chop fine to make 1 cup and add at the end of Step 2.

Per serving: 242 calories, 3 g fat, 0 g saturated fat, 0% calories from saturated fat, 51 g carbohydrate, 11 g dietary fiber, 243 mg sodium
Exchanges: 2 Starch, 4 Vegetable

Low Carb
Per serving: 168 calories, 2 g fat, 0 g saturated fat, 0% calories from saturated fat, 35 g carbohydrate, 8 g dietary fiber, 241 mg sodium
Exchanges: 1 Starch, 4 Vegetable

Resolve-to-Double-the-Serving Stew

SERVING SIZE: 1/6 of recipe, SERVES: 6

2 Tbsp all-purpose flour
3/4 tsp salt
1/2 tsp ground black pepper
1 lb lean beef stew meat, cut into 1-inch cubes
1 Tbsp vegetable oil
3 cups low-fat, low-sodium beef broth, plus more as needed
2 medium onions

2 stalks celery
2 medium potatoes
2 medium turnips
4 carrots
1/2 tsp dried thyme
2 cloves garlic, chopped
1/2 cup fresh parsley, chopped

1 In a plastic bag, combine flour, salt, and pepper. Add meat and shake to coat. Heat oil in large saucepan or Dutch oven. Add meat and brown. Prepare the vegetables by cutting one onion, two celery stalks, one potato, one turnip and two carrots into large chunks. Add the vegetables to the meat along with the garlic and thyme. Stir in broth and bring to boil. Reduce heat and cover. Simmer for about 40 minutes or until meat is tender.

2 While meat is cooking, prepare remaining vegetables by cutting the onion, celery, potato, turnip, and carrot into 1-inch cubes. Remove simmered vegetables (onion, celery, potatoes, turnips, carrots) and whiz in a blender until smooth. Return vegetable puree to pot. Thin with beef broth or water, if necessary. Add remaining uncooked onions, celery, potato, turnips, and carrots to the pot. Bring to simmer and cover. Cook for an additional 30 minutes or until vegetables are tender. Add parsley just before serving.

Per serving: 308 calories, 7 g fat, 2 g saturated fat, 10% calories from saturated fat, 15 g carbohydrate, 2 g dietary fiber, 572 mg sodium, 20 g protein, 45 mg cholesterol
Exchanges: 1/2 Starch, 2 Lean Meat, 2 Vegetable

Beef Stew with Pears

SERVING SIZE: 1/4 of recipe, SERVES: 4

	1/2	lb beef bottom round, cut in 1/2-inch pieces
	1 1/2	tsp non-aromatic olive oil, divided
<C	2	cups thickly sliced onions
	5	Tbsp tomato paste
	2	cloves garlic, bashed and chopped
	1/4	cup nonalcoholic red wine
	3	cups low sodium beef broth
<C	1	lb carrots, peeled and cut into 1-inch pieces
<C	12	tiny red potatoes
<C	2	pears, or chayote squash peeled and cut in 1-inch pieces
<C	2	cups frozen peas
	2	Tbsp cornstarch or arrowroot mixed with 1/4 cup nonalcoholic red wine (slurry)
	2	Tbsp chopped fresh parsley
	1/4	tsp freshly ground black pepper
	1/4	tsp salt

1 Heat 1 tsp of the oil on medium high in a high-sided skillet. Dry the meat on paper towels and brown the meat on one side without disturbing; about 3 minutes. Remove and set aside.

2 In the same skillet, heat the remaining oil and cook the onions 1 minute. Add the tomato paste and cook until it darkens. Stir in the garlic and cook another minute. Add the reserved meat, wine, and broth. Bring to a boil, reduce the heat, and simmer 30 minutes or until the meat is nearly tender.

3 Add the carrots, potatoes, and pears or chayote and simmer 30 minutes longer, or until the vegetables are tender. Stir in the peas and slurry and bring to a boil to thicken and become glossy. Add the parsley, pepper, and salt.

<C **To Cut Carb**

<C Onions: reduce to 1 cup.

<C Carrots: reduce to 8 oz.

<C Potatoes: reduce to 8 small.

<C Pears: reduce to only 1.

<C Peas: reduce to 1 cup.

+> Increase vegetable of your choice. You'll need to increase with low-carb plants by 2 cups.

Per serving: 466 calories, 6 g fat, 1 g saturated fat, 0% calories from saturated fat, 78 g carbohydrate, 14 g fiber, 387 mg sodium
Exchanges: 3 Starch, 1 Lean Meat, 5 Vegetables, 1/2 Fruit, 1/2 Fat

Low Carb

Per serving: 343 calories, 6 g fat, 1 g saturated fat, 0% calories from saturated fat, 50 g carbohydrate, 9 g dietary fiber, 337 mg sodium
Exchanges: 2 Starch, 1 Lean Meat, 3 Vegetable, 1/2 Fruit. 1/2 Fat

Desserts

Meringue Islands with Plum Sauce

SERVING SIZE: 1/6 of recipe, SERVES: 6

Meringue

1/4 cup plus 6 Tbsp granulated sugar
  4 large egg whites, at room
    temperature
1/4 tsp cream of tartar

1/2 tsp vanilla extract
 12 low-fat ladyfingers or Italian
    savoiardi biscuits

Plum Sauce

    4 mammees or dark red plums, such as Friar (1 lb)
    1 cup slightly sweet white wine (I prefer nonalcoholic Ariel blanc)
1 1/2 Tbsp brown sugar
    1 tsp fresh lemon juice

Garnish

Fresh mint leaves

To Prepare the Meringue

1. Make sure the egg whites are at room temperature before beginning the recipe. Preheat the oven to 350°F and position a rack in the center of the oven. Spray a 6-cup capacity loaf pan (either glass or nonstick metal) with cooking spray.

2. Melt 1/4 cup of the sugar in a small saucepan over medium-high heat, shaking the pan occasionally, until the sugar melts and turns brown, about 3 minutes. Pour the caramel into the bottom of the prepared loaf pan and quickly tip the pan back and forth until the bottom is completely covered. The caramel will harden almost immediately.

3. Make sure the mixing bowl and whip are perfectly clean and grease-free. Beat the whites on low speed until frothy, then add the cream of tartar. Increase the speed to high and beat until soft peaks begin to form. Gradually sprinkle in the sugar, 1 Tbsp at a time, until all 6 Tbsp have been added. Beat on high speed until stiff peaks form, about 2 minutes. Beat in the vanilla.

4 Spread a third of the meringue over the caramel in the bottom of the prepared baking pan. Trim the ends of 6 of the ladyfingers or savoiardis so that
they will fit across the width of the pan. Lay them side-by-side on top of the
meringue layer. Spread half the remaining meringue over the cookies, using
a rubber spatula to fill the crevices between the cookies. Rap the loaf pan on
the counter to release any air bubbles. Repeat the cookie layer with the
remaining 6 whole cookies, which should fit across the top of the pan without cutting. Spread the remaining meringue over the cookies for the final
layer, again pressing into the crevices and tapping to release air.

5 Place a large baking pan in the oven and partially fill with boiling water to
create a water bath for the meringue. Set the loaf pan in the center of the
baking pan and adjust the water level to reach halfway up the sides. Bake
the meringue for 30 minutes, then take a look in the oven. If the top is
getting too brown, cover loosely with foil. Bake for an additional
15 minutes, for a total of 45 minutes.

6 Remove the pan from the oven and run a wet knife along the sides of the
pan to loosen the meringue. Invert onto a large plate and allow to cool.
When ready to serve, cut into 6 pieces with a wet knife.

To Prepare the Plum Sauce

7 Cut the plums into quarters and discard the pits. Combine the plums and
wine in a large saucepan and roughly mash the fruit with a fork. Bring the
mixture to a boil over high heat. Continue to mash the plums occasionally
while the sauce is coming to the boil, which should take 2 or 3 minutes.
Reduce the heat and simmer, uncovered, for about 15 minutes.

8 Pour the sauce into a blender and process for 1 minute. Press the purée
through a strainer into a medium saucepan, discarding any remaining pulp.
Add the brown sugar and lemon juice and cook over low heat until the
sugar dissolves.

To Serve

9 Spoon a puddle of plum sauce onto a dessert plate and top with a slice of the
baked meringue. Garnish with mint leaves.

Per serving: 194 calories, 1 g fat, 0 g saturated fat, 0% of calories from saturated
fat, 44 g carbohydrate, 1 g dietary fiber, 58 mg sodium
Exchanges: 3 Carbohydrate

Apple and Pear Crisp

SERVING SIZE: 1 piece, SERVES: 9

Fruit

3 cooking apples (Jonagold, Winesap, Northern Spy, or other tart flavorful apple)

3 Bosc pears

<c 1/2 cup golden raisins

2 cups nonalcoholic fruity white wine (I like Ariel blanc)

1/8 tsp ground cloves

1/2 cup low-fat vanilla yogurt

Topping

1/2 cup old-fashioned oats

1/2 cup low-fat graham crackers crumbs, or flour

3 Tbsp sliced almonds

<c 1/2 cup brown sugar

1 tsp cinnamon

1/4 tsp nutmeg

3 Tbsp butter flavored stick margarine

Directions

1 Preheat the oven to 350°F. Peel and core the apples and cut into eighths. Peel and core the pears and cut into quarters. Place in a large skillet, add the raisins, wine, and cloves, and cover with a piece of waxed paper cut to fit. Bring to a boil, lower the heat and poach gently 15 minutes or until tender but not mushy. Drain, reserving the liquid, and lay the fruit in an 8-inch × 8-inch baking dish.

2 Combine the oats, almonds, graham cracker crumbs, sugar, cinnamon and nutmeg in a bowl. Stir in the margarine until the mixture holds together in a crumble. Scatter over the fruit and bake, uncovered, in the preheated oven 30 minutes or until golden and crisp on top.

3 Pour the reserved liquid back into the skillet and boil vigorously until reduced to about 2 Tbsp. Take off the heat and stir in the yogurt. Cut the crisp into 9 pieces and serve with the yogurt sauce.

<c **To Cut Carb**

<c Raisins: reduce to 1/4 cup.

<c Brown sugar: reduce to 1 Tbsp and add 2 Tbsp Splenda.

Per serving: 226 calories, 6 g fat, 1 g saturated fat, 4% calories from saturated fat, 41 g carbohydrate, 4 g dietary fiber, 72 mg sodium
Exchanges: 1/2 Fat, 3 Carbohydrate

Low Carb
Per serving: 175 calories, 6 g fat, 1 g saturated fat, 5% calories from saturated fat, 30 g carbohydrate, 3 g dietary fiber, 90 mg sodium
Exchanges: 1/2 Fat, 2 Carbohydrate

Blackberry Warm Egg Custard

SERVING SIZE: 1/8 of recipe, SERVES: 8

1 lb fresh or frozen and thawed blackberries
1 1/2 cups nonalcoholic fruity white wine
3 Tbsp real maple syrup
1/4 tsp almond extract
1/4 tsp vanilla extract
2 Tbsp cornstarch mixed with 1/4 cup nonalcoholic fruity white wine
1/2 cup sugar
1 cup egg substitute

1 Divide 1 1/4 cups of the blackberries among 8 wine glasses (10 oz). Press the rest of the blackberries through a sieve. Discard the seeds and set the juice aside.

2 Bring the wine to a boil in a medium saucepan. Add the maple syrup, almond, and vanilla extracts. Stir in the slurry, bring back to a boil, and stir 30 seconds while it thickens. Set aside to cool slightly.

3 Heat a small amount of water in a medium saucepan. Set a round copper or other metal bowl on top to create a double boiler. Reduce the heat to a simmer. Pour the sugar and egg substitute into the bowl and beat over the simmering water until frothy, thick, creamy, and more than tripled in volume, about 3 minutes.

4 Pour the wine syrup into the egg mixture in a thin stream, whisking all the time. Add 3/4 of the blackberry puree, mixing well. Spoon the pudding over the blackberries in the glasses. Swirl the remaining puree on top of each dessert.

Per serving: 124 calories, 0 g fat, 0 g saturated fat, 0% calories from saturated fat, 27 g carbohydrate, 3 g fiber, 55 mg sodium
Exchanges: 2 Carbohydrate

Fresh Berries with Sweet Vinegar Sauce

SERVING SIZE: 1/4 of recipe, SERVES: 4

Sweet Vinegar Sauce

1/4 cup raspberry vinegar or balsamic vinegar
1/4 cup sugar
3 drops vanilla extract

1/4 cup plain, nonfat yogurt
1 cup blueberries
1 cup blackberries

1 Combine vinegar and sugar in a small saucepan and bring to a boil. Boil for 4 minutes, stirring often. (Be prepared—the mixture will smell unpleasant as some of the vinegar's acid boils off, and it will reduce a little bit.) Turn off heat. Add vanilla, and slowly whisk in yogurt. Toss with berries and serve.

Per serving: 115 calories, 0 g fat, 0 g saturated fat, 0% calories from saturated fat, 27 g carbohydrate, 3 g dietary fiber, 22 mg sodium, 2 g protein, 0 mg cholesterol
Exchanges: 1 Fruit, 1 Carbohydrate

Molded Rhubarb Strawberry Dessert

SERVING SIZE: 1 slice or square, SERVES: 8

1 lb rhubarb, fresh or frozen
1/4 cup orange juice
5 Tbsp brown sugar

2 packets unflavored gelatin
1 cup strawberries, sliced

1 Cut the rhubarb in 1/2-inch chunks or use frozen rhubarb as is. Place in a saucepan and pour on the orange juice. Bring to a boil, reduce the heat, and simmer 8 minutes or until soft. Stir in the brown sugar.

2 Sprinkle the gelatin over 1/2 cup cold water to soften for 10 minutes. Stir into the hot fruit to dissolve. Add the strawberries and mix gently. Pour into a mold or glass 8-inch × 8-inch baking pan and chill.

3 Unmold the dessert by setting in hot water for 30 seconds or until it loosens. Tip onto a plate. Cut into 8 wedges and serve. If you've chosen the glass pan, cut into 8 squares and serve.

Per serving: 60 calories, 0 g fat, 0 g saturated fat, 0% calories from saturated fat, 13 g carbohydrate, 1 g dietary fiber, 8 mg sodium, 2 g protein
Exchanges: 1/2 Fruit, 1/2 Carbohydrate

Baked Apples

SERVING SIZE: 1 apple, SERVES: 4

<C 4 baking apples (Jonagold, Northern Spy, Rome, or Winesap)
<C 1 cup apple juice or water
     1/2 tsp ground cinnamon
     1/4 tsp allspice
          pinch ground cloves
<C 1/4 cup brown sugar
     1/4 cup low-fat vanilla yogurt

1 Preheat the oven to 350°F. Core the apples with a spoon or apple corer. Set in a baking pan and pour on the juice or water. Lay a sheet of aluminum foil on top and bake 40 to 50 minutes or until the apples are tender.

2 Set the apples on dessert plates and pour the juice into a small saucepan. Stir in the cinnamon, allspice, cloves, and brown sugar. Bring to a boil and cook down until the sauce is a thick syrup. Pour over the apples and serve with a dollop of the yogurt.

<C To Cut Carb

<C Apples: choose smaller apples.
<C Apple juice: use water instead.
<C Brown sugar: reduce to 1 Tbsp and add 2 Tbsp Splenda.

Per serving: 186 calories, 1 g fat, 0 g saturated fat, 0% calories from saturated fat, 47 g carbohydrate, 4 g dietary fiber, 18 mg sodium
Exchanges: 2 Fruit, 1 Carbohydrate

Low Carb
Per serving: 93 calories, 1 g fat, 0 g saturated fat, 0% calories from saturated fat, 23 g carbohydrate, 3 g dietary fiber, 12 mg sodium
Exchanges: 1 1/2 Fruit

Boston Cream Pie

SERVING SIZE: 1 slice, SERVES: 8

Sponge Cake

1/3 cup sifted cake flour
3 Tbsp cornstarch
3 large eggs at room temperature
3 large egg whites at room
    temperature

1 tsp non-aromatic olive oil
1 tsp vanilla extract
1 tsp vanilla extract
<C 1/2 cup + 1 Tbsp granulated sugar
1/2 tsp cream of tartar

Filling

1 cup vanilla low-fat yogurt cheese
    (page 475)
1/3 cup toasted sliced almonds

<C 1 Tbsp maple syrup
1/3 cup toasted sliced almonds

Glaze

<C 1 cup powdered sugar
3 Tbsp Dutch cocoa

<C 3 Tbsp strong coffee
+> 1/2 tsp vanilla

1 Preheat the oven to 425°F. Spray two 9-inch cake pans. Cut parchment or wax paper to fit the bottom of each, spray, and dust with flour.

2 Combine the flour and cornstarch in a small bowl. Using 2 mixing bowls, place the 3 egg whites in one and 2 of the whole eggs in the other. Separate the third egg and put the yolk with the whole eggs and the white with the whites, where you now have 4 egg whites. Add the oil, vanilla, and 1/2 cup of the sugar to the whole eggs and beat for a full 5 minutes. The mixture will be thick and creamy. Fold in the flour mixture half at a time.

3 Beat the egg whites, adding the cream of tartar when foamy. Add the remaining Tbsp of sugar when soft peaks form and continue beating until stiff and shiny. Spoon 1/4 of the beaten whites into the batter and stir to lighten. Fold in the rest. Divide between the 2 prepared pans. Bake for 6 minutes in the preheated oven or until set and golden in color. Cool for 10 minutes on a rack then loosen and remove from the pans to cool completely.

4 While the cake is cooling make the filling and the glaze. Stir the yogurt cheese and maple syrup together to mix thoroughly. Combine the powdered sugar, cocoa, coffee, and vanilla in a small bowl. Cover so it doesn't form a crust.

5 To assemble the pie, lay one of the cake layers on a serving plate. Cover with the filling and scattered toasted almonds. Lay the second cake layer on top. Drizzle on the glaze starting in the center. Try to keep most of it on top of the cake so when you cut it, the glaze will dribble attractively down the sides of each wedge.

<C **To Cut Carb (and caffeine)** ═══════════════

<C Sponge cake sugar: reduce to 1/4 cup and add 1/4 cup Splenda.

<C Maple syrup: replace with 1 Tbsp Splenda.

<C Glaze sugar: replace with 3/4 cup Splenda.

<C Strong coffee: replace with water.

+> Vanilla: increase by 1/2 teaspoon.

Per serving: 262 calories, 5 g fat, 2 g saturated fat, 5% calories from saturated fat, 48 g carbohydrate, 1 g dietary fiber, 73 mg sodium
Exchanges: 1 Fat, 3 Carbohydrate

Low Carb
Per serving: 181 calories, 5 g fat, 2 g saturated fat, 8% calories from saturated fat, 26 g carbohydrate, 1 g dietary fiber, 70 mg sodium
Exchanges: 1 Fat, 2 Carbohydrate

Blueberry and Chocolate Pudding

SERVING SIZE: 1/4 of recipe, SERVES: 4

1 package nonfat, sugar-free chocolate pudding mix

2 cups fresh or frozen unsweetened blueberries

2 Tbsp toasted sliced almonds

1/4 cup low-fat vanilla yogurt

1 Prepare the chocolate pudding according to package directions with nonfat milk. When it has thickened, stir in the blueberries and almonds.

2 Divide among 4 dessert dishes, add a dollop of vanilla yogurt and serve.

Per serving: 167 calories, 3 g fat, 0 g saturated fat, 0% calories from saturated fat, 27 g carbohydrates, 3 g dietary fiber, 404 mg sodium
Exchanges: 1/2 Fat, 2 Carbohydrate

Warm Apples and Oranges in Syrup

SERVING SIZE: 1/4 of recipe, SERVES: 4

2 red apples
2 navel oranges
1/2 cup unsweetened orange juice

1/2 cup unsweetened apple juice
1 Tbsp arrowroot or cornstarch
1/4 tsp ground cinnamon

1 Peel the oranges and pull them apart into sections. Quarter the apples, core, and cut in half. The fruit pieces should be about the same size.

2 Combine the juices in a saucepan and stir in the arrowroot or cornstarch before it gets warm. Bring to a boil and stir until thickened, about 30 seconds. Add the fruit and cinnamon and heat through.

Per serving: 107 calories, 0 g fat, 0 g saturated fat, 0% calories from saturated fat, 27 g carbohydrate, 4 g dietary fiber, 2 mg sodium
Exchanges: 2 Carbohydrate

Pumpkin Cheesecake Pudding

SERVING SIZE: 1/6 of recipe, SERVES: 6

1 packet unflavored gelatin
1/2 cup cold water
3 cups canned puréed pumpkin or
    frozen winter squash
3/4 cup brown sugar

1 1/2 cups low-fat cottage cheese
1/2 tsp cinnamon
1/2 tsp ground ginger
1/4 tsp ground cloves
3/4 cup low-fat plain yogurt

1 Soften the gelatin in the cold water in a small saucepan for 1 minute. Turn the heat to medium high and heat to dissolve completely.

2 Pour into a food processor with the pumpkin, brown sugar, cottage cheese, cinnamon, ginger, and cloves. Blend until smooth. Stir in the yogurt and pour into 6 individual custard cups.

3 Chill in the refrigerator until set.

Per serving: 175 calories, 1 g fat, 1 g saturated fat, 7% calories from saturated fat, 31 g carbohydrate, 4 g dietary fiber, 267 mg sodium
Exchanges: 1 Very Lean Meat, 2 Carbohydrate

Mango Yogurt Dessert

SERVING SIZE: 1/4 of recipe, SERVES: 4

    2 mangoes, peeled and cut in chunks   1 Tbsp chopped pistachio nuts
<C 2 cups low-fat vanilla yogurt

1. Mash the mango pieces with a fork. Stir into the yogurt. Divide among 4 dessert dishes and scatter pistachio nuts over the top. (You can also try this with 1 cup soaked dried apricots or 2 cut up fresh pears.)

<C **To Cut Carb**
<C Vanilla yogurt: replace with plain non-fat yogurt and add 2 Tbsp of Splenda.

Per serving: 197 calories, 3 g fat, 1 g saturated fat, 5% calories from saturated fat, 39 g carbohydrates, 2 g dietary fiber, 85 mg sodium
Exchanges: 1/2 Fat, 2 1/2 Carbohydrate

Low Carb
Per serving: 157 calories, 2 g fat, 0 g saturated fat, 0% calories from saturated fat, 31 g carbohydrate, 2 g dietary fiber, 103 mg sodium
Exchanges: 1 1/2 Fruit, 1/2 Fat-Free Milk, 1/2 Fat

Fruit on a Stick

SERVING SIZE: 1 popsicle, SERVES: 8

    2 nectarines
    2 cups orange juice
1 1/2 cup raspberries

1. Remove the seeds from the nectarines and cut in chunks. Puree with the orange juice in a blender.

2. Pour into plastic popsicle molds or ice cube trays. Divide the whole raspberries among the molds and freeze.

3. Lots of other combinations are possible depending on your family's preferences. You could try pears pureed in apple juice with blueberries, or how about a banana pureed in pineapple juice with grapes?

Per serving: 50 calories, 0 g fat, 0 g saturated fat, 0% calories from saturated fat, 12 g carbohydrate, 2 g dietary fiber, 1 mg sodium
Exchanges: 1 Fruit

Broiled Apricots with Almonds

SERVING SIZE: 4 apricot halves, SERVES: 4

4 tsp brown sugar
1/4 tsp ground cardamom
8 plump fresh apricots, pitted and halved

4 tsp sliced almonds
1/2 cup low-fat yogurt

1 Preheat your broiler. Combine the brown sugar with the cardamom. Lay the apricot halves on a broiler pan and sprinkle with the sugar mixture. Scatter the almonds over the top.

2 Broil about 6 inches away from the heat source until the sugar bubbles and the almonds turn brown, about 2 or 3 minutes. Watch carefully because the almonds turn black in the wink of an eye.

3 Serve 4 halves on each of 4 plates with a dollop of vanilla yogurt.

Per serving: 89 calories, 2 g fat, 0 g saturated fat, 0% calories from saturated fat, 17 g carbohydrate, 2 g dietary fiber, 23 mg sodium
Exchanges: 1/2 Fat, 1 Carbohydrate

Broiled Bananas with an Orange & Apple Sauce

SERVING SIZE: 1/4 of recipe, SERVES: 4

2 firm bananas, peeled
2 navel oranges, peeled and segmented
3/4 cup unsweetened orange juice

3/4 cup unsweetened apple juice
1/4 tsp cardamom
1 Tbsp arrowroot mixed with 2 Tbsp water (slurry)

1 Preheat the broiler. Lay the whole, peeled bananas on the sprayed rack of the broiler pan. Set the pan about 3 inches away from the element and broil for 10 minutes or until golden brown on top.

2 While the bananas are broiling, pour 1/4 cup of the combined juices into a high-sided skillet on high heat. When it has reduced down to syrupy bubbles, add the orange segments and toss to coat.

3 Pour in the rest of the juice and stir in the cardamom. Bring to a boil and stir in the slurry. When the bananas are ready, slice each one into 6 pieces and add to the sauce. Serve warm.

Per serving: 135 calories, 1 g fat, 0 g saturated fat, 0% calories saturated fat, 34 g carbohydrate, 3 g dietary fiber, 2 mg sodium, 2 g protein
Exchanges: 2 1/2 Fruit

Cherry Custard

SERVING SIZE: 1/4 of recipe, SERVES: 4

2 cups pitted fresh or frozen sweet cherries (no sugar added)	<C 1/4 cup brown sugar
<C 1 cup evaporated fat-free milk	1/2 tsp almond extract
<C 1 cup 2% milk	1 cup egg substitute

1 Preheat the oven to 325°F. Divide the cherries among 4 8-oz custard cups. Combine the evaporated milk, 2% milk, and sugar in a small saucepan, stirring to dissolve the sugar. Take off the heat, stir in the almond extract and egg substitute. Pour over the cherries.

2 Set the bowls in a baking pan and add hot water to come 3/4 of the way up the sides. Bake in the preheated oven 1 hour or until firm. Cool and serve.

3 You can slip these out of the bowls onto dessert plates to dress them up. Garnish with fresh mint leaves or edible flowers such as pansies, bachelor buttons, or primroses.

<C To Cut Carb

<C Evaporated milk: reduce to 2/3 cup.	<C Brown sugar: reduce to 1 Tbsp and add 2 Tbsp Splenda.
<C 2% milk: reduce to 2/3 cup.	

Per serving: 216 calories, 2 g fat, 1 g saturated fat, 4% calories from saturated fat, 37 g carbohydrate, 2 g dietary fiber, 230 mg sodium
Exchanges: 1/2 Fat, 2 1/2 Carbohydrates

Low Carb
Per serving: 153 calories, 2 g fat, 1 g saturated fat, 4% calories from saturated fat, 24 g carbohydrate, 2 g dietary fiber, 190 mg sodium
Exchanges: 1/2 Fat, 1 1/2 Carbohydrates

Greek Islands Bread Pudding

SERVING SIZE: 1 wedge, SERVES: 6

<C   3 whole-wheat, Greek style, pitas
<C   6 Tbsp currants
    1 1/2 cups light soy milk or evaporated
        skim milk
    1 1/2 cups 1% milk
       1 orange

       2 tsp dried rosemary
<C   5 Tbsp honey
    1 1/2 cups egg substitute
       1 tsp vanilla
     1/4 tsp cinnamon
       2 Tbsp sliced almonds

1 Lay the 3 pitas on top of each other, having first scattered each with 3 Tbsp of currants and cut into 6 wedges. Lay the stacks of wedges in a circle in a chef's pan or round baking dish deep enough to hold the liquid.

2 Cut the orange part of the orange peel (zest) off the orange by starting at the top and cutting around in a spiral. Cut the white part off and segment the orange for garnish. Bruise the orange zest with the back of a knife and lay it in a medium saucepan. Add the 2 milks, rosemary, and 3 Tbsp of the honey and let the herb and zest infuse like tea, over medium heat, 10 minutes.

3 Stir in the vanilla and cinnamon and pour over the bread through a strainer. Preheat the oven to 350°F. Let the bread soak for 30 minutes. Sprinkle each Island (stack of wedges) with a few of the almonds and drizzle with 1 Tbsp of the honey.

4 Bake in the preheated oven for 45 minutes or until a toothpick inserted into the custard comes out clean. Cut into 6 wedges, scatter the remaining 1 Tbsp of currants over the top and drizzle on the remaining honey. Serve warm or at room temperature with sliced oranges on the side.

<C To Cut Carb

<C Pitas: reduce to 1 1/2, cut the whole one in half horizontally, the height will be changed, reduced by half, but the flavor will increase.

<C Honey: reduce to 2 Tbsp and add 1 Tbsp of Splenda and 2 Tbsp water.

<C Currants: reduce to 4 Tbsp.

Per serving: 315 calories, 4 g fat, 1 g saturated fat, 2 % calories from saturated fat, 57 g carbohydrate, 5 g dietary fiber, 409 mg sodium
Exchanges: 1/2 Fat-Free Milk, 3 Carbohydrate

Low Carb
Per serving: 192 calories, 3 g fat, 1 g saturated fat, 5% calories from saturated fat, 30 g carbohydrate, 2 g dietary fiber, 202 mg sodium
Exchanges: 1/2 Fat-Free Milk, 1/2 Fat, 1 1/2 Carbohydrate

Honey Cake

SERVING SIZE: 1 slice, SERVES: 8

2 cups whole-wheat pastry flour
1 tsp baking powder
1/2 tsp baking soda
1 tsp ground cinnamon
1/2 tsp ground ginger
1/4 tsp ground nutmeg
1/8 tsp ground cloves
1/4 cup chopped walnuts
1/4 cup chopped dates
2 Tbsp finely chopped candied orange peel

2 Tbsp non-aromatic olive oil
3 Tbsp fruit fat replacement, such as Lighter Baking
1/2 cup egg substitute
1/4 cup honey
1/2 cup firmly packed light brown sugar
2 Tbsp instant coffee crystals or powder dissolved in 1/2 cup hot water
1 1/2 cups peeled and diced pear (about 1 large)

1 Set the rack in the middle of the oven and preheat to 350°F. Coat a 1 1/2 quart loaf pan with pan spray and sprinkle with flour. Tap off the excess flour and set aside.

2 Combine the flour, baking powder, soda, cinnamon, ginger, nutmeg, and cloves in a bowl with a whisk. Add the walnuts, dates, and orange peel. Mix thoroughly.

3 In another bowl, beat the oil, fat replacement, egg substitute, honey, and brown sugar together with a whisk until smooth. Stir in the coffee then add the diced pears.

4 Gently combine the flour mixture with the liquid until just wet. Pour into the prepared pan and bake for 1 hour or until a toothpick inserted in the center comes out clean. Let cool slightly, loosen, and tip out onto a rack. Slice into 8 pieces and serve warm or at room temperature.

Per serving: 308 calories, 6 g fat, 1 g saturated fat, 2% calories from saturated fat, 60 g carbohydrate, 6 g dietary fiber, 162 mg sodium, 5 g protein
Exchanges: 1/2 Fat, 4 Carbohydrate

Indian Pudding

SERVING SIZE: 18 of recipe, SERVES: 8

Pudding

2 tsp molasses
1/4 cup whole hazelnuts, divided
1/2 cup dried apples, roughly chopped
scant 1/2 tsp ginger
scant 1/2 tsp cinnamon
<C 2 1/2 cups 1% milk
<C 5 Tbsp yellow cornmeal

pinch salt
<C 1/4 cup maple syrup
1/4 cup + 2 Tbsp dried
cranberries, divided
1/2 cup egg substitute
1 Tbsp arrowroot

Sauce

1 cup nonfat yogurt cheese (page 475)
<C 2 Tbsp maple syrup

1/8 tsp cinnamon
1/8 tsp ginger

1 Preheat the oven to 350°F. Grease a 6-cup loaf pan with pan spray. Spoon the molasses into the bottom of the pan and set aside. Roast the hazelnuts in a small metal pan for 5 minutes in the preheated oven. Rub the hot roasted nuts in a kitchen towel to remove some of the skins. Chop roughly and set aside. Reduce the oven heat further to 300°F.

2 Heat the milk in a large saucepan on medium high until bubbles appear around the edge. Whisk in the cornmeal and cook until the mixture boils then remove from the heat. Add the salt, cinnamon, ginger, maple syrup, 2 Tbsp of the nuts, 1/4 cup of the cranberries, and the apple pieces. Combine the egg substitute and arrowroot and stir into the milk mixture.

3 Pour into the prepared loaf pan. Set into a larger pan and put in the oven. Pour hot water into the larger pan until the water comes about half way up the pudding pan to make a water bath. Lay a piece of oiled foil over the top and bake 2 hours.

4 Make the sauce by combing the yogurt cheese, maple syrup, cinnamon, and ginger. Refrigerate until ready to serve. When the pudding is done, cool on a rack. Tip out of the pan and cut in 8 slices. Serve with a dollop of the sauce and a sprinkle of the reserved nuts and cranberries.

<C Yellow cornmeal: reduce to 4 Tbsp.

<C Milk: reduce to 2 cups.

<C Maple syrup (for pudding): reduce to 2 Tbsp and add 2 Tbsp of Splenda.

<C Maple syrup (for sauce): reduce to 1 Tbsp and add 1 Tbsp Splenda.

Per serving: 185 calories, 3 g fat, 1 g saturated fat, 4% calories from saturated fat, 32 g carbohydrate, 2 g dietary fiber, 108 mg sodium, 8 g protein
Exchanges: 1/2 Fat, 2 Carbohydrate

Low Carb
Per serving: 157 calories, 3 g fat, 1 g saturated fat, 3% calories from saturated fat, 26 g carbohydrate, 2 g dietary fiber, 100 mg sodium
Exchanges: 1/2 Fat, 2 Carbohydrate

Sweet Potato Dessert

SERVING SIZE: 1/4 of recipe, SERVES: 4

<C   1 lb orange sweet potatoes
<C 1/3 cup raisins
     1 (8 oz) carton low-fat vanilla yogurt

<C   2 Tbsp brown sugar
   1/2 tsp allspice

1 Preheat the oven to 350° F. Peel and boil or steam the sweet potatoes until soft, about 14 minutes. Mash and stir in raisins and yogurt. Spoon into a small baking dish, smoothing the surface.

2 Combine the brown sugar and allspice and spread evenly over the top. Bake 20 minutes or until heated through.

<C **To Cut Carb**
<C Sweet Potatoes: reduce to 8 oz.
<C Raisins: reduce to 1/4 cup.

<C Brown sugar: reduce to 2 tsp and add 1 Tbsp Splenda.

Per serving: 199 calories, 1 g fat, 1 g saturated fat, 4% calories from saturated fat, 45 g carbohydrate, 2 g dietary fiber, 55 mg sodium
Exchanges: 3 Carbohydrate

Low Carb
Per serving: 131 calories, 1 g fat, 0 g saturated fat, 0% calories from saturated fat, 28 g carbohydrate, 1 g dietary fiber, 46 mg sodium
Exchanges: 2 Carbohydrate

Black Rice Pudding

SERVING SIZE: 1/4 of recipe, SERVES: 4

1/2 cup Thai black rice (see sidebar)	2 Tbsp brown sugar
1 1/2 cups water	1/2 cup coconut cream

1 Bring the black rice and water to a boil in a small saucepan. Reduce the heat, cover, and simmer 30 minutes or until the rice is tender but still chewy.

2 Stir in the sugar and coconut cream and serve warm or chilled.

> Watch your post-prandial glucose level on this dish. If it goes beyond 180 you could simply cut the portion; self-restraint is a wonderful gift!

Per serving: 150 calories, 2 g fat, 1 g saturated fat, 6% calories from saturated fat, 30 g carbohydrate, 0 g dietary fiber, 11 mg sodium
Exchanges: 2 Starch, 1 1/2 Fat

Mixed Fruit with a Surprise

SERVING SIZE: 1/4 of recipe, SERVES: 4

2 cups quartered strawberries (cantaloupe, papaya, or?)
2 cups peeled kiwi chunks (watermelon, orange sections, or?)
1 star fruit (or other new fruit you are curious about)
1/2 cup ginger ale
2 Tbsp chopped fresh mint or 1 tsp lime zest

1 Combine the strawberries, kiwis, star fruit, ginger ale, and mint. Let sit 30 minutes to mingle the flavors. Serve and enjoy!

Per serving: 86 calories, 1 g fat, 0 g saturated fat, 0% calories from saturated fat, 19 g carbohydrate, 4 g dietary fiber, 5 mg sodium
Exchanges: 1 1/2 Fruit

Oranges and Kiwis with a Glossy Glaze

SERVING SIZE: 1/4 of recipe, SERVES: 4

2 medium navel oranges or grapefruit
2 kiwi fruit
1/2 cup cranberry juice cocktail or white grape juice
1/4 cup dried cranberries
1 Tbsp honey
1 tsp cornstarch mixed with 1 Tbsp cranberry juice (slurry)

1 Peel the oranges with a knife to take off the white membrane underneath. Cut into 1-inch chunks. Peel the kiwis and cut into 1-inch chunks. Chill the fruit in a medium sized bowl.

2 Combine the cranberry juice, dried cranberries, honey, and slurry in a small saucepan. Bring to a boil to thicken and clear. Cool.

3 Pour the glaze over the chilled fruit and serve.

Per serving: 115 calories, 0 g fat, 0 g saturated fat, 0% calories from saturated fat, 29 g carbohydrate, 3 g dietary fiber, 3 mg sodium
Exchanges: 2 Fruit

Sparkling Grape Dessert

SERVING SIZE: 1/4 of recipe, SERVES: 4

1 cup red (Flame) seedless grapes, removed from stems
1 cup green (Thompson) seedless grapes, removed from stems
1 cup sparkling white grape juice, ginger ale, or tonic
12 leaves rolled and cut mint

1 Combine the grapes, sparkling beverage, and mint in a bowl. Chill for at least an hour. Spoon into stemmed glasses with the juice and serve. Top with a sprig of fresh mint.

Per serving: 79 calories, 0 g fat, 0 g saturated fat, 0% calories from saturated fat, 20 g carbohydrate, 1 g dietary fiber, 6 mg sodium
Exchanges: 1 1/2 Fruit

Koko Tapioca with Bananas and Crystallized Ginger

SERVING SIZE: 1/6 of recipe, SERVES: 6

1/2 cup small pearl tapioca
<C 1/4 cup firmly packed brown sugar
1/4 cup Dutch-process or European-style cocoa
2 cups 2% milk
1/4 cup egg substitute

1/2 tsp vanilla extract
<C 1/4 cup finely chopped crystallized ginger
<C 3 ripe bananas
2 Tbsp toasted almond slices

1 Soak tapioca in 3 cups water for 1 hour. Drain and set aside.

2 Combine sugar and cocoa in the top of a double boiler over hot water. When well mixed, add 1/3 cup boiling water, and whisk until smooth.

3 Add milk, and cook over medium heat until temperature reaches 140°F. Cook for 5 minutes more, not letting temperature rise above 155°F.

4 Whisk in drained tapioca and egg substitute. Turn up heat and cook over boiling water, stirring often, until tapioca is tender and pudding is thick, about 15 minutes.

5 Stir in vanilla and ginger. Remove pudding from heat and set aside to cool.

6 Peel and slice bananas and layer with tapioca in six wine or champagne glasses that hold about 1 cup each. Sprinkle tops with almonds. Serve chilled or at room temperature.

<C **To Cut Carb**

<C Brown sugar: reduce to 1 Tbsp and add 2 Tbsp Splenda.
<C Ginger: reduce to 1 Tbsp.
<C Bananas: reduce to 2 bananas.

Per serving: 217 calories, 2 g fat, 1 g saturated fat, 4% calories from saturated fat, 48 g carbohydrate, 3 g dietary fiber, 65 mg sodium.
Exchanges: 3 Carbohydrate

Low Carb
Per serving: 156 calories, 2 g fat, 1 g saturated fat, 6% calories from saturated fat, 32 g carbohydrate, 2 g dietary fiber, 62 mg sodium
Exchanges: 2 Carbohydrate

Pineapple Nieve

SERVING SIZE: 1/6 of recipe, SERVES: 6

1 whole fresh pineapple	1/4 cup granulated sugar
1/4 cup fresh lime juice	

1 Either peel or core the pineapple depending upon whether you want to use the shell as a serving dish for the nieve. If it is to be used, immediately put the hollowed husk in the freezer.

2 Chop the fruit into rough chunks. Process them in a food processor for about 2 minutes, or until there are no whole pieces left. Add the lime juice and sugar and blend for another 15 seconds, until well mixed. If you can still see thin strings of pineapple pulp, press or rub the mixture through a mesh strainer.

3 Freeze the fruit sauce in an ice cream machine, following the manufacturer's directions. If you don't have an ice cream machine, freeze the liquid in a shallow baking pan in your freezer until it is almost solid. This will take an hour or two depending on your freezer. Once it is frozen, remove from the freezer and break into small pieces. Put the pieces in the large bowl of an electric mixer and beat until smooth. Return the mixture to the shallow pan and refreeze. Repeat the freezing and beating process until you are satisfied with the consistency of the ice. The more times you beat, the smoother the texture will be. One short beating will produce a granita. Several beatings will result in a richer, smoother texture.

4 When you are satisfied with the texture, let the ice ripen in the freezer for 30 minutes. Then it is ready to serve or pack into the frozen pineapple shell.

5 To serve, scoop the ice into small-stemmed dessert dishes or present in the frozen husk. Serve with cinnamon chips and a cup of warm chocolate drink.

Per serving: 74 calories, 0 g fat, 0 g saturated fat, 0% calories from saturated fat, 19 g carbohydrate, 1 g dietary fiber
Exchanges: 1/2 Fruit, 1/2 Carbohydrate

Lady Baltimore on a Roll

SERVING SIZE: 1/12 recipe, SERVES: 12 (Treena has 1/2 a serving.)

Cake (*Almond Sponge Roll from* Let Them Eat Cake *by Susan Purdy*)

1/2 cup sifted cake flour
1/4 cup sifted cornstarch
1 tsp baking powder
2 large eggs, separated plus
  2 large egg whites
1/4 tsp cream of tartar

1/2 cup plus 2 Tbsp sugar, divided
1 Tbsp non-aromatic olive oil
1 tsp vanilla extract
1 tsp almond extract
1/4 cup powdered sugar

Filling

2 cups low-fat yogurt cheese
1/4 cup toasted pecans, chopped
1/4 cup Grape Nuts

6 figs cut in thin strips
1/2 cup chopped raisins, chopped
1/2 tsp almond extract

Frosting (*from* The New Basics *by Rosso and Lukins*)

1 egg white
1/2 cup sugar
1/8 tsp baking powder

1 Tbsp freshly squeezed lemon juice
1 Tbsp freshly squeezed orange juice
1 tsp finely grated orange zest

1. Preheat oven to 350°F. Spray 10 1/2-inch × 15 1/2-inch jelly roll pan and line with parchment or waxed paper. Spray the paper, and dust lightly with flour. Sift together flour, cornstarch, and baking powder, and set aside.

2. Beat egg whites until foamy, add cream of tartar, and gradually sprinkle in 6 Tbsp sugar while beating until stiff but not dry. Set aside. Without washing the beaters, whip together egg yolks, oil, extracts, and remaining 1/4 cup sugar. Beat on high speed 3 or 4 minutes until batter forms a ribbon falling back on itself when the beater is lifted.

3. Fold a third of the beaten whites into batter, then fold in a few Tbsp flour mixture. Fold rest of whites and flour, alternately, into the batter 1/3 of each at a time. Keep it smooth, light, and airy. Pour into prepared pan and smooth all the way to the edges. Bake 11–13 minutes or until top is golden and feels springy to the touch.

4. Sift 1/4 cup powdered sugar on a clean tea towel covering a 10-inch × 15-inch rectangle. When cake is done, set the sugared towel over the cake and invert. Lift off the pan, and remove the paper on the bottom of the cake.

Trim edges a little if they are dry or thin. Fold edge of towel over long side of cake and roll up while still quite hot. Set seam-side down to cool.

5 Combine pecans, Grape Nuts, figs, and raisins with almond extract in a small bowl. When cake is cool, unroll, and spread with yogurt cheese, leaving 3-inch strip bare on the far edge. Scatter fruit and nut mix evenly over the yogurt. Roll tightly and set seam side down on a long serving plate. Trim each end.

6 Combine egg white, sugar, baking powder, orange juice, lemon juice, and orange zest in the top of a double boiler. Set over boiling water and beat constantly with a handheld electric mixer for 7 minutes or until frosting is satiny and fluffy. Remove from heat, and spread over rolled cake. Cut into 12 servings with a wet knife.

Per serving: 242 calories, 5 g fat, 1 g saturated fat, 4% calories from saturated fat, 44 g carbohydrate, 2 g dietary fiber, 111 mg sodium
Exchanges: 1/2 Fat, 3 Carbohydrate

Rhubarb and Strawberries

SERVING SIZE: 1/6 of recipe, SERVES: 6

1 lb rhubarb (about 2 cups), sliced	2 packets plain gelatin
1/4 cup water or orange juice	1 cup strawberries, washed and
<C 5 Tbsp brown sugar	sliced

1 In a medium saucepan, simmer rhubarb and water or juice for about 8 minutes or until soft. Stir in brown sugar and gelatin. Add strawberries. Pour mixture into bowl and chill.

<C **To Cut Carb**
<C Brown sugar: reduce to 2 Tbsp and add 3 Tbsp of Splenda.

Per serving: 70 calories, 0 g fat, 0 g saturated fat, 0% calories from saturated fat, 15 g carbohydrate, 2 g dietary fiber, 11 mg sodium, 3 g protein
Exchanges: 1 Carbohydrate

Low Carb
Per serving: 47 calories, 0 g fat, 0 g saturated fat, 0% calories from saturated fat, 9 g carbohydrate, 2 g dietary fiber, 9 mg sodium, 3 g protein
Exchanges: 1/2 Carbohydrate

Promised Land Meringue Cake

SERVING SIZE: 1 slice, SERVES: 6

Meringue Shell

5 large egg whites, at room temperature
2/3 cup sugar
1 tsp vanilla extract

1 tsp distilled vinegar
2 tsp cornstarch

Fruit Wine Sauce

1 Tbsp honey
2 nectarines, peeled, fruit reserved
for filling
1 tsp lemon zest from 1/2 lemon
1/8 tsp ground cardamom

1 cup fruity white wine (I prefer
nonalcoholic Ariel Blanc)
2 tsp arrowroot
4 tsp water

Fruit Filling

2 kiwi fruit, peeled and sliced
2 nectarines, sliced

12 fresh strawberries, stemmed and sliced
Other soft fruit or berries in season

To Prepare the Shell

1 Preheat the oven to 300°F. Make sure the egg whites are at room temperature before beginning the recipe.

2 Cut a piece of baking parchment to fit a baking sheet. Draw a 9-inch circle on the parchment, turn it over, and place on top of the baking sheet.

3 Make sure that the bowl and whip attachment of your electric mixer are perfectly clean and grease-free. Beat the egg whites on low speed until frothy, then increase the speed to high and beat until soft peaks begin to form. Gradually sprinkle the sugar over the top, 1 Tbsp at a time, continuing to beat at high speed. When all the sugar is beaten in, add the vanilla, vinegar, and cornstarch. Beat until the egg whites are stiff but not dry, about 2 to 3 minutes.

4 Spoon the meringue into a large pastry bag fitted with a large open star tip. Pipe a scalloped circle of meringue around the drawn circle on the parchment. Pipe another scalloped circle inside the first one. Then pipe a third circle on top of the seam of the first two, forming a tiered rim.

5 Bake the meringue in the preheated oven for 15 minutes. Reduce the heat to 205°F and continue to bake for 1 hour. The meringue will be crisp on the outside and soft in the middle. Set aside on a wire rack to cool. Once the meringue is completely cool, you can store it in an airtight container.

To Prepare the Sauce

6 Warm the honey in a small saucepan over high heat. When it is thick and bubbly, add the nectarine skins and lemon zest. Cook, stirring constantly, for about 2 minutes to extract all the flavorful oils.

7 Stir in the cardamom and 1/4 cup of the wine. Keep at a boil to reduce the wine, then add 1/4 cup more wine. Reduce that, then add the remaining 1/2 cup and simmer for 5 minutes. Strain the sauce, discarding the debris. Rinse the pan and pour in the strained liquid.

8 Mix the arrowroot with 4 tsp of water to make a slurry. Add the slurry to the sauce and stir over medium heat until it thickens and clears.

To Serve

9 Arrange the fruit artfully in the center of the meringue. Pour the sauce over the fruit to give it gloss. Slice into 6 wedges and serve at the table.

Per serving: 194 calories, 1 g fat, 0 g saturated fat, 0% calories from saturated fat, 45 g carbohydrate, 3 g dietary fiber, 51 mg sodium
Exchanges: 1 Fruit, 2 Carbohydrate

Strawberry Sunshine

SERVING SIZE: 1/4 of recipe, SERVES: 4

3 cups strawberries, cut in half   4 tsp brown sugar
1 cup low-fat vanilla yogurt

1 Mix ingredients together and enjoy.

Per serving: 103 calories, 1 g fat, 1 g saturated fat, 9% calories from saturated fat, 21 g carbohydrate, 3 g dietary fiber, 43 mg sodium
Exchanges: 1 1/2 Carbohydrate

Potted Wattleseed Custard

SERVING SIZE: 1 custard cup, SERVES: 6

1 1/2 cups evaporated skim milk
1 1/2 cups 2% milk
   2 Tbsp wattleseeds or 2 Tbsp Postum
     and 1 Tbsp instant coffee

1/4 cup brown sugar
1/2 tsp vanilla extract
  1 cup egg substitute

1 Preheat the oven to 325°F.

To Prepare the Custard Using Wattleseeds

2 Combine the two kinds of milk, brown sugar, and wattleseeds in a large saucepan.

3 Cook the mixture over medium heat just to the point of boiling. Remove from heat and set aside for 10 or 15 minutes to allow the milk to absorb as much flavor as possible.

4 Strain through cheesecloth into another saucepan and stir in the vanilla and egg substitute.

5 Pour the custard into 6 6-ounce custard cups. Arrange the cups in a baking dish and set in the oven. Pull the rack out slightly and pour enough hot water into the baking dish to come about 3/4 of the way up the sides of the cups.

6 Bake for 50 to 60 minutes or until a knife inserted into the center of each custard comes out perfectly clean. As soon as they are cool enough to handle, take them out of the water bath and allow to cool on a rack.

To Prepare the Custard Using Postum

7 Combine the two kinds of milk in a large saucepan and heat until almost boiling.

8 Add the Postum and instant coffee, stirring to dissolve. Add the brown sugar, stirring until it is completely dissolved. Stir in the vanilla and egg substitute.

9 Proceed with step 5 of the method above.

To Serve

10 The custards can be served at room temperature or chilled. Attractive 6-ounce containers, like small French soufflé dishes or custard cups, help a great deal with the presentation.

Per serving: 111 calories, 1 g fat, 1 g saturated fat; 10% of calories from saturated fat, 14 g carbohydrate, 0 g dietary fiber, 12 g protein
Exchanges: 1 Very Lean Meat, 1 Fat-Free Milk

Key Lime Pie

SERVING SIZE: 1 piece, SERVES: 8

1/2 recipe Basic Pie Crust (page 479)
  4 tsp lime zest
1/2 cup freshly squeezed lime juice
  4 egg yolks
  1 (14 oz) can nonfat sweetened condensed milk

  2 egg whites
1/4 tsp cream of tartar
1/4 cup sugar
1/4 tsp vanilla

1 Preheat oven to 425°F. Roll out pie crust to fit an 8-inch pie tin. Lay rolled dough in the pan without stretching it, and crimp the edge. Prick with a fork. Lay a piece of parchment or waxed paper in the pie shell and pour in enough beans to cover the bottom. These weights keep it from bubbling up while baking. Bake for 8 minutes or until golden brown.

2 Reduce heat to 350°F. Combine lime zest, juice, egg yolks, and milk in a bowl with a whisk. Pour into baked shell, and bake 15 minutes. When pie is done, raise oven temperature back to 425°F.

3 While the pie is baking, make the meringue. Beat the egg whites until foamy. Add cream of tartar. When soft peaks appear, sprinkle in sugar, and continue to beat until the meringue holds stiff peaks. Beat vanilla in at the end. Spoon the meringue around the sides of the pie, and seal to prevent it from shrinking. Scoop the rest into the center and smooth it over all. Pick up peaks with the back of a spoon, and bake for 4 minutes or until golden brown.

Per serving: 249 calories, 7 g fat, 2 g saturated fat, 6% calories from saturated fat, 39 g carbohydrate, 0 g dietary fiber, 131 mg sodium
Exchanges: 1 1/2 Fat, 2 1/2 Carbohydrate

Sweet Potato Mousse

SERVING SIZE: 1/6 of recipe, SERVES: 6

<C 1/2 cup fresh orange juice
<C 1/3 cup raisins
<C   3 Tbsp brown sugar
    3/8 tsp ground allspice
<C   3 lb sweet potatoes, peeled
    and roughly chopped

1/8 tsp salt
1/2 cup nonfat yogurt cheese
  (page 475)
1/2 tsp freshly grated orange zest
  1 Tbsp slivered almonds

Garnish

1 Edible flowers such as pansies, nasturtiums, or bachelor buttons.

2 Preheat the oven to 400°F.

3 Warm the orange juice in a small saucepan over medium heat. Add the raisins, 2 Tbsp of the brown sugar, and 1/8 tsp of the allspice to the warm juice. Set aside and let the raisins soak while the potatoes are cooking.

4 Put the potatoes and salt in a large saucepan, cover with water, and bring to a boil. Cook for 15 minutes, or until very soft. Drain the cooking liquid and return the potatoes to the pan. Cover the potatoes with a clean dishtowel and place over low heat for 5 to 10 minutes, or until the potatoes have a dry, floury appearance.

5 Mash with a potato masher and add the yogurt cheese, remaining 1/4 tsp of allspice, and orange zest.

6 Drain the raisins and set aside to use for garnish. Add their marinade to the potatoes and stir until smooth.

7 Spray a 10-inch round ovenproof baking dish with cooking spray and spread the potatoes in the dish. Set aside until ready to bake.

8 To bake, texturize the potatoes with the tines of a fork and sprinkle the remaining Tbsp of brown sugar and the almonds over the top. Bake in the preheated oven for 15 minutes.

9 To serve, scoop a portion of the potato mousse onto a dessert plate and top with a few of the plumped raisins. Set an edible flower alongside.

<c Orange juice: reduce to 1/4 cup.
<c Raisins: reduce to 1 Tbsp.
<c Brown sugar: reduce to 1 Tbsp plus 1 Tbsp Splenda.

Per serving: 255 calories, 1 g fat, 0 g saturated fat, 0% calories from saturated fat, 58 g carbohydrate, 5 g dietary fiber, 94 mg sodium
Exchanges: 3 1/2 Carbohydrate

Low Carb
Per serving: 214 calories, 1 g fat, 0 g saturated fat, 0% calories from saturated fat, 47 g carbohydrate, 3 g dietary fiber, 92 mg sodium
Exchanges: 3 Carbohydrate

Poached Canned Pears with Ginger Walnut Yogurt Sauce

SERVING SIZE: 1/4 of recipe, SERVES: 4

8 canned pear halves water packed with reserved juice
2 Tbsp chopped walnuts

<c 2 Tbsp chopped crystallized ginger
1 cup low-fat vanilla yogurt

1 Lay the pear halves round side down in a heavy skillet. Pour a little of the can juices over the top. Bring to a boil, lower the heat, and boil the liquid until the syrup is thick and caramelized and the pear half is golden.

2 Lay 2 halves on each plate. Toss the nuts and ginger into the pan with the remaining juice and heat through. Spoon a pool of yogurt around the pears then pour the sauce with the nuts and ginger over the top.

<c **To Cut Carb**
<c Ginger: reduce to 1 Tbsp.

Per serving: 139 calories, 3 g fat, 1 g saturated fat, 5% calories from saturated fat, 27 g carbohydrate, 3 g dietary fiber, 51 mg sodium
Exchanges: 1/2 Fat, 1 1/2 Carbohydrate

Low Carb
Per serving: 130 calories, 3 g fat, 1 g saturated fat, 5% calories from saturated fat, 24 g carbohydrate, 3 g dietary fiber, 45 mg sodium
Exchanges: 1/2 Fat, 1 1/2 Carbohydrate

Sweet Potato Pie

SERVING SIZE: 1 piece, SERVES: 8

1/2 Basic Pie Crust Recipe (page 479)

Filling

<C 2 cups mashed sweet potatoes
    1 Tbsp butter-flavored margarine
+> 1/2 cup egg substitute
<C 1/4 cup firmly packed brown sugar
<C 1 Tbsp molasses

3/4 cup low-fat evaporated milk
1/4 tsp ground nutmeg
1/4 tsp ground cinnamon
1/4 tsp ground ginger

Topping

1 1/2 cup low fat yogurt cheese
    1 Tbsp molasses syrup

1 Preheat the oven to 425°F. Roll out the piecrust to fit a 9-inch pie tin. Lay the rolled dough in the pan without stretching it and crimp the edge. Prick with a fork. Lay a piece of parchment or waxed paper in the pie shell and pour in enough beans to cover the bottom. These will act as pie weights to keep it from bubbling up while baking. Bake for 8 minutes or until golden brown. Reduce the heat to 350°F.

2 Combine the mashed sweet potatoes, margarine, egg substitute, brown sugar, molasses, milk, nutmeg, cinnamon, and ginger. Pour into the baked crust and smooth. Cover the rim of the piecrust with strips of aluminum foil. Bake 45–55 minutes or until a knife inserted in the center comes out clean. Cool slightly before serving.

3 Stir the maple syrup into the yogurt cheese and refrigerate until ready to use. Cut the pie into 8 pieces and serve with a dollop of yogurt topping.

<C **To Cut Carb**
<C Sweet potato: reduce to 1 1/2 cups.
+> Egg substitute: increase by 1/4 cup.
<C Brown sugar: replace with 4 Tbsp Splenda.
<C Molasses (filling): reduce to 2 tsp.

Per serving: 299 calories, 8 g fat, 3 g saturated fat, 9% calories from saturated fat, 48 g carbohydrate, 2 g dietary fiber, 190 mg sodium
Exchanges: 1 1/2 Fat, 3 Carbohydrate

Low Carb
Per serving: 256 calories, 8 g fat, 3 g saturated fat, 10% calories from saturated fat, 37 g carbohydrate, 1 g dietary fiber, 199 mg sodium
Exchanges: 1 Fat, 2 1/2 Carbohydrate

Cantaloupe Slush with Mango

SERVING SIZE: 1/4 of recipe, SERVES: 4

1 medium-sized cantaloupe   <C 2 tsp honey
  Juice of half a lemon

1 Peel and seed cantaloupe. Cut into 1-inch pieces. It should be about 6 cups.

2 Place in blender or food processor with lemon juice and honey, and puree until very smooth. Pour mixture into a shallow 9-inch × 12-inch glass pan and set in the freezer for 2 hours.

3 With a fork, chip and stir the icy mixture and return it to the freezer for 2 to 4 hours.

4 Peel and cut mango into long, thin, attractive slices, avoiding the pit (which is shaped like a large almond).

5 Again with a fork, chip the frozen cantaloupe mixture so it resembles a snow cone or shaved ice. Spoon it into clear bowls, and top with mango slices. Serve.

<C **To Cut Carb** ═══════════════════════════
<C Honey: delete and replace with 2 tsp Splenda.

Per serving: 134 calories, 1 g fat, 0 g saturated fat, 0% calories from saturated fat, 33 g carbohydrate, 3 g dietary fiber, 24 mg sodium
Exchanges: 2 Fruit

Low Carb
Per serving: 125 calories, 1 g fat, 0 g saturated fat, 0% calories from saturated fat, 31 g carbohydrate, 3 g dietary fiber, 24 mg sodium
Exchanges: 2 Fruit

Trifle Style Summer Pudding

SERVING SIZE: 1/10 of recipe, SERVES: 10

1 1/2 cups fresh or frozen unsweetened raspberries

1 1/2 cups fresh or frozen unsweetened blackberries

1 1/2 cups fresh or frozen unsweetened strawberries, sliced

1 1/2 cups fresh or frozen blueberries

<C 1/2 cup sugar

1 packet unflavored gelatin

3 Tbsp cold water

3 Tbsp boiling water

<C 20 Italian lady fingers (savoiardi)

Custard

3 Tbsp arrowroot

<C 6 Tbsp granulated sugar

2 cups 2% milk

1 tsp vanilla

1 cup egg substitute

1. Combine the berries in a large saucepan, add the sugar, and bring just to a boil to break out the juice and dissolve the sugar. Set aside to cool. Sprinkle the gelatin over the cold water in a small bowl to soften for a few minutes. Add the boiling water to completely dissolve the gelatin. Stir into the berries.

2. Arrange 2 lady fingers in each of 10 individual dessert dishes. Divide the berry mixture among the dessert dishes with the cookies sticking out. Leave about an inch space in the top of each dish for the custard.

3. Combine the arrowroot and sugar in a small bowl. Stir in 1/2 cup of the milk to make a slurry. Heat the remaining milk in a heavy saucepan until small bubbles form around the edge or a skin starts forming on the top. Add the slurry and vanilla and stir constantly while it comes to a boil. Take off the heat and stir in the egg substitute. Pour the custard on top of the berry mixture in each dish and chill until set, 2 hours or more. Garnish with a mint sprig or an edible flower such as a pansy or violet.

<C **To Cut Carb**

<C Sugar and granulated sugar: replace both with Splenda using just a little less (1/2 cup less 1 Tbsp and 5 Tbsp)

+> Grated zest of one lemon (I tsp): add to the custard *after* the egg substitute.

<C Lady fingers: reduce to 10 pieces.

Per serving: 191 calories, 2 g fat, 1 g saturated fat, 2% calories from saturated fat, 40 g carbohydrate, 4 g dietary fiber, 87 mg sodium
Exchanges: 2 1/2 Carbohydrate

Low Carb
Per serving: 114 calories, 2 g fat, 1 g saturated fat, 2% calories from saturated fat, 21 g carbohydrate, 4 g dietary fiber, 80 mg sodium
Exchanges: 1 1/2 Carbohydrate

Jordan Rice Pudding

SERVING SIZE: 1/8 of recipe, SERVES: 8

1 1/2 cups light soy milk or evaporated skim milk
2 cups mango nectar
1 cup water
1 1/3 cups uncooked short-grain white rice
1/8 tsp cardamom

1 mango, peeled and chopped in 1/4-inch pieces
4 dates, pitted and chopped in 1/4-inch pieces
1 cup low-fat vanilla yogurt
3 Tbsp coarsely chopped almonds

Authentic Flavors

Almonds can be replaced by pistachio nuts, a great green color as a garnish and typical of the region.

---

1 Stir the milk, mango nectar, water, rice, and cardamom together in an oven-proof high-sided skillet or 3-quart saucepan and heat slowly on medium. Stir occasionally and don't worry when small particles of the milk start to form around the edges, the end result will be smooth and creamy. Preheat the oven to 350ºF. When the liquid comes to a boil, stir one last time and set the pan, uncovered, into the preheated oven and bake 30 minutes.

2 Cool for 10 minutes then stir the chopped mango, dates, and yogurt into the hot pudding. Scatter the chopped pistachios over the top and serve.

Per serving: 247 calories, 3 g fat, 1 g saturated fat, 1% calories from saturated fat, 51 g carbohydrates, 3 g dietary fiber, 39 mg sodium, 5 g protein
Exchanges: 3 1/2 Carbohydrate

Strawberry Banana Fruit Leather

SERVING SIZE: 1 piece, SERVES: 8

3 cups strawberries
1 ripe banana
2 Tbsp honey

2 Tbsp frozen orange juice concentrate
1 tsp lemon juice

1 Cover a 12-inch × 17-inch baking pan with sides in plastic wrap.

2 Whiz the strawberries, banana, orange juice concentrate, honey, and lemon juice in a blender until very smooth. You can do this in batches if need be. You should have 2 cups of puree.

3 Pour into the prepared pan and spread with a spatula making the edges thicker than the middle. Bake in a 140°F oven with the door slightly open for about 6 hours or until just barely sticky. Cool, roll the long way, and cut into 8 2-inch pieces. Store in the fridge for up to a week—but your kids will probably eat it before the week is through.

Per serving: 52 calories, 0 g fat, 0 g saturated fat, 0% calories from saturated fat, 13 g carbohydrate, 2 g dietary fiber, 1 mg sodium
Exchanges: 1 Fruit

Cantaloupe with Fresh Ginger

SERVING SIZE: 1/4 dish, SERVES: 4

1 cantaloupe, peeled, seeded, and cut into balls or chunks
1 Tbsp freshly grated ginger root

1 Combine the cantaloupe with the grated ginger in a glass bowl. Cover and chill for at least 1 hour. Serve for dessert or as a side dish to ham or chicken.

Per serving: 99 calories, 0 g fat, 0 g saturated fat, 0% calories from saturated fat, 25 g carbohydrates, 4 g dietary fiber, 62 mg sodium
Exchanges: 1 1/2 Fruit

Almost Heaven Brownies

SERVING SIZE: 1 brownie, SERVES: 24

1/4 cup pitted prunes	4 large egg whites
1/4 cup hot water	1 cup sugar
1/2 cup cocoa	1 cup cake flour
1 tsp vanilla extract	1/4 tsp salt
3 Tbsp non-aromatic olive oil	1 tsp baking soda
1/2 cup buttermilk	1 cup crisp rice cereal

1 Preheat the oven to 350°F. Grease a 9-inch × 13-inch baking pan with pan spray. Cut a piece of waxed paper to fit the bottom and spray again. Soak the prunes in hot water for 15 minutes to soften. Puree in a food processor or blender.

2 Combine pureed prunes, cocoa, vanilla, and oil in a medium bowl and mix well. Add the buttermilk and whisk until the mixture is smooth. Whisk in the egg whites until light.

3 Mix the sugar, flour, salt, and soda in a large mixing bowl. Fold in the chocolate mixture and then stir in the rice cereal. Pour into the prepared pan and bake 25 minutes or until a toothpick inserted in the middle comes out clean. Cool and cut into 24 pieces.

Per serving: 81 calories, 2 g fat, 0 g saturated fat, 0% calories from saturated fat, 15 g carbohydrate, 1 g dietary fiber, 102 mg sodium
Exchanges: 1 Carbohydrate

Grape Yogurt Dessert

SERVING SIZE: 1/4 of recipe, SERVES: 4

2 cups red seedless (Flame) grapes, removed from stems	2 cups low-fat vanilla yogurt
	4 tsp wheat germ

1 Layer grapes and yogurt in pretty stemmed wine glasses. Top with a sprinkling of wheat germ. Chill and serve.

Per serving: 142 calories, 2 g fat, 1 g saturated fat, 6% calories from saturated fat, 27 g carbohydrate, 1 g dietary fiber, 81 mg sodium, 4 g protein
Exchanges: 1 Fruit, 1 Carbohydrate

Raspberry Fool

SERVING SIZE: 1/4 of recipe, SERVES: 4

2 cups fresh or frozen raspberries   2 cups low-fat vanilla yogurt
1/2 tsp almond extract (optional)   2 Tbsp toasted sliced almonds

1   Purée the berries in a blender or with a potato masher. Strain out the seeds if you want a perfectly smooth dessert.

2   Stir almond extract into the yogurt. Swirl the raspberry puree into the yogurt so it stays in red stripes not stirred in to make a pink pudding. Scoop into dessert bowls and scatter almond slices over the top.

Per serving: 170 calories, 4 g fat, 1 g saturated fat, 5% calories from saturated fat, 28 g carbohydrate, 5 g dietary fiber, 87 mg sodium, 6 g protein
Exchanges: 1/2 Fruit, 1/2 Fat, 1 1/2 Carbohydrate

Fungi Foster Cornmeal Pudding with Caramel Crunch

SERVING SIZE: 1/6 of recipe, SERVES: 6

Pudding

<C 3/4 cup evaporated skim milk   2 tsp cornstarch
1 1/4 cups 2% milk   1 Tbsp sugar
1 cinnamon stick, about 2 1/2 inches long   1/4 cup egg substitute
<C 6 Tbsp yellow cornmeal   <C 1/4 cup raisins

Sauce

1 cup low-fat vanilla yogurt

Caramel

1/2 cup sugar   2 tsp hot water
1/8 tsp ground cinnamon

To Prepare the Pudding

1 In a large saucepan, combine the evaporated milk with 3/4 cup of the 2% milk and the cinnamon stick. Warm over medium-high heat until small bubbles rise around the edge of the pan or a skin starts to form on top of the milk.

2 Combine another 1/4 cup of the 2% milk with the cornmeal and whisk into the hot milk. Stir often until the cornmeal is thick enough for a spoon to stand upright, about 5 minutes.

3 Combine the cornstarch with the remaining 1/4 cup of 2% milk to make a slurry.

4 Add the sugar, egg substitute, and raisins to the cornmeal mixture. Remove from the heat and add the slurry. Return to the burner and stir over medium heat until the mixture thickens again. The pudding is ready when you can move a spoon across the bottom of the pan without the path behind it filling in. This might take up to 5 more minutes, depending on the heat and your pan. Remove and discard the cinnamon stick. Cover the cornmeal mixture to prevent the surface from hardening and set aside until ready to serve.

To Prepare the Sauce

5 Stir the yogurt with a spoon in a small bowl. Do this just before you serve to avoid separation.

To Prepare the Caramel

6 Melt the sugar in a small, heavy-bottomed saucepan over medium-high heat, stirring frequently. When the sugar has melted and turned golden, pull the pan off the heat and add the cinnamon and hot water. Stand back because the water will make the melted sugar bubble vigorously.

7 Turn off the heat and return the pan to the warm burner. You will need to move quickly now, before the caramel sets like hard toffee in the pan.

To Serve

8 Place a generous spoonful of yogurt onto each dessert plate. Scoop 1/4 cup or so of the corn pudding into the center of each puddle of yogurt. (An ice cream scoop with a clicker makes this easy.) Using a pointed teaspoon, swirl the caramel over the top in a decorative way. The caramel will harden as soon as it hits the pudding. If the caramel should become too hard, simply warm it again over low heat.

(Continued)

<c Evaporated skim milk: reduce to 1/2 cup.　　<c Raisins: reduce to 2 Tbsp.
<c Yellow corn meal: reduce to 5 Tbsp.

Per serving: 214 calories, 2 g fat, 1 g saturated fat, 4% calories from saturated fat, 43 g carbohydrate, 1 g dietary fiber, 113 mg sodium, 8 g protein
Exchanges: 3 Carbohydrate

Low Carb
Per serving: 191 calories, 2 g fat, 1 g saturated fat, 4% calories from saturated fat, 38 g carbohydrate, 1 g dietary fiber, 100 mg sodium, 7 g protein
Exchanges: 2 1/2 Carbohydrate

Orange Ice

SERVING SIZE: 1/2 cup, SERVES: 6

3 cups orange juice　　　　　1 tsp orange zest
2 Tbsp lemon juice　　　　<c 3/4 cup sugar

1 Combine the orange juice, lemon juice, orange zest, and sugar. Stir until the sugar is completely dissolved. Pour into an ice cream machine and freeze according to the manufacturer's instructions. Allow to ripen in the deep freeze for an hour before serving.

2 If you don't have an ice cream freezer, pour into a 9-inch × 13-inch baking dish and place in the freezer. When it is just frozen (up to 2 hours), break up with a wooden spoon and place in a large bowl. Beat with an electric mixer until slushy and refreeze. You can serve it at this point or continue beating and freezing until it reaches the smoothness you desire.

<c **To Cut Carb**
<c Sugar: reduce to 1/4 cup and add 2 Tbsp Splenda.

Per serving: 154 calories, 0 g fat, 0 g saturated fat, 0% calories from saturated fat, 38 g carbohydrate, 0 g dietary fiber, 2 mg sodium
Exchanges: 1 Fruit, 1 1/2 Carbohydrate

Low Carb
Per serving: 90 calories, 0 g fat, 0 g saturated fat, 0% calories from saturated fat, 22 g carbohydrate, 0 g dietary fiber, 2 mg sodium
Exchanges: 1 Fruit, 1/2 Carbohydrate

Kiwis with Mango Sauce

SERVING SIZE: 1/4 of recipe, SERVES: 4

4 kiwis   <C 1/2 cup orange juice
2 mangoes

1   Cut kiwis in half around the middle. Run a spoon under the peel to remove the fruit whole, or peel the kiwi with a potato peeler, and then cut in half.

2   Peel mangoes, slice, and drop into a blender. Whiz, using just enough orange juice to allow mango slices to move, until smooth. Add rest of orange juice to make sauce pourable.

3   Divide sauce among 4 dessert plates. Set kiwis, 1 half down and 1 half with seeds showing, in mango sauce.

<C To Cut Carb
<C Orange juice: reduce to 1/4 cup.

Per serving: 147 calories, 1 g fat, 0 g saturated fat, 0% calories from saturated fat, 37 g carbohydrate, 5 g dietary fiber, 8 mg sodium
Exchanges: 2 1/2 Fruit

Low Carb
Per serving: 140 calories, 1 g fat, 0 g saturated fat, 0% calories from saturated fat, 35 g carbohydrate, 5 g dietary fiber, 7 mg sodium
Exchanges: 2 1/2 Fruit

Peach Raspberry Dessert

SERVING SIZE: 1/4 of recipe, SERVES: 4

2 fresh peaches or 4 canned halves   1 cup low-fat vanilla, peach, or
1 cup fresh or frozen raspberries   raspberry yogurt

1   Peel the fresh peaches, cut in half, and discard the seed. Lay a peach half in a dessert bowl. Spoon 1/4 cup raspberries into the hollow of each. Top the raspberries with yogurt and serve.

Per serving: 60 calories, 1 g fat, 0 g saturated fat, 0% calories from saturated fat, 13 g carbohydrate, 20 g dietary fiber, 3 mg sodium
Exchanges: 1/2 Fruit, 1/2 Carbohydrate

Fiji Fruit Baskets

SERVING SIZE: 1 fruit basket, SERVES: 6

Fruit Salad

1/2 fresh pineapple, peeled, cored, and cut into 1/2-inch dice

<C 2 bananas, peeled and cut into 1/2-inch dice

1 mango, peeled, seeded, and cut into 1/2-inch dice

1 tsp finely grated lime zest

<C 1 1/2 cups tonic water

Cookie Cups

1/4 cup packed dark brown sugar

1/4 cup dark corn syrup

2 tsp unsulfured molasses

2 Tbsp butter

2 Tbsp light olive oil

1/4 cup unsweetened apple juice

1/2 tsp ground ginger

1/4 tsp ground cinnamon

2/3 sifted all-purpose flour

Cream Filling

<C 1 1/4 cups low-fat vanilla yogurt

To make small cookies instead of cups, drop the batter by teaspoonfuls several inches apart. Using the back of a spoon, spread the batter into thin rounds and bake as above.

To Prepare the Salad

1 Combine the diced pineapple, bananas, and mango in a glass bowl. Sprinkle with the lime zest and cover with tonic water. Refrigerate until you are ready to use, but no longer than overnight.

To Prepare the Cookie Cups

2 Preheat the oven to 400°F. Coat 3 or 4 cookie sheets with cooking spray.

3 Set out 4 to 6 small juice glasses, large spice jars, or other cylindrical objects about 1 3/4 inches in diameter and at least 3 inches tall. You will use

these to shape the warm cookies. (You don't really need all 6 because you can only bake two cookies at a time and they cool quite quickly.)

4 In a large saucepan, combine the sugar, corn syrup, molasses, butter, oil, apple juice, ginger, and cinnamon. Bring to a boil over medium-high heat, stirring constantly, and boil vigorously for 1 minute. Remove from the heat and stir in the flour with a wire whisk. Beat until smooth.

5 Drop 1 Tbsp of the batter in a puddle on each half of a greased cookie sheet. (You will only be able to cook two cookies per sheet.) Using the back of a spoon, spread the batter into two smooth, thin circles 5 1/4 inches in diameter. Make sure there is plenty of space between the circles.

6 Bake for 7–8 minutes, or until the cookies are a dark golden brown. Watch carefully as they will burn easily. I set my timer for 5 minutes and add time depending on their color. Set the baking sheet on a wire rack and allow the wafers to cool for about 2 minutes.

7 Use a metal spatula to loosen and lift the wafers and drape them atop the inverted glasses. This is the tricky part. If the wafers are too hot, they will tear. If they are too cool, they won't form into cups. As you start loosening around the edges, you will be able to tell if they are ready. If they get too cool, you can reheat them in the oven. There is enough batter to make at least 10 cups, so you can do a little experimenting. The bent and broken bits make splendid snacks.

8 As the cookies firm up (this will happen very quickly), set them on a wire rack to cool completely. If the batter should get too thick to work easily, just rewarm it on the stove. When completely cool, the cups can be carefully stored in an airtight container, where they will keep up to a week.

To Serve

9 Drain the fruit in a colander and discard the juice—or drink it. Stir the yogurt with a spoon to liquefy it and spoon about 2 Tbsp into each cookie cup. Divide the fruit among the cups and top with a dollop of yogurt.

<c **To Cut Carb**
<c Bananas: replace with your favorite low-carb fruit.
<c Tonic water: remove entirely or replace with Diet Tonic.
<c Yogurt: replace with the aerosol light whipped cream.

Per serving: 258 calories, 6 g fat, 2 g saturated fat, 8% calories from saturated fat, 50 g carbohydrate, 2 g dietary fiber, 73 mg sodium
Exchanges: 1 1/2 Fruit, 1 Fat, 1 1/2 Carbohydrate

(Continued)

Low Carb
Per serving: 213 calories, 7 g fat, 2 g saturated fat, 10% calories from saturated fat, 40 g carbohydrate, 3 g dietary fiber, 50 mg sodium
Exchanges: 1 Fruit, 1 Fat, 1 1/2 Carbohydrate

Tarte Tatin

SERVING SIZE: 1 wedge, SERVES: 8

1/2 recipe Basic Pie Crust (page 479)	1/3 cup sugar
4 1/2 Jonagold or other soft cooking apples	1/4 cup butter flavored margarine
1/4 cup water	1 tsp lemon zest

1 Roll out dough for 1 pie crust into a 9-inch circle. Lay a cloth over it and set aside. Core, peel, and halve the apples. Lay them on a plate the same size as the pan you are going to use and trim the apples to fit together in a circle of 8 halves with 1 in the center. Set aside.

2 Preheat the oven to 425°F. Combine the water, sugar, and margarine in a chef's pan or heavy-bottomed skillet. Bring to a boil on high heat and stir until it turns golden brown. Pull off the heat and lay the apples in the pan round side down. Scatter the lemon zest over the top. Reduce the heat to medium. Place a lid, 1 size smaller than the lip of the pan, right down on top of the apples. Cook, shaking occasionally, 15 minutes or until the apples are tender. Remove from the heat and cool 10 minutes.

3 Fold the rolled out crust in quarters and lay on the top of the apples, unfolding to cover completely. Tuck the edges down around the hot apples and prick the crust a few times with a fork. Bake 20–30 minutes or until the crust is golden brown. Set on a rack and cool slightly, 10 minutes. Place a large inverted plate on top of the crust. Hold with a cloth in both hands and smartly turn it upside down (you *can* do it, *really!*). Then cut in wedges and serve with really good coffee.

Per serving: 191 calories, 10 g fat, 2 g saturated fat, 9% calories from saturated fat, 26 g carbohydrate, 1 g dietary fiber, 100 mg sodium
Exchanges: 2 Fat, 1 1/2 Carbohydrate

Spicy Coconut Pudding

SERVING SIZE: 1/4 of recipe, SERVES: 4

Coconut Cream

3/4 cup 2% milk
1/2 tsp sugar
  2 Tbsp desiccated coconut

1 Tbsp cornstarch mixed with
  2 Tbsp 2% milk (slurry)
1/2 tsp coconut essence

Syrup

1/4 cup firmly packed dark brown sugar
1/2 cup water
  3-inch cinnamon stick

1/2 tsp cardamom seeds
1/4 tsp whole cloves
1/8 tsp ground nutmeg

Custard

1 cup egg substitute
1/3 cup 2% milk

1/2 tsp coconut essence
  2 Tbsp firmly packed brown sugar

1 Preheat the oven to 350°F. Combine the milk, sugar, and coconut in a small saucepan and simmer 10 minutes. Strain and discard the coconut. Stir the slurry and coconut essence into the warm milk. Heat on medium, stirring until thickened. Set aside to cool.

2 Stir 1/4 cup of the brown sugar, water, and spices together in a small saucepan and bring to a boil. Reduce the heat and simmer for 5 minutes. Strain and set aside to cool.

3 When the syrup has cooled to room temperature, beat it together with the egg substitute until it's light in color. Add the milk, coconut essence, and coconut cream and mix well. Pour into ramekins or custard cups, set into a pan of hot water, and bake for 30 minutes or until a knife plunged into the center comes out clean. Chill.

4 A few hours before serving, sprinkle the brown sugar evenly over the custards. Place under the broiler and cook until all the sugar is bubbly, about 2 minutes. The sugar burns very easily so watch it carefully. Remove and cool.

Per serving: 150 calories, 2 g fat, 1 g saturated fat, 6% calories from saturated fat, 26 g carbohydrate, 0 g dietary fiber, 129 mg sodium, 7 g protein
Exchanges: 2 Carbohydrate

Orange Chocolate Yogurt Cake

SERVING SIZE: 1 slice, SERVES: 8

Cake

1/3 cup Dutch-process or European-style cocoa
1/2 cup firmly packed brown sugar
1/4 cup boiling water
1/2 cup plain nonfat yogurt
1 1/2 Tbsp light olive oil
1 1/2 Tbsp corn syrup
1 1/2 Tbsp unsweetened applesauce
1 large egg yolk
1 1/2 tsp vanilla extract

1 tsp grated orange zest (optional)
3/4 cup unsifted cake flour
1 Tbsp cornstarch
1 tsp baking powder
1/2 tsp baking soda
Pinch of salt
2 large egg whites, at room temperature
2 Tbsp granulated sugar

Orange Sauce

1 cup yogurt cheese (page 475)
1/4 cup 1% soy milk or skim milk
1/4 cup frozen orange juice concentrate

2 Tbsp pure maple syrup
1 tsp grated orange zest
1 tsp fresh lemon juice

Garnish

2 oranges, peeled and segmented (18 segments)
6 mint sprigs

To Prepare the Cake

1 Preheat the oven to 350°F. Make sure the egg whites are at room temperature before beginning the recipe.

2 Spray an 8-inch round cake pan with cooking spray. Cut a round piece of parchment or waxed paper to fit the bottom of the pan. Smooth the paper into the pan, spray with cooking spray, and coat the bottom and sides with flour. Set aside.

3 Combine the cocoa and brown sugar in a small bowl. Pour in the boiling water and stir until smooth. Set aside to cool.

4 In a large bowl, whisk together the yogurt, oil, corn syrup, applesauce, egg yolk, vanilla, and orange zest. Add the chocolate mixture and mix thoroughly.

5 In a separate bowl, combine the cake flour, cornstarch, baking powder, soda, and salt. Stir the dry ingredients gently into the chocolate mixture.

6 Make sure the bowl and whip attachment of your electric mixer are perfectly clean and grease-free. Beat the egg whites until soft peaks form. Sprinkle the sugar slowly over the top, one Tbsp at a time, and continue to beat until the whites are stiff but not dry.

7 Stir a large spoonful of beaten egg whites into the batter to lighten it. Gently fold in the rest of the egg whites in two steps.

8 Pour the batter into the prepared pan and bake for 35 to 40 minutes, or until a toothpick or cake tester inserted in the center comes out clean. Cool on a rack for 20 minutes, then tip out of the pan onto another rack to cool completely. The cake will fall slightly as it cools. This cake is best served the same day it is baked, but if you allow it to cool completely and then wrap it carefully, it will be fine the next day.

To Prepare the Sauce

9 In a medium bowl, whisk together the yogurt cheese, milk, orange juice concentrate, syrup, orange zest, and lemon juice. Keep whisking until the sauce is perfectly smooth. This sauce can be made ahead and refrigerated.

To Serve

10 Cut the cake into eight wedges. Place a wedge on each dessert plate and top with a spoonful of sauce. Lay a few orange segments and a sprig of mint on the side. (Leftover cake will keep for a few days if wrapped in plastic.)

Per serving: 296 calories, 4 g fat, 1 g saturated fat, 3% calories from saturated fat, 55 g carbohydrate, 2 g dietary fiber, 280 mg sodium, 12 g protein
Exchanges: 1/2 Fat, 4 Carbohydrate

Honeydew with Raspberry Sauce

SERVING SIZE: 1/4 of recipe, SERVES: 4

1 honeydew melon
3 cups fresh raspberries or 1 (10 oz) package
    frozen without sugar

2 Tbsp sugar
1 Tbsp cornstarch

(Continued)

1   Peel the melon by cutting off both ends. Stand the melon on one of its flat ends and cut away the rind from top to bottom. Now cut the melon in half lengthwise. Scoop out the seeds and pulp. Cut each half in two and each quarter into 3 or 4 wedges. Set aside.

2   Make the sauce by pressing the berries through a sieve into a saucepan. (Thaw the frozen berries in a sieve over a saucepan to catch the juice and push them through when completely thawed.) Stir the sugar and cornstarch into the juice and bring to a boil. Boil gently 30 seconds to cook the cornstarch. The sauce will be thick and clear.

3   Chill or serve warm over the honeydew wedges.

Per serving: 121 calories, 0 g fat, 0 g saturated fat, 0% calories from saturated fat, 30 g carbohydrate, 8 g dietary fiber, 19 mg sodium
Exchanges: 1 1/2 Fruit, 1/2 Carbohydrate

Pineapple Mint Dessert

SERVING SIZE: 1/8 of recipe, SERVES: 8

 1 whole fresh pineapple
20 fresh mint leaves

1   Twist the leaves off the top of the pineapple. Slice off the top and bottom, leaving a fat cylinder. Cut off the skin in wide strips from top to bottom. (Leaving some of the "eyes" won't hurt.) Now cut the pineapple in quarters lengthwise. Remove the core (it's great to chew on) and you're ready to cut it into chunks. Cut each quarter in thirds lengthwise then across into bite size pieces.

2   Make 4 neat piles of the mint leaves. Roll each pile lengthwise into a short cigar. Cut across into thin strips called *chiffonade*. Treating the mint this way will allow the mint to stay green and pretty. Mint, like basil, has tender leaves and doesn't like to be chopped. Stir the mint into the pineapple chunks and serve. Leftovers will keep in the refrigerator for 2 to 3 days.

Per serving: 38 calories, 0 g fat, 0 g saturated fat, 0% calories from saturated fat, 9 g carbohydrate, 1 g dietary fiber, 1 mg sodium
Exchanges: 1/2 Fruit

Raspberry (or other fruit) Smoothie

SERVING SIZE: 1 smoothie, SERVES: 1

1/4 cup nonfat plain yogurt
1/2 cup nonfat milk
1/2 cup fresh or frozen raspberries, strawberries, peaches, or whichever fruit you like

<C 1/2 banana sliced
2 Tbsp frozen orange juice concentrate

Whiz the yogurt, milk, fruit, bananas, and orange juice concentrate in a blender until smooth.

<C **To Cut Carb**
<C Banana: delete.

Per serving: 220 calories, 1 g fat, 1 g saturated fat, 5% calories from saturated fat, 46 g carbohydrate, 6 g dietary fiber, 116 mg sodium
Exchanges: 2 Fruit, 1 Fat-Free Milk

Low Carb
Per serving: 162 calories, 1 g fat, 0 g saturated fat, 0% calories from saturated fat, 32 g carbohydrate, 4 g dietary fiber, 115 mg sodium
Exchanges: 1 Fruit, 1 Fat-Free Milk

Melon Berry Sparkler

SERVING SIZE: 1/4 of recipe, SERVES: 4

1 1/3 cups cantaloupe chunks
1 1/3 cups honeydew chunks
1 1/3 strawberry halves

zest of 1 lime, 1/2 teaspoon
1 cup ginger ale

Combine the cantaloupe, honeydew, strawberries, and lime zest in a bowl. Pour over the ginger ale and serve in a wine glass or glass bowl.

Per serving: 80 calories, 0 g fat, 0 g saturated fat, 0% calories from saturated fat, 20 g carbohydrate, 2 g dietary fiber, 15 mg sodium
Exchanges: 1 1/2 Fruit

Baked Pineapple with an Orange Ginger Sauce

SERVING SIZE: 1/6 of recipe, SERVES: 6

1 whole fresh pineapple or 1 (20 oz) can sliced pineapple in juice, drained
1 cup orange juice
5 quarter-size slices ginger root
1 tsp arrowroot or cornstarch mixed with 2 Tbsp orange juice, slurry

1 Preheat the oven to 350°F. Cut off both ends of the pineapple. Cut lengthwise into sixths and remove the core. Run a knife blade between the flesh and skin of each pineapple wedge, leaving the flesh sitting on the skin. Slice the flesh crosswise at 1/2-inch intervals then make one cut lengthwise from end to end. Set into a 9-inch × 13-inch glass baking dish and bake 15 minutes or until heated through. If you are using canned pineapple, lay the slices in a glass baking dish and heat through the same way you would the fresh.

2 Bring the orange juice and ginger root to a boil in a small saucepan. Simmer 5 minutes. Remove the ginger and stir in the slurry. Heat to thicken and clear.

3 Divide the pineapple among 4 dessert plates and spoon the sauce over the top.

Per serving: 101 calories, 1 g fat, 0 g saturated fat, 0% calories from saturated fat, 25 g carbohydrate, 2 g dietary fiber, 1 mg sodium
Exchanges: 1 1/2 Fruit

The Basics—Sauces, Stocks, and Condiments

Super Salsa

SERVING SIZE: 1/6 of recipe, SERVES: 6

  1 (15 oz) can reduced-sodium black beans
1 1/2 cups prepared chunky salsa (plain tomato, roasted garlic, chipotle, peach, or mango)
  garnishes to taste (garlic, green onions, corn, cilantro, a few sliced green olives, cumin, chili powder, or cayenne)

1 Drain and rinse the beans. Stir into the salsa and add any garnishes you think your family would like.

2 Serve as an appetizer with baked tortilla chips, as a side dish at a barbecue, on a baked potato, or as an omelet filling.

Per serving: 49 calories, 0 g fat, 0 g saturated fat, 0% calories from saturated fat, 11 g carbohydrate, 4 g dietary fiber, 586 mg sodium
Exchanges: 1/2 Starch

Passion Fruit Vinaigrette

SERVING SIZE: 1/6 of recipe, SERVES: 6

  4 passion fruit
  1 shallot, finely chopped
  1 clove garlic, bashed and chopped
1/2 tsp honey

  1 tsp lemon juice
1/2 tsp Worcestershire sauce
  3 Tbsp rice vinegar
1/2 tsp arrowroot

1 Cut the passion fruit in half and scoop the pulp and seeds into a small bowl. Put the shallot, garlic, honey, lemon juice, and Worcestershire sauce in a blender and whiz until smooth. Add the vinegar.

2 Pour over the passion fruit. Stir and press with a rubber spatula to rinse the seeds and separate them from the pulp. Pour through a medium sieve, pressing to release as much pulp as you can. Stir in the arrowroot, heat until thickened, and pour over spinach or other salad greens.

Per serving: 14 calories, 0 g fat, 0 g saturated fat, 0% calories from saturated fat, 4 g carbohydrate, 0 g dietary fiber, 5 mg sodium
Exchanges: Free Food

Raspberry Sauce

SERVING SIZE: 1/4 of recipe, SERVES: 4

1 (10 oz) package of frozen raspberries with no sugar
2 tsp cornstarch mixed with 2 Tbsp water

1 Defrost the raspberries in a sieve over a saucepan. The juice will drip out as they thaw, doing some of the work for you! Press the rest through the sieve and discard the seeds. You should have 1 cup of juice.

2 Stir in the slurry and bring to a boil to thicken and clear. Cool and pour into a plastic squirt bottle like the ones they sell for mustard or ketchup. When you want to use it, squirt nice zig-zags of raspberry sauce across a bowl of frozen yogurt or on a plate with angel food cake.

Per serving: 34 calories, 0 g fat, 0 g saturated fat, 0% calories from saturated fat, 8 g carbohydrate, 1 g dietary fiber, 0 mg sodium
Exchanges: 1/2 Fruit

Okra for Soups, Stews, and Gumbos

SERVING SIZE: 1/4 of recipe, SERVES: 4

1/4 cup flour
1/2 tsp salt
1/2 tsp pepper
2 cups fresh or frozen okra, trimmed and sliced in 1/2-inch pieces
1 1/2 tsp olive oil

1 Combine the flour, salt, and pepper in a bag. Add the okra and shake to coat.

2 Heat the oil in a large skillet on medium high. Tip the okra into a sieve to shake off the extra flour. Drop the okra into the heated oil and cook until nicely browned. Drop into a gumbo style soup or stew and enjoy.

Per serving: 62 calories, 2 g fat, 0 g saturated fat, 0% calories from saturated fat, 10 g carbohydrate, 2 g dietary fiber, 144 mg sodium
Exchanges: 1/2 Starch, 1 Vegetable

Apple Butter

SERVING SIZE: 1/6 of recipe, SERVES: 6

3 cooking apples (Jonagold, Macintosh, Rome, or Winesap)	1/8 cup raisins
	1/4 cup brown sugar
1/4 cup unsweetened apple juice	1/8 tsp ground cinnamon
1/4 cup water	pinch cloves

1 Wash, core, and slice the apples. Place in a saucepan with the juice, water, and raisins. Bring to a boil, reduce the heat and simmer until the apples are soft, about 20 minutes.

2 Whiz in a blender until smooth and return to the pan. Add the brown sugar, cinnamon, and cloves and simmer another 30 minutes or until dark brown and thick. Spread on toast or spoon over low-fat frozen yogurt.

Per serving: 89 calories, 0 g fat, 0 g saturated fat, 0% calories from saturated fat, 23 g carbohydrate, 2 g dietary fiber, 4 mg sodium
Exchanges: 1 1/2 Fruit

Nectarine Salsa

SERVING SIZE: 1/4 of recipe, SERVES: 4

4 ripe but firm nectarines or papayas	3 Tbsp lime juice
1/3 cup thinly sliced green onions	1/4 cup chopped cilantro
1 jalapeño pepper, finely chopped with the seeds if you like it hot	1/4 tsp salt
	1 tsp brown sugar

1 Cut the nectarines in half and remove the seeds. Cut into 1/4-inch pieces and mix with the green onion, jalapeño pepper, lime juice, cilantro, and salt. Add the brown sugar if you need it. Let it sit to mellow the flavors while you prepare the rest of the meal.

2 Serve over grilled white fish, chicken breasts, or pork.

Per serving: 68 calories, 1 g fat, 0 g saturated fat, 0% calories from saturated fat, 16 g carbohydrate, 2 g dietary fiber, 145 mg sodium
Exchanges: 1 Fruit

Basic Chicken, Turkey, or Duck Broth

SERVING SIZE: 1/4 of recipe, SERVES: 4

1 tsp non-aromatic olive oil	1 bay leaf
1 onion, peeled and chopped	2 sprigs fresh thyme or 1 tsp dried
1/2 cup coarsely chopped celery	2 sprigs fresh parsley
1 cup coarsely chopped carrots	6 black peppercorns
2 lb chicken, turkey, or duck backs and necks or 1 carcass with scraps	2 whole cloves
	8 cups water

1 Pour the oil into a large stockpot over medium heat. Add the onion, celery tops, and carrots and fry to release their volatile oils, about 5 minutes. Add the chicken and seasonings and cover with 8 cups water.

2 Bring to a boil, skimming off foam that rises to the top. Reduce the heat, and simmer 2 to 4 hours, skimming occasionally as needed.

3 Pour through a fine sieve and skim off all fat. You can chill, letting the fat harden before you skim it off or use a fat strainer to make it easier.

Per serving: 11 calories, 0 g fat, 0 g saturated fat, 0% calories from saturated fat, 0 g carbohydrate, 0 g dietary fiber, 20 mg sodium
Exchanges: Free Food

Nectarine Sauce

SERVING SIZE: 1/4 of recipe, SERVES: 4

2 nectarines, pitted	1/2 cup orange juice
pinch nutmeg	

1 Cut up the nectarines and place in blender jar. Add the orange juice and nutmeg and whiz until smooth. Pour over sliced bananas, raspberries, or pears for a beautiful and tasty dessert.

Per serving: 48 calories, 0 g fat, 0 g saturated fat, 0% calories from saturated fat, 11 g carbohydrate, 1 g dietary fiber, 0 mg sodium
Exchanges: 1 Fruit

Tomato Herb Salad Dressing

SERVING SIZE: 1/6 of recipe, SERVES: 6

1 cup low-sodium tomato juice
1 Tbsp lemon juice
4 1/2 tsp extra virgin olive oil
1/2 tsp dry mustard
1/2 tsp dried tarragon

1 1/2 tsp chopped fresh basil
   or 1/2 tsp dried basil
1/4 tsp salt
   pinch cayenne pepper

1 Whiz together tomato juice, lemon juice, oil, mustard, tarragon, basil, salt, and cayenne pepper in a blender. Serve as a dressing for salad greens.

Per serving: 39 calories, 3 g fat, 0 g saturated fat, 0% calories from saturated fat, 2 g carbohydrate, 0 g dietary fiber, 97 mg sodium
Exchanges: 1/2 Fat

Red Plum Sauce for Meat

SERVING SIZE: 1/4 of recipe, SERVES: 4

1/2 tsp non-aromatic olive oil
1/2 cup chopped sweet onion
  2 cups chopped red or purple plums
1/4 tsp dried oregano

<C 1 cup pear nectar or apple juice
1/4 tsp salt
1/4 tsp freshly ground black pepper

1 Heat the oil in a high-sided skillet on medium high. Sauté the onion until it wilts and turns translucent. Add the plums, thyme, and juice. Bring to a boil, reduce the heat, and simmer 20 minutes.

2 Press through a sieve, season with salt and pepper, and serve with pork, turkey, or duck. You can skip the sieving and it will be a lovely chutney to serve with meats or curries.

<C **To Cut Carb** ─────────────────────
<C Pear nectar: replace with 1 cup of nonalcoholic Merlot (red wine).

Per serving: 96 calories, 1 g fat, 0 g saturated fat, 0% calories from saturated fat, 22 g carbohydrate, 2 g fiber, 149 mg sodium
Exchanges: 1 1/2 Fruit

Per serving: 71 calories, 1 g fat, 0 g saturated fat, 0% calories from saturated fat, 15 g carbohydrate, 2 g dietary fiber, 150 mg sodium
Exchanges: 1 Fruit

Coconut Cream

SERVING SIZE: 1 Tbsp, SERVES: 16

3/4 cup 2% milk
1/2 tsp sugar
2 Tbsp unsweetened desiccated coconut

1 Tbsp cornstarch mixed with
2 Tbsp 2% milk (slurry)
1/2 tsp coconut essence

1 Combine milk, sugar, and coconut in a small saucepan, and simmer 10 minutes. Strain and discard the coconut.

2 Stir the slurry and coconut essence into the warm milk. Heat on medium, stirring until thickened. Set aside to cool.

Per serving: 14 calories, 1 g fat, 0.6 g saturated fat, 4% calories from saturated fat, 1 g carbohydrate, 0 g dietary fiber, 7 mg sodium
Exchanges: Free food

No Bake Fig Crust

SERVING SIZE: 1 9-inch crust, SERVES: N/A

18 white or black figs, stemmed
1 cup broken graham crackers, chocolate wafers or gingersnaps depending on filling

1 Place the figs and crackers in a food processor and whiz until it forms a ball.

2 Press evenly into a pie tin or spring form pan with wet fingers. Fill with filling that doesn't need to bake.

Per serving: 78 calories, 1 g fat, 0 g saturated fat, 0% calories from saturated fat, 17 g carbohydrate, 2 g dietary fiber, 68 mg sodium
Exchanges: 1/2 Starch, 1/2 Fruit

Basic Beef Stock

SERVING SIZE: 1 cup, SERVES: 4

1 lb beef bones, fat trimmed off
1 tsp non-aromatic olive oil
1 onion, coarsely chopped
1/2 cup coarsely chopped leaves and
    tops of celery
1 cup coarsely chopped carrots

1 bay leaf
1 tsp dried thyme
6 black peppercorns
2 whole cloves
8 cups water

1 Preheat the oven to 375°F. Place the beef bones in a roasting pan and cook until nicely browned, about 25 minutes. The browning produces a richer flavor and deeper color in the final stock.

2 Pour the oil into a large stockpot over medium heat. Add the onion, celery, and carrots and fry to release their volatile oils, about 5 minutes. Add the bones, bay leaf, thyme, peppercorns, and cloves. Pour in the water, bring to a boil, reduce the heat, and simmer 4 to 8 hours, adding more water if necessary. Skim off any foam as it rises to the surface.

3 Pour through a fine strainer, discard the solids, skim off all the fat. The stock can be frozen for up to 6 months.

Per serving: 12 calories, 0 g fat, 0 g saturated fat, 0% calories from saturated fat, 0 g carbohydrate, 0 g dietary fiber, 18 mg sodium
Exchanges: Free Food

Lime Brightener for Vegetables

SERVING SIZE: 1/2 cup, SERVES: 4

2 Tbsp fresh lime juice
1 1/2 tsp olive oil

1 tsp chopped fresh oregano
2 cups cooked vegetables

1 Combine lime juice, oil, and oregano with a whisk, and pour over hot steamed vegetables, broiled tomato halves, or sliced raw tomatoes.

Per serving (with 2 cups cooked broccoli): 39 calories, 2 g fat, 0 g saturated fat, 0% calories from saturated fat, 5 g carbohydrate, 2 g dietary fiber, 20 mg sodium
Exchanges: 1 Vegetable, 1/2 Fat

Apricot Cilantro Sauce for Chicken or Fish

SERVING SIZE: 1/6 of recipe, SERVES: 6

1 cup dried apricots
1 tsp light olive oil
1 cup chopped sweet onion
1 Tbsp finely chopped ginger root
2 pounds plum tomatoes, seeded
 and diced
 pinch cloves

1/2 tsp ground cinnamon
1/4 tsp ground coriander
1/4 tsp salt
1/4 tsp black pepper
 2 Tbsp chopped cilantro
 2 Tbsp apricot preserves

1 Soak the apricots in enough hot water to cover for 1 hour. Drain and chop.

2 Heat the oil in a saucepan on medium high. Cook the onion and ginger 2 minutes. Add the tomatoes, apricots, cloves, cinnamon, coriander, salt, and pepper. Cook 10 minutes.

3 Stir in the cilantro and apricot preserves. Spoon over cooked chicken breasts or white fish fillets.

Per serving: 101 calories, 1 g fat, 0 g saturated fat, 0% calories from saturated fat, 23 g carbohydrate, 4 g dietary fiber, 97 mg sodium
Exchanges: 2 Vegetable, 1 Fruit

Bouquet Garni

SERVING SIZE: N/A, SERVES: N/A

1 bay leaf
2 sprigs fresh thyme or 1 tsp dried
6 peppercorns

2 whole cloves
3 sprigs parsley

1 Tie all the ingredients in a square of cheesecloth and use to flavor soups and stews.

Per serving: 0 calories, 0 g fat, 0 g saturated fat, 0% calories from saturated fat, 0 g carbohydrate, 0 g dietary fiber, 0 mg sodium
Exchanges: Free Food

Basic Fish or Shrimp Stock

SERVING SIZE: 1 cup, SERVES: 4

1 tsp non-aromatic olive oil
1 onion, peeled and chopped
1/2 cup coarsely chopped celery tops
2 sprigs fresh thyme or 1 tsp dried thyme
1 bay leaf

1 lb fish bones (no heads) or
    shrimp shells
6 black peppercorns
2 whole cloves
5 cups water

1 Pour the oil into a large saucepan and sauté the onion, celery tops, thyme, and bay leaf until onion is translucent, about 5 minutes. To ensure a light colored stock, be careful not to brown.

2 Add the fresh bones or shrimp shells, peppercorns, and cloves, cover with 5 cups water, bring to a boil, reduce the heat, and simmer for 25 minutes.

3 Strain through a fine-mesh sieve and cheesecloth.

Per serving: 13 calories, 1 g fat, 0 g saturated fat, 0% calories from saturated fat, 0 g carbohydrate, 0 g dietary fiber, 6 mg sodium
Exchanges: Free Food

Mushroom Smother

SERVING SIZE: 1/4 of recipe, SERVES: 4

1/2 lb brown or white button
    mushrooms, sliced (2 cups)
2 Tbsp lemon juice

1/4 tsp salt
1/4 tsp pepper
2 Tbsp chopped parsley, dill, or chives

1 Wash the mushrooms under cold water and dry immediately with paper towels. Slice into 1/4-inch pieces, stems and all. Toss the mushroom slices with lemon juice, salt, and pepper. Heat a high-sided skillet on high and add the mushrooms. Sauté until nice and brown. Stir in the chopped herbs.

2 Serve over broiled chicken breasts, lamb chops, or thick wedges of baked winter squash.

Per serving: 17 calories, 0 g fat, 0 g saturated fat, 0% calories from saturated fat, 3 g carbohydrate, 1 g dietary fiber, 143 mg sodium
Exchanges: 1 Vegetable

Apricot Sauce

SERVING SIZE: 1/4 of recipe, SERVES: 4

1/2 cup dried apricots	1/4 tsp ground cinnamon
1 1/2 cups apple juice	1 Tbsp cornstarch

1 Bring the apricots and apple juice to a boil. Turn off the heat and let soak for about 30 minutes. Stir in the cinnamon and cornstarch. Pour into a blender and whiz until very smooth, adding more juice if it is too thick. Pour back into the saucepan.

2 Heat until the sauce becomes smooth and glossy. Serve hot or cold over low fat frozen yogurt.

Per serving: 95 calories, 0 g fat, 0 g saturated fat, 0% calories from saturated fat, 24 g carbohydrate, 0 g dietary fiber, 5 mg sodium
Exchanges: 1 1/2 Fruit

Basic Lamb Stock

SERVING SIZE: 1 cup, SERVES: 4

1 tsp non-aromatic olive oil	2 cloves garlic, bashed and chopped
trim from the lamb steaks	3-inch sprig rosemary
1/2 large onion, roughly chopped	4 cups water

1 Heat the oil in a chef's pan or deep skillet. Toss in the rim and stir to brown 1 or 2 minutes. Add the onion, garlic, and rosemary, stirring until the ingredients start to brown. Pour in the water, bring to a boil, reduce the heat, and simmer while you prepare the rest of the stew. You will get a lot of flavor in just 15 or 20 minutes. Strain into a fat separator and pour 3 cups into the stew.

2 You can make more by returning the stock ingredients to the pan and adding 4 cups more water. Simmer another 20 minutes, de-fat, and freeze for another time.

Per serving: 16 calories, 1 g fat, 0 g saturated fat, 0% calories from saturated fat, 0 g carbohydrate, 0 g dietary fiber, 2 mg sodium
Exchanges: Free Food

Savory Cherry Relish

SERVING SIZE: 1/4 of recipe, SERVES: 4

     1 tsp olive oil
     2 Tbsp finely chopped shallots or onions
     1 cup chopped fresh or canned sweet cherries
     1 cup chopped fresh pie cherries or 1/2 cup dried tart cherries
1/2 cup orange juice
     1 tsp cornstarch or arrowroot mixed with 1 Tbsp orange juice (slurry)
     2 Tbsp chopped parsley
1/4 tsp salt
1/4 tsp pepper

1 Heat the oil in a saucepan on medium high. Sauté the shallots 2 minutes being careful not to brown. Add all the cherries and the orange juice and bring to a boil. Reduce the heat and simmer 10 minutes.

2 Stir in the slurry to thicken, 30 seconds. Add the parsley, salt, and pepper. Spoon on to a small serving (3 oz) of beef or pork. It will greatly enhance the meat and make it seem like there is a lot more of it!

Per serving: 79 calories, 2 g fat, 0 g saturated fat, 0% calories from saturated fat, 16 g carbohydrate, 2 g dietary fiber, 142 mg sodium
Exchanges: 1 Fruit, 1/2 Fat

Strawberry Jalapeño Salsa

SERVING SIZE: 1/4 of recipe, SERVES: 4

3 cups sliced fresh strawberries
1 apple, cored and chopped
1 jalapeño, chopped (leave the seeds in if you like it hot)
1 Tbsp brown sugar

1 Just before serving, combine the strawberries, apples, jalapeño, and brown sugar. Serve with cold meats.

Per serving: 71 calories, 1 g fat, 0 g saturated fat, 0% calories from saturated fat, 18 g carbohydrate, 3 g dietary fiber, 3 mg sodium
Exchanges: 1 Fruit

Roasted Garlic and Green Pea Pasta Sauce

SERVING SIZE: 1/4 of recipe, SERVES: 4

1 head garlic
1 lb frozen peas
1 cup nonfat evaporated milk

1/4 tsp salt
 2 Tbsp grated Parmesan cheese
 2 Tbsp chopped parsley

1 Preheat the oven to 350°F. Cut off the stem end of the head of garlic exposing the cloves inside. Wrap in foil and bake in the preheated oven 1 hour or until very soft. Unwrap and allow to cool.

2 Drop the peas into boiling water and cook 2 minutes. Drain and toss into a blender. Squeeze the garlic head toward the cut end to collect all the soft flesh. Add to the peas in the blender along with the evaporated milk and salt. Whiz until smooth.

3 Push through a sieve and reheat. Serve over pasta with Parmesan cheese and chopped parsley on top.

Per serving: 167 calories, 1 g fat, 1 g saturated fat, 5% calories from saturated fat, 27 g carbohydrate, 6 g dietary fiber, 372 mg sodium, 12 g protein
Exchanges: 1 1/2 Starch, 1/2 Fat-Free Milk

Mango Dessert Sauce

SERVING SIZE: 1/4 of recipe, SERVES: 4

 2 fresh mangoes
1/4 tsp nutmeg

1 cup orange, pineapple or other fruit juice

1 Peel and cut the mangoes then toss them into your blender. Start the blender and pour in just enough juice to start the mango pieces moving. Whiz until smooth. Add the rest of the juice, whiz to mix, and pour over fresh raspberries, pears, or vanilla frozen yogurt.

Per serving: 96 calories, 0 g fat, 0 g saturated fat, 0% calories from saturated fat, 24 g carbohydrate, 2 g dietary fiber, 3 mg sodium, 0 g protein
Exchanges: 1 1/2 Fruit

Green Enchilada Sauce

SERVING SIZE: 2 cups, SERVES: 1

1 lb tomatillos
1/2 cup chopped sweet onion
1 jalapeño pepper, chopped with seeds (hot), without seeds (milder)
2 cloves garlic, chopped
1 Tbsp chopped cilantro
1 1/2 cups low-sodium chicken broth

1 Remove the husks, and rinse the tomatillos. Place in a saucepan barely covered with water, and simmer until soft, about 3 minutes. Pour into a bowl through a sieve with the cooking liquid. Press to puree the pulp.

2 Combine with the onion, garlic, jalapeño, and cilantro. Blend until smooth.

3 Pour into a saucepan with the chicken broth, and bring to a boil. Boil softly until the volume is reduced and the flavors, concentrated—about 15 minutes.

4 Use as sauce on chicken or cheese enchiladas, to poach chicken breasts, or add zest to Tex-Mex soups and stews.

Per serving: 57 calories, 1 g fat, 16% calories from fat, 0 g saturated fat, 0% calories from saturated fat, 10 g carbohydrate, 3 g dietary fiber, 147 mg sodium
Exchanges: 2 Vegetable

Mango Chutney

SERVING SIZE: 1/4 of recipe, SERVES: 4

1 mango, peeled and cut in small chunks
2 Tbsp chopped sweet onion
1 tsp grated fresh ginger
1/8 tsp cayenne pepper
1/2 cup grape juice

1 Combine the mango, onion, ginger, cayenne, and grape juice in a saucepan. Bring to a boil, reduce the heat, and simmer 10 minutes. Serve as a condiment or sauce with chicken, white fish, or pork.

Per serving: 48 calories, 0 g fat, 0 g saturated fat, 0% calories from saturated fat, 12 g carbohydrate, 1 g dietary fiber, 2 mg sodium, 0 g protein
Exchanges: 1 Fruit

Basic Vegetable Stock

SERVING SIZE: 1 cups, SERVES: 4

1 tsp non-aromatic olive oil
1 onion, peeled and chopped
2 cloves garlic, peeled and bashed
1/2 tsp freshly grated ginger root
1/2 cup coarsely chopped carrot
1 cup coarsely chopped celery
1 cup coarsely chopped turnip
1/4 cup coarsely chopped leeks, white and light green parts only
3 sprigs fresh parsley
1/2 tsp black peppercorns
5 cups water

1 Pour the oil into a large stockpot over medium heat, add the onion and garlic, and sauté for 5 minutes. Add the rest of the ingredients and cover with 5 cups water.

2 Bring to a boil, reduce the heat, and simmer 30 minutes.

3 Strain through a fine-mesh sieve and cheesecloth.

Per serving: 12 calories, 1 g fat, 0 g saturated fat, 0% calories from saturated fat, 0 g carbohydrate, 0 g dietary fiber, 1 mg sodium
Exchanges: Free Food

Berry Vinegar

SERVING SIZE: 2 Tbsp, SERVES: 16

2 cups fresh blackberries or raspberries
1 pint rice vinegar

1 Combine the berries and vinegar and pour into a quart jar. Close and let set in the refrigerator for 2 weeks.

2 Strain, discard the berries, and use the vinegar in salads and sauces.

Per serving: 5 calories, 0 g fat, 0 g saturated fat, 0 % calories from saturated fat, 1 g carbohydrate, 0 g fiber, 0 mg sodium
Exchanges: Free Food

Boiled Lentils

(*To have on hand to add to soups and stews*)

SERVING SIZE: 1/2 cup, SERVES: 6

1 cup red or brown lentils, rinsed
  and sorted
1 onion
3 to 4 cups low-sodium chicken or
  vegetable stock (pages 463, 473)
  Bouquet Garni

1 bay leaf
1/2 tsp dried thyme or 2 sprigs fresh
2 cloves
6 black peppercorns
3 sprigs parsley

1 Place the lentils in a large saucepan with the whole onion. Pour 3 cups of the stock over the top and bring to a boil. Tie the bouquet garni ingredients in a piece of cheesecloth and drop into the pot.

2 Reduce the heat and simmer 30 minutes or until tender. Add more stock if it starts getting dry. Remove and discard the onion and bouquet garni. Chill and store in the refrigerator or freezer to use in soups or stews.

Per serving: 114 calories, 0 g fat, 0 g saturated fat, 0% calories from saturated fat, 18 g carbohydrate, 10 g fiber, 38 mg sodium
Exchanges: 1 Starch, 1 Very Lean Meat

Sweet Pea Guacamole

SERVING SIZE: 1/4 of recipe, SERVES: 4

2 cups fresh or frozen peas
2 Tbsp fresh lemon or lime juice
1/2 tsp chili powder or to taste
1/8 tsp cayenne pepper or to taste

1/4 to 1/2 cup salsa
1 Tbsp minced onion
1 garlic clove, minced

1 In medium saucepan, bring 3 cups water to a boil. Add fresh or frozen peas and cook 5–8 minutes or until soft. Drain. In blender or bowl, mash peas, juice, chili powder, cayenne, salsa, onion, and garlic. Serve with baked tortilla chips or pita wedges.

Per serving: 71 calories, 0 g fat, 0 g saturated fat, 0% calories from saturated fat, 13 g carbohydrate, 5 g dietary fiber, 125 mg sodium, 4 g protein
Exchanges: 1 Starch

Yogurt Cheese

SERVING SIZE: 1 Tbsp, SERVES: 16

The Wonders of Yogurt Cheese

I'm loath to overstate any one food or idea. However, the consistent use of yogurt cheese instead of butter, margarine, or cream has made a huge difference in our consumption of calories from fat. In our case, the actual savings over one year amounts to just over 40,000 calories, or over 11 pounds of body fat—just with one food!

---

1 Find a 32-oz tub of plain, nonfat yogurt that contains *no* thickeners, such as gelatin or starch (just check the ingredients). Avoid a yogurt with cornstarch or thickeners, which stop the yogurt from separating. I've found that Dannon does one that's almost always readily available.

2 The method is so simple—it only takes 28 seconds! Use a yogurt strainer or a colander with absorbent kitchen toweling. Pour the yogurt into the strainer and place in the refrigerator for at least 8 hours or overnight. During this time, 50% of the whey drains away and you are left with yogurt cheese. The conversion to cheese (straining off the whey) takes about 12 hours. The "cheese" becomes quite firm and the small lumps disappear, which makes it ideal for use in sauces. You don't have to worry about it or watch it. I've once left it for a week without a problem.

3 Add a soft tub light margarine (with no trans fatty acids) in equal proportions to create a cup of spread (you can also use 2/3 strained yogurt and 1/3 margarine proportion for even less fat and calories).

4 Other ways to use yogurt cheese:

- Mix with maple syrup to serve alongside a slice of pie.
- Substitute for sour cream on a baked potato, adding fresh ground pepper and chives.
- Serve as a sauce with poached chicken, using the yogurt cheese and chicken stock thickened with cornstarch and garnished with capers and pimento and a dash of parsley on the top.

Per serving (yogurt cheese only): 12 calories, 0 g fat, 0 g saturated fat, 0% calories from saturated fat, 2 g carbohydrate, 0 g dietary fiber, 17 mg sodium
Exchanges: Free Food

Around the Globe Ethmix

SERVING SIZE: N/A, SERVES: N/A

Scandinavian Ethmix

4 1/2 tsp horseradish powder (wasabi)	2 1/4 tsp dried seaweed
2 1/4 tsp caraway seeds	1 tsp ground white pepper
3 Tbsp dried parsley	1/2 tsp ground allspice
2 1/4 tsp wild mushroom powder	4 1/4 tsp sea salt

Grind all above to a fine powder and add: 1/2 tsp dried dill weed

Northern France Ethmix

10 tsp dried tarragon	1/2 tsp ground cloves
1 1/4 tsp powdered bay leaf	10 tsp dried chervil
5 tsp dried thyme	

Grind to a fine powder.

Northwest Italy Ethmix

8 tsp dried oregano	4 tsp rubbed sage
4 tsp dried basil	2 tsp dried rosemary
4 tsp ground fennel seeds	

Grind to a fine powder.

Southern France Ethmix

2 1/2 tsp dried rosemary	1 1/4 tsp powdered bay leaf
2 1/2 tsp dried basil	5 tsp dried marjoram
5 tsp rubbed sage	5 tsp dried oregano

Grind to a fine powder.

Germany Ethmix

16 whole juniper berries	2 tsp horseradish powder (wasabi)
1 tsp dried Cascade hops	2 tsp caraway powder
1 tsp mushroom powder	8 tsp dried marjoram
4 tsp dried chives	2 tsp white pepper

Grind to a fine powder.

Shanghai Coastline Ethmix

7 Tbsp crushed red pepper flakes
2 3/4 tsp ground ginger

2 3/4 tsp ground anise

Grind to a fine powder.

Poland Ethmix

4 tsp caraway powder
1 1/2 tsp dried marjoram
3 whole juniper berries

1/8 tsp ground cloves
3/4 tsp white pepper

Grind to a fine powder.

Thailand Ethmix

10 tsp dried lemon grass
5 tsp galangal
1 1/2 tsp ground red pepper (cayenne)

1 1/4 tsp dried spearmint
5 tsp dried cilantro
2 1/2 tsp dried basil

Grind to a fine powder.

India Ethmix

5 tsp turmeric
2 1/2 tsp dry mustard
5 tsp ground cumin
5 tsp ground coriander

1 1/4 tsp ground red pepper (cayenne)
2 1/2 tsp dill seeds
2 1/2 tsp cardamom seeds
2 1/2 tsp fenugreek seeds

Grind to a fine powder.

Morocco Ethmix

5 tsp grated nutmeg
5 tsp ground cumin
5 tsp ground coriander
2 1/2 tsp ground allspice

2 1/2 tsp ground ginger
1 1/4 tsp ground red pepper (cayenne)
1 1/4 tsp ground cinnamon

Grind to a fine powder.

Bali Ethmix

3/4 tsp ground bay leaves
4 tsp ground ginger
3 tsp turmeric
1 1/2 tsp dried onion

1 1/2 tsp dried garlic
1 1/2 tsp freshly ground black pepper
6 tsp crushed red pepper flakes

Grind to a fine powder.

Greek Islands Ethmix

4 Tbsp oregano	6 tsp dried lemongrass
6 tsp ground fennel seeds	3/4 tsp black pepper

Grind to a fine powder.

Exchanges (For All): Free Food

Roasted Tomato Salsa

(*Copyright Rick Bayless's* Mexican Kitchen)

SERVING SIZE: 1/2 cup, SERVES: 4

1 lb Italian plum tomatoes, such as Roma	1/2 tsp salt
2 fresh jalapeño peppers	1/3 cup sweet onion, finely chopped
3 cloves garlic, unpeeled	1/2 cup loosely packed cilantro, chopped

1 Preheat the broiler.

2 Line a shallow baking pan with aluminum foil and lay the whole tomatoes on it. Broil the tomatoes until their skins are blistered and blackened, about 6 minutes. Turn and blacken the other side. Cool and peel, reserving the juices.

3 Heat a heavy frying pan over medium heat. Lay the peppers and garlic in the dry pan and turn occasionally until soft, 5 to 10 minutes for the peppers and up to 15 minutes for the garlic. A quick pinch will tell you if they are ready. They should be softened and yield to slight pressure. Cool, peel the garlic, and remove the stems from the peppers.

4 Pulse the peppers, garlic, and salt in a blender or food processor. Add the tomatoes and their reserved juice and pulse a few times more, until coarsely chopped. Pour the mixture into a bowl, stir in the onion and cilantro, and set aside until ready to serve. This salsa will keep in the refrigerator for one or two days.

Per serving: 28 calories, 0 g fat, 0 g saturated fat, 0% calories from saturated fat, 6 g carbohydrate, 1 g dietary fiber, 1 g protein
Exchanges: 1 Vegetable

Blackberry Sauce Sweet or Savory

SERVING SIZE: 1/4 of recipe, SERVES: 4

2 cups fresh or frozen blackberries
1 cup apple juice

2 Tbsp arrowroot or cornstarch mixed
with 1/4 cup apple juice (slurry)

1 Combine the berries and apple juice in a saucepan and bring to a boil.
Reduce the heat and simmer 5 minutes. Press through a sieve to get rid of
the seeds and return the liquid to the pan.

2 Stir in the slurry and heat to thicken and clear. Serve over low fat frozen
yogurt or add 1/4 tsp each salt and pepper and serve over lamb or pork.

Per serving: 99 calories, 0 g fat, 0 g saturated fat, 0% calories from saturated fat,
24 g carbohydrate, 4 g fiber, 3 mg sodium
Exchanges: 1 1/2 Starch

Basic Pie Crust

SERVING SIZE: 1 slice, SERVES: 16

1 1/2 cups cake flour
1 tsp sugar
1/8 tsp salt
2 Tbsp non-aromatic olive oil

1/4 cup hard margarine or butter,
frozen for 15 minutes
1 tsp vinegar
4 Tbsp ice water

1 Combine the flour, sugar, and salt in a food processor. Pour in the oil and
pulse until mixed. Cut the margarine or butter into small pieces and add to
the flour mixture. Pulse 10 times or until the mixture is full of lumps the size
of small peas.

2 Pour in the vinegar and ice water. Pulse 10 more times or until the dough
begins to hold together. Gather into 2 equal balls, wrap separately, and
refrigerate at least 30 minutes before rolling out.

3 This dough can, of course, be made by hand. Combine the flour, sugar, and
salt and stir in the oil. Add the margarine and mix with a pastry cutter or
2 knives until the size of small peas. Add the vinegar and ice water and mix
with a fork just until it starts to hold together. Gather into 2 balls, wrap, and
refrigerate as above.

(Continued)

Per serving: 88 calories, 5 g fat, 1 g saturated fat, 11% calories from saturated fat, 10 g carbohydrate, 0 g dietary fiber, 52 mg sodium
Exchanges: 1/2 Starch, 1 Fat

Vegetable Puree (for soup base)

SERVING SIZE: 1 1/2 cups, SERVES: 8

1 tsp non-aromatic olive oil	1 cup chopped celery
1 1/2 cups chopped onion	3 medium turnips (3/4 lb), peeled
2 cloves garlic, bashed and	and chopped
chopped	2 sprigs parsley
1 tsp grated ginger root	1/4 tsp pepper
1 cup chopped carrots	5 cups water

1 Heat the oil in a Dutch oven on medium-high. Sauté the onion 2 minutes. Add the garlic and ginger and cook 1 minute more. Toss in the carrots, celery, turnips, parsley, and pepper.

2 Pour in the water. Bring to a boil, reduce the heat, and simmer 25 minutes or until the vegetables are tender. Drain the vegetables reserving the liquid.

3 Puree the vegetables in batches with just enough liquid to keep the vegetables moving. Combine all the pureed vegetables with all the remaining liquid.

4 This is a wonderful base for soup. It can be used immediately or frozen in zip-top plastic freezer bags.

Per serving: 78 calories, 1 g fat, 0 g saturated fat, 0% calories from saturated fat, 15 g carbohydrate, 4 g dietary fiber, 101 mg sodium
Exchanges: 3 Vegetable

Index

Recipe Index

Date _____ Deep Breathing _____ Sleep _____
HOURS

Water 🥛 🥛 🥛 🥛 🥛 🥛 🥛 🥛   Blood Pressure _____

F O O D

BREAKFAST
Time _____   Total Carb_____

	Serving Size	Food and Drinks
Grain		
Vegetable		
Protein		
Fruit		
Milk		
Fat		

SNACK
Time _____   Total Carb_____

LUNCH
Time _____   Total Carb_____

	Serving Size	Food and Drinks
Grain		
Vegetable		
Protein		
Fruit		
Milk		
Fat		

SNACK
Time _____   Total Carb_____

DINNER
Time _____   Total Carb_____

	Serving Size	Food and Drinks
Grain		
Vegetable		
Protein		
Fruit		
Milk		
Fat		

TOTALS

VEGETABLES   FRUIT   NUTS   WHOLE GRAINS

| FUN | EMOTIONS | MOOD | ILLNESS | STRESS |

Energy Level 1   2   3   4   5   6   7   8   9   10

MOVEMENT

Time of Day   Comments

Walking _____ steps/minutes

Weights _____ lbs, _____ reps

Stretches _____ minutes

Laughter _____

Other _____   **Weight** _____

BLOOD GLUCOSE NUMBERS

| Time | Breakfast | | Lunch | | Dinner | | Bedtime |
	Before	After	Before	After	Before	After	

MEDICATIONS

Time	Type

Six Ways to Prevent Heart Disease

1. Stop smoking.
2. Lose weight.
3. Lower high blood pressure.
4. Get regular daily exercise, such as a 30 to 60 minute walk.
5. Lower cholesterol.
6. Take 1 baby aspirin or 1/2 a regular aspirin a day.

Diabetes puts your heart at risk. Heart disease can be prevented with lifestyle, exercise, and medications. And even when you have heart disease, the risk can be greatly reduced with careful attention to your risk factors, such as high blood pressure. With this effort, you can enjoy more years—and they will be quality years.

—**Barry Effron, MD**
Chief of Cardiology, University Hospitals of Cleveland
Professor at Case Western Reserve University School
of Medicine